# Laparoscopic Urologic Oncology

# Current Clinical Urology

Eric A. Klein, Series Editor

*Laparoscopic Urologic Oncology,* edited by **Jeffrey A. Cadeddu,** 2004

*Essential Urology: A Guide to Clinical Practice,* edited by **Jeannette M. Potts,** 2004

*Management of Benign Prostatic Hypertrophy,* edited by **Kevin T. McVary,** 2004

*Pediatric Urology*, edited by **John P. Gearhart,** 2003

*Essential Urologic Laparoscopy: The Complete Clinical Guide,* edited by **Stephen Y. Nakada,** 2003

*Urologic Prostheses: The Complete Guide to Devices, Their Implantation, and Patient Followup,* edited by **Culley C. Carson, III,** 2002

*Male Sexual Function: A Guide to Clinical Management,* edited by **John J. Mulcahy,** 2001

*Prostate Cancer Screening,* edited by **Ian M. Thompson, Martin I. Resnick, and Eric A. Klein,** 2001

*Bladder Cancer: Current Diagnosis and Treatment,* edited by **Michael J. Droller,** 2001

*Office Urology: The Clinician's Guide,* edited by **Elroy D. Kursh and James C. Ulchaker,** 2001

*Voiding Dysfunction: Diagnosis and Treatment,* edited by **Rodney A. Appell,** 2000

*Management of Prostate Cancer,* edited by **Eric A. Klein,** 2000

# LAPAROSCOPIC UROLOGIC ONCOLOGY

*Edited by*

JEFFREY A. CADEDDU, MD

*University of Texas Southwestern Medical Center, Dallas, TX*

Springer Science+Business Media, LLC

ISBN 978-1-4684-9803-5 ISBN 978-1-59259-425-2 (eBook)
DOI 10.1007/978-1-59259-425-2


Originally published by Humana Press Inc. in 2004
999 Riverview Drive, Suite 208
Totowa, New Jersey 07512
**www.humanapress.com**
Softcover reprint of the hardcover 1st edition 2004



Production Editor: Robin B. Weisberg

Cover Illustration: From Fig. 5 in Chapter 14, "Laparoscopic Radical Prostatectomy," by Michael D. Fabrizio, Douglas Soderdahl, and Paul F. Schellhammer.

Cover design by Patricia F. Cleary.

This publication is printed on acid-free paper. ◯
ANSI Z39.48-1984 (American National Standards Institute) Permanence of Paper for Printed Library Materials.

For additional copies, pricing for bulk purchases, and/or information about other Humana titles, contact Humana at the above address or at any of the following numbers: Tel.: 973-256-1699; Fax: 973-256-8341, E-mail: humana@humanapr.com; or visit our Website: humanapress.com



Library of Congress Cataloging-in-Publication Data

Laparoscopic urologic oncology / edited by Jeffrey A. Cadeddu.
p. ; cm. — (Current clinical urology)
Includes bibliographical references and index.

1. Genitourinary organs—Cancer—Endoscopic surgery. 2. Laparoscopic surgery. I. Cadeddu, Jeffrey A. II. Series.
[DNLM: 1. Laparoscopy—methods. 2. Urogenital Neoplasms—surgery. WJ 160 L199 2003]
RD670.L37 2003
616.99'46059—dc21

2003042322

# Preface

Minimally invasive urologic surgery is revolutionizing how physicians treat many urologic diseases. Laparoscopy in particular has reduced the pain, morbidity, and recovery time for many procedures traditionally performed through an open incision. Since laparoscopy is now the preferred modality for many benign conditions, the indications have expanded with the technique, so that it is now applied to the management of most urologic cancers.

The aim of *Laparoscopic Urologic Oncology* is to provide the first comprehensive textbook dedicated to the minimally invasive management of urologic cancers. The book is not intended to review the biology of urologic tumors, which is well covered in other texts, but rather their management. In particular, it focuses on surgical technique and the role of laparoscopic surgery in the management of these tumors. It also addresses patient conditions for which a minimally invasive alternative does not exist. The book is not a surgical atlas, but it does provide a balanced insight into its indications, contraindications, and results. Furthermore, the authors compare results to conventional open surgery, discuss controversies, and identify the shortcomings of minimally invasive procedures. In particular, such issues as the adequacy of oncologic results and their morbidity are compared to those experienced with conventional open techniques.

*Laparoscopic Urologic Oncology* focuses on educating both general urologists and urologic oncologists on the current and future role of laparoscopy and other minimally invasive techniques in urologic oncology. It is also intended to serve as a valuable reference to practicing laparoscopic and endoscopic urologic surgeons.

This book is dedicated to my wife Marlo, and children, Arianna and Duncan, without whose support this would not be possible.

***Jeffrey A. Cadeddu, MD***

# Contents

Preface ........ v
List of Contributors ........ ix

PART I: RENAL CELL CARCINOMA

1 Standard Transperitoneal and Retroperitoneal Laparoscopic Nephrectomy for Clinical T1-3a, N0, and M0 Tumors ........ 3
***David I. Lee and Ralph V. Clayman***

2 Role of Laparoscopic Nephrectomy in Metastatic Renal Cell Carcinoma ........ 27
***Stephen E. Pautler and McClellan M. Walther***

3 Morcellation vs Intact Specimen Removal: *Clinical Implications and Risk of Tumor Recurrences* ........ 37
***Steve Y. Chung and Timothy D. Averch***

4 Hand-Assisted Laparoscopic Radical Nephrectomy ........ 51
***Patrick S. Lowry and Stephen Y. Nakada***

5 Laparoscopic Management of the Complex Renal Cyst ........ 71
***Ryan F. Paterson, Tibério M. Siqueira, Jr., and Arieh L. Shalhav***

6 Laparoscopic Partial Nephrectomy ........ 93
***D. Brooke Johnson and Jeffrey A. Cadeddu***

7 Laparoscopic and Minimally Invasive Renal Tumor Ablation: *Cryotherapy and Radiofrequency Techniques* ........ 111
***Steven M. Baughman and Jay T. Bishoff***

8 Percutaneous Radiofrequency Tumor Ablation ........ 135
***Francis J. McGovern, Debra A. Gervais, and Peter R. Mueller***

PART II: TRANSITIONAL CELL CARCINOMA OF THE URETER AND RENAL PELVIS

9 Laparoscopic Nephroureterectomy ........ 155
***Herkanwal S. Khaira and J. Stuart Wolf, Jr.***

PART III: TESTICULAR CANCER

10 Laparoscopic Retroperitoneal Lymph Node Dissection for Nonseminomatous Germ Cell Tumors of the Testis ............... 177
*David S. Wang and Howard N. Winfield*

PART IV: ADRENAL ADENOMA AND CARCINOMA

11 Laparoscopic Adrenalectomy for Benign Disease ............................ 195
*D. Duane Baldwin and S. Duke Herrell*

12 Laparoscopic Adrenalectomy for Carcinoma ................................... 235
*Paul K. Pietrow and David M. Albala*

PART V: PROSTATE CANCER

13 Role of Laparoscopic Pelvic Lymph Node Dissection in Adenocarcinoma of the Prostate .............................................. 251
*Matthew T. Gettman*

14 Laparoscopic Radical Prostatectomy ................................................ 273
*Michael D. Fabrizio, Douglas Soderdahl, and Paul F. Schellhammer*

PART VI: BLADDER CANCER

15 Laparoscopic Radical Cystectomy .................................................... 297
*Sidney C. Abreu and Inderbir S. Gill*

16 Laparoscopic Urinary Diversion ...................................................... 305
*James Borin and Stephen J. Savage*

PART VII: COMPLICATIONS OF LAPAROSCOPIC SURGERY

17 Management of Intra- and Postoperative Complications .................. 329
*James R. Porter*

Index ......................................................................................... 357

# Contributors


SIDNEY C. ABREU, MD, *Urologic Institute, Cleveland Clinic Foundation, Cleveland, OH*

DAVID M. ALBALA, MD, *Division of Urology, Duke University Medical Center, Durham, NC*

TIMOTHY D. AVERCH, MD, *Department of Urology, University of Pittsburgh Medical Center, Pittsburgh, PA*

D. DUANE BALDWIN, MD, *Division of Urology, Department of Surgery, Vanderbilt University Medical Center, Nashville, TN*

STEVEN M. BAUGHMAN, MD, *Department of Urology, Wilford Hall Medical Center, Lackland AFB, Lackland, TX*

JAY T. BISHOFF, MD, FACS, *Department of Urology, Wilford Hall Medical Center, Lackland AFB, Lackland, TX*

JAMES BORIN, MD, *Department of Urology, Mount Sinai Medical Center, New York, NY*

JEFFREY A. CADEDDU, MD, *Department of Urology, University of Texas Southwestern Medical Center, Dallas, TX*

STEVE Y. CHUNG, MD, *Department of Urology, University of Pittsburgh Medical Center, Pittsburgh, PA*

RALPH V. CLAYMAN, MD, *Department of Urology, University of California at Irvine, Irvine, CA*

MICHAEL D. FABRIZIO, MD, *Department of Urology, Eastern Virginia Medical Center, Virginia Beach, VA*

DEBRA A. GERVAIS, MD, *Department of Radiology, Massachussetts General Hospital, Harvard Medical School, Boston, MA*

MATTHEW T. GETTMAN, MD, *Department of Urology, Mayo Clinic, Rochester, MN*

INDERBIR S. GILL, MD, MCh, *Urologic Institute, Cleveland Clinic Foundation, Cleveland, OH*

S. DUKE HERRELL, MD, *Department of Urologic Surgery, Vanderbilt University Medical Center, Nashville, TN*

D. BROOKE JOHNSON, MD, *Department of Urology, University of Texas Southwestern Medical Center, Dallas, TX*

HERKANWAL S. KHAIRA, MD, *Department of Urology, University of Michigan Medical School, Ann Arbor, MI*

David I. Lee, MD, *Department of Urology, University of California at Irvine, Irvine, CA*
Patrick S. Lowry, MD, *Division of Urology, University of Wisconsin Medical School, Madison, WI*
Francis J. McGovern, MD, *Department of Urology, Massachussetts General Hospital, Harvard Medical School, Boston, MA*
Peter R. Mueller, MD, *Department of Radiology, Massachussetts General Hospital, Harvard Medical School, Boston, MA*
Stephen Y. Nakada, MD, *Division of Urology, University of Wisconsin Medical School, Madison, WI*
Stephen E. Pautler, MD, FRCSC, *Urologic Oncology Branch, National Cancer Institute, National Institutes of Health, Bethesda, MD*
Ryan F. Paterson, MD, *Department of Urology, Indiana University Medical Center, Indianapolis, IN*
Paul K. Pietrow, MD, *Division of Urology, Duke University Medical Center, Durham, NC*
James R. Porter, MD, *Department of Urology, University of Washington Medical Center, Seattle, WA*
Stephen J. Savage, MD, *Department of Urology, Memorial Sloan-Kettering Cancer Center, New York, NY*
Paul F. Schellhammer, MD, *Department of Urology, Eastern Virginia Medical Center, Virginia Beach, VA*
Arieh L. Shalhav, MD, *Section of Urology, Department of Surgery, University of Chicago Pritzker School of Medicine, Chicago, IL*
Tibério M. Siqueira, Jr., MD, *Department of Urology, Indiana University Medical Center, Indianapolis, IN*
Douglas Soderdahl, MD, *Department of Urology, Eastern Virginia Medical Center, Virginia Beach, VA*
McClellan M. Walther, MD, FACS, *Urologic Oncology Branch, National Cancer Institute, National Institutes of Health, Bethesda, MD*
David S. Wang, MD, *Department of Urology, University of Iowa Hospitals and Clinics, Iowa City, IA*
Howard N. Winfield, MD, *Department of Urology, University of Iowa Hospitals and Clinics, Iowa City, IA*
J. Stuart Wolf, Jr., MD, *Department of Urology, University of Michigan Medical School, Ann Arbor, MI*

# I

# Renal Cell Carcinoma

# 1 Standard Transperitoneal and Retroperitoneal Laparoscopic Nephrectomy for Clinical T1-3a, N0, and M0 Tumors

*David I. Lee,* MD *and Ralph V. Clayman,* MD

*CONTENTS*

INTRODUCTION
OVERVIEW OF SURGICAL TECHNIQUE
TRANSPERITONEAL RADICAL/TOTAL NEPHRECTOMY: SURGICAL TECHNIQUE
RETROPERITONEAL RADICAL NEPHRECTOMY
SURGICAL TECHNIQUE
RESULTS
MORBIDITY
COSTS
CONCLUSIONS
REFERENCES

## INTRODUCTION

Laparoscopic nephrectomy for a renal tumor was introduced by Clayman, Kavoussi, and associates in 1990 *(1)*; in experienced hands, this approach has become an accepted alternative to traditional open radical nephrectomy (ORN) for small and medium-sized ( 13 cm) renal masses without evidence of renal vein or inferior vena caval involvement (i.e., T1, T2, and T3a renal tumors). Tumors that are staged T3b by evidence of renal vein or minimal inferior vena caval involvement may rarely be treated laparoscopically but extensive laparoscopic experience and availability of specialized laparoscopic vascular equipment

From: *Laparoscopic Urologic Oncology*
Edited by: J. A. Cadeddu © Humana Press Inc., Totowa, NJ

(e.g., laparoscopic Satinsky clamp) are necessary. Extensive vena caval involvement and tumors that appear very locally aggressive should be handled in an open fashion.

## OVERVIEW OF SURGICAL TECHNIQUE

An antibiotic bowel preparation is not performed; but a light mechanical bowel preparation is thought to be helpful. Usually a clear liquid diet is advised for the day prior to the procedure and a Dulcolax suppository or bottle of magnesium citrate is given on the day prior to surgery. One gram of cefazolin (Ancef) is administered immediately preoperatively. In the obese patient or the individual with a history of deep venous thrombosis, 5000 units of heparin are administered subcutaneously 2 h prior to the procedure and continued on a 12-h basis postoperatively until the patient is ambulatory. At the outset of the procedure, just prior to any skin incision, 30 mg of ketorolac (Toradol) is given intravenously.

General endotracheal anesthesia is induced and the patient's stomach and bladder are decompressed with an orogastric tube and a Foley catheter, respectively. Pneumatic compression stockings are applied to both legs. The patient is carefully positioned on a well-padded operating table (e.g., foam egg crate) in a 70° flank position with the affected kidney on the upside. The operating table is fully flexed and the kidney rest is fully raised beneath the iliac crest. The downside leg is flexed at the knee and separated from the extended upside leg by pillows; the upside leg is placed on a sufficient number of pillows until it is level with the flank, thereby precluding any strain on the upside leg. The downside heel, hip, and knee are cushioned. The downside arm is padded and an axillary roll is carefully positioned. The upside arm is placed on a well-padded arm-board; the arm-board is positioned such that there is no tension on the brachial plexus. Once the patient has been properly positioned, he or she is secured to the operating table by padded safety straps that are passed over the chest, hip, and knee.

## TRANSPERITONEAL RADICAL/TOTAL NEPHRECTOMY: SURGICAL TECHNIQUE

### *Access*

For right or left renal access (Figs. 1 and 2) a 12-mm incision is made approx 2 fingerbreadths medial and cranial to the anterior superior iliac spine. Other potential sites for initial access, include a midclavicular line subcostal approach (Stoller) or, in the thin patient, a transumbilical placement. The subcutaneous tissue is spread with a Kelly clamp, and the anterior rectus fascia is secured with two Allis clamps. A Veress

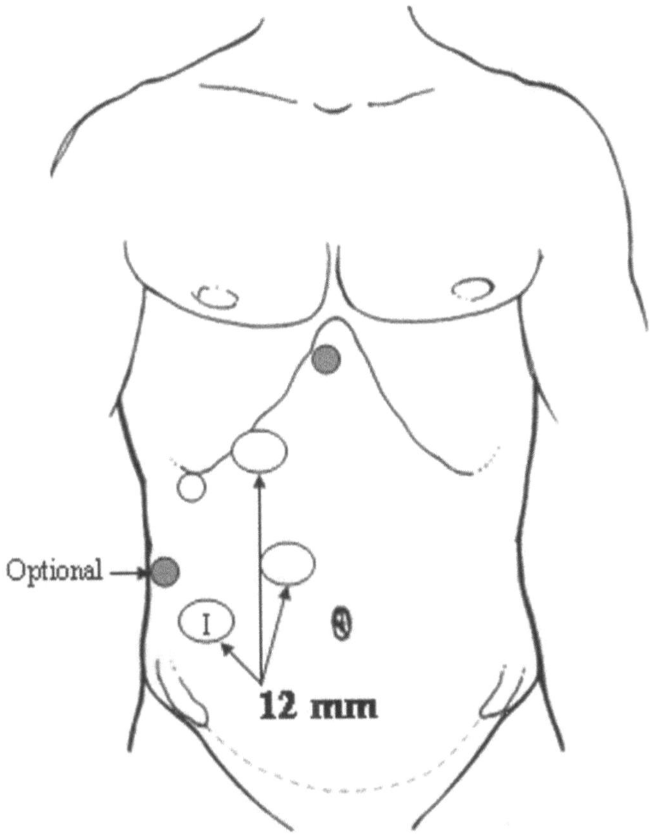


**Fig. 1.** Diagram demonstrating port sites used for right transperitoneal nephrectomy. I = insufflation port. Large circles represent 12-mm port sites. Small circles represent 5-mm port sites. Optional ports are in gray: the upper gray port may be used for liver retraction, while the lower gray port is only used if there is difficulty with specimen entrapment in a LapSac.

needle pneumoperitoneum of 25 mm Hg is obtained. Alternatively, the pneumoperitoneum may be obtained using an open or endoscopic cannula technique. A 12-mm blunt-tip trocar is placed at this same site (Fig. 1—port site I), and the abdominal pressure is reduced to 15 mm Hg. A 10-mm 30° laparoscope is inserted and the underlying bowel is closely inspected for any injury that may have occurred during Veress needle or trocar placement. Subsequently, two additional 12-mm blunt-tip trocars are placed under direct endoscopic vision; 2 cm below the costal margin in the midclavicular line, and immediately lateral to the margin of the rectus abdominus muscle approx 3–5 fingerbreadths above the umbilicus. Finally, after mobilization of the colon from the abdominal sidewall,

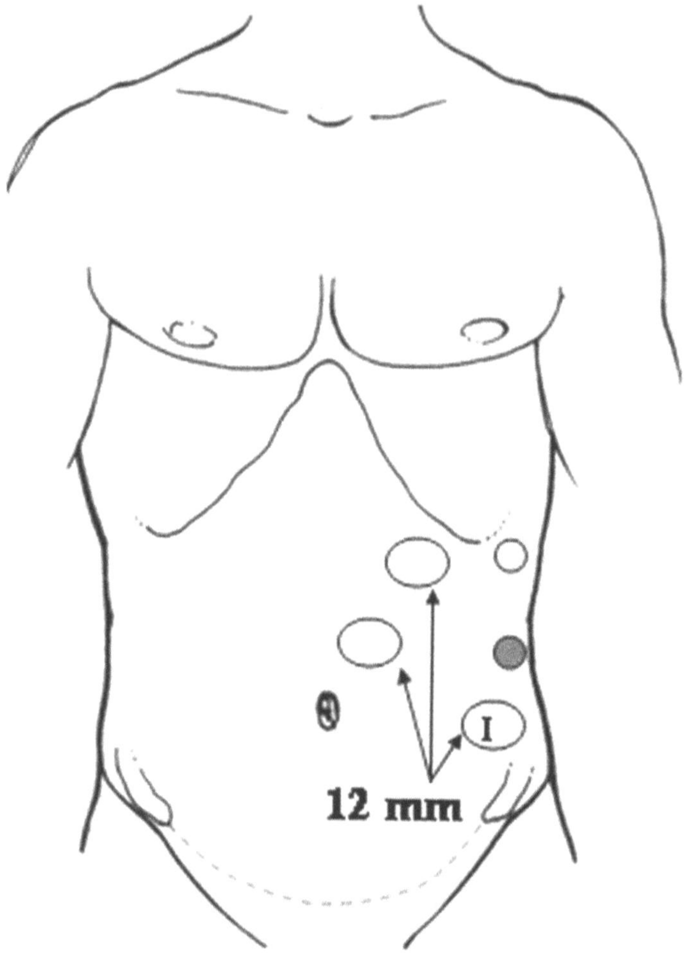


**Fig. 2.** Diagram demonstrating port sites used for left transperitoneal nephrectomy. I = insufflation port. Large circles represent 12-mm port sites. Small circles represent 5-mm port sites. Gray port site is optional; it is only placed if there is difficulty with specimen entrapment in a LapSac.

a fourth blunt-tip trocar (5 mm) is commonly placed subcostal in the posterior axillary line. For right-sided nephrectomies, a fifth blunt-tip trocar may be placed in the midline approx 2–4 cm below the xiphoid (optional) to help with liver retraction (Fig. 1). Similarly, if at the end of the procedure there is difficulty entrapping the specimen, another blunt-tip port (5 mm) can be placed just above the iliac crest.

With regard to trocars, presently, only nonbladed trocars are used at our institution. The design of these trocars eliminates the need to use any suture to fix them in place and precludes fascial closure of nonmidline 12 mm ports at the end of the procedure.

## *Operative Technique: Transperitoneal Laparoscopic Radical Nephrectomy*

### Right Side

The peritoneal cavity is closely inspected. The liver is visualized for mass lesions. The outline of the kidney within Gerota's fascia is commonly visible behind the ascending colon.

**Step 1: Peritoneal Incisions and Pararenal Dissection.** The key to en bloc resection of the kidney within Gerota's fascia lies in defining the borders of the dissection. On the right side, the dissection follows an anatomic template with a "wedge-shaped" configuration (Fig. 3). The apical edge of the wedge is the line of Toldt. The dissection is initiated using a 5-mm curved harmonic forceps and atraumatic grasping forceps for counter-traction. The harmonic forceps is preferred for the majority of the dissection as it provides excellent hemostasis with minimal associated peripheral thermal injury to surrounding tissues, especially the ascending colon. The line of Toldt is incised beginning at the pelvic brim 2–3 cm away from the colon; this line of incision is continued straight cephalad, lateral to the kidney, and up to the level of the diaphragm; the triangular ligament of the liver is also incised at this time. This defines the thin edge of the wedge. Next, the mobilization of the colon is continued by dissecting it from the anterior surface of the kidney, all of the time staying 2–3 cm lateral to the colon itself; this is done until the hepatic flexure overlying the mid-upper portion of the medial half of the kidney has been freed and dropped medially. This part of the dissection defines the lower border of the wedge as well as the uppermost portion of the broad medial side of the wedge.

The broad side of the wedge comprises three distinct levels of dissection along the medial aspect of the kidney (Fig. 3): (1) the upper portion of the mobilized ascending colon, (2) Kocher maneuver on the duodenum to move it medially (Fig. 3), and (3) dissection of the anterior and lateral surfaces of the inferior vena cava (IVC).

The duodenum may appear flattened against the medial aspect of the kidney; the surgeon should be cognizant that the duodenum must always be dissected away from the kidney before the anterior surface of the vena cava can be identified (Fig. 4). To facilitate development of the third and deepest plane of dissection (i.e., the IVC dissection), it is helpful to first define the superior side of the wedge by incising the posterior coronary hepatic ligament. This is done by "T"ing off of the

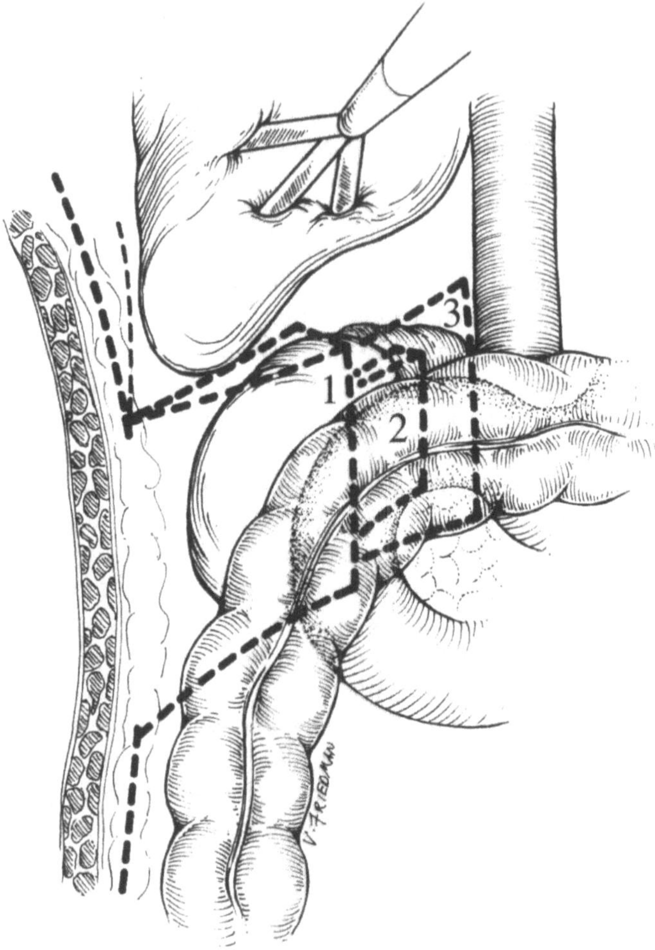


**Fig. 3.** Diagram of the right-sided nephrectomy demonstrating the wedge-shaped configuration. The numbers refer to the three distinct levels of dissection along the medial aspect of the kidney: colon, duodenum, and IVC. Note that on the right side the lateral border of the kidney is left intact; this is done to preclude the kidney from falling medial and obscuring the renal hilum.

initial vertical incision lateral to the kidney which was extended up to the diaphragm; the incision begins at the lateral edge of the lower border of the liver and is extended medially to the level of the IVC. The incision should stay approx 2–3 cm away from the liver parenchyma. The surgeon will thus come directly onto the lateral and anterior surface of the IVC well above the duodenum and the adrenal gland. At this point, the en bloc area of dissection of the specimen has been completely defined,

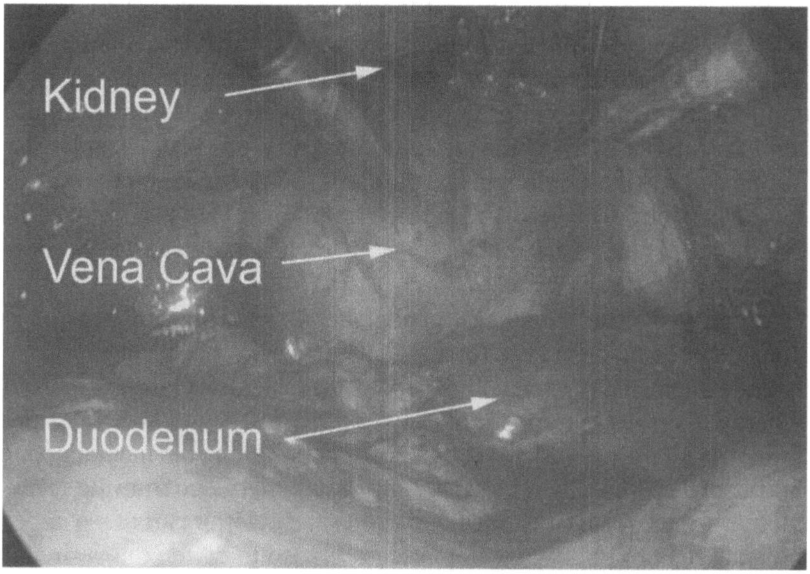


**Fig. 4.** Laparoscopic view of the duodenum Kocherized. The dissection of the IVC, which is in the center of the figure is next. At this point, the ascending colon and hepatic flexure, which were initially mobilized, lie medial to the duodenum.

ensuring removal of the kidney within Gerota's fascia, along with the pararenal and perirenal fat, the adrenal gland, and an anterior patch of peritoneum.

**Step 2: Securing the Gonadal Vein.** The dissection on the IVC is continued caudally until the entry of the gonadal vein is identified. This vein is circumferentially dissected free from surrounding tissue, secured with four 9-mm vascular clips, and divided between the second and third clips. Alternatively, the 10-mm Ligasure device can be used to divide the gonadal vein.

**Step 3: Securing the Ureter.** The gonadal vein can be traced distally from the vena cava. The right ureter usually lies just posterior and lateral to the right gonadal vein. We prefer to divide the ureter at the end of the procedure with four clips to provide a good length of ureter to which a grasping forceps can be affixed to facilitate subsequent specimen entrapment. Other surgeons prefer to secure and divide the ureter at this juncture, which allows greater retraction of the kidney and may thereby facilitate the subsequent hilar dissection. At this point, all of the caudal retroperitoneal attachments to Gerota's fascia can be dissected thereby freeing the specimen inferiorly.

**Step 4: Securing the Adrenal Vein.** Continued cephalad dissection of the IVC exposes the renal hilum and adrenal vein. The adrenal vein is dissected from the surrounding tissue and secured with either three 9-mm clips leaving two clips on the cava, or with the 10-mm Ligasure device. Alternatively, if the supra-adrenal area has been cleanly dissected down to the diaphragm and the lateral border of the supra-adrenal IVC has been identified, an Endo-GIA vascular load can be used to secure all of the tissue medial to the adrenal and lateral to the IVC including the adrenal vein.

If one wishes to spare the adrenal gland, then the upper dissection is considerably modified. A formal incision in the posterior coronary hepatic ligament is no longer needed. Instead, Gerota's fascia is incised where it overlies the upper pole of the kidney. The upper pole of the kidney is identified and dissection is continued along the medial upper border of the kidney thereby separating the adrenal gland from the specimen. Once the renal capsule of the medial and anterior part of the upper pole is seen, an Endo-GIA stapler can be used to divide the perirenal fatty tissue between the adrenal gland and the kidney.

**Step 5: The Renal Hilum.** Placement of a 5-mm Jarit PEER retractor attached to an Endoholder on the kidney at the level of the hilum can provide lateral retraction facilitating the upcoming hilar dissection. If the IVC has been cleanly dissected, the take off of the renal vein is usually quite evident. The PEER retractor is opened such that it straddles the renal hilum; lateral pressure is applied on either side of the hilum as the kidney is pulled laterally by the retractor. Once adequate tension has been achieved, the Endoholder is secured, thereby locking the retractor in place. The right renal artery is subsequently identified behind the renal vein and dissected circumferentially to allow placement of five 9-mm clips in order to leave three clips on the aorta side. The use of the hook dissector is quite helpful as tissue can be engaged and lifted away from the underlying vessels prior to its being cut. In this regard, we prefer to use a hook electrode that has active electrode monitoring (Encision Inc., Boulder, CO) in order to limit the chance of any inadvertent spread of current to the bowel or other structures; with this device, any break in the insulation on the shaft of the hook electrode results in its being disabled. The renal vein is then dissected circumferentially and secured with an Endo-GIA vascular stapler (3-cm load).

One modification described by Chan and colleagues is to just free the anterior, medial, and lateral borders of the renal artery and then secure it with an Endo-GIA vascular load; however, when doing this it is important for the surgeon to develop the plane of dissection deeply along the upper and lower borders of the renal artery until the muscles of the retroperitoneum can be clearly seen in order to insure that the entire width of the artery is secured in the stapler (2).

Occasionally, an adequate length of the renal artery cannot be exposed due to the width of the overlying renal vein. In this situation, one or two clips can be applied across the artery to occlude the artery without transection. Now that the main renal artery is occluded, the renal vein is divided with the Endo-GIA stapler. The artery is then further dissected and divided after five clips are applied as previously described; again leaving three clips on the aortic stump of the renal artery.

Rarely, the artery cannot be accessed from the anterior approach. It is then necessary to dissect the kidney laterally, flip the entire specimen medially, and approach the artery posteriorly. In this case, the artery is often dissected further medially, where it crosses beneath the posterior surface of the IVC. Great care must be used in dissecting the anterior surface of the renal artery in this location in order to not inadvertently injure the IVC.

A third approach to the hilum is along its inferior surface. The ureter is transected and pulled lateral and cephalad. The ureter is followed up to the level of the renal pelvis. Just in front of the pelvis the renal vein and artery can be identified and dissected. This type of dissection often results in the renal vein being taken very close to the kidney rather than at its origin from the cava.

**Step 6: Freeing the Specimen and Securing the Ureter.** The specimen, within Gerota's fascia, is then freed from the retro-peritoneum using electrocautery, the harmonic dissector, and blunt dissection. At this time, the lateral attachments of the kidney to the abdominal sidewall, which were kept intact at the beginning of the procedure, are incised. After the ureter is secured with four clips, the ureter is grasped with a locking grasping forceps passed via the 5-mm subcostal posterior axillary line port and the entire specimen is moved cephalad until it rests on the anterior surface of the liver. Once in this position, the shaft of the grasping forceps is fixed in place by attaching it to the Endoholder.

**Step 7a: Entrapment for Morcellation.** If specimen morcellation is planned, a LapSac is used. Morcellation should not be performed with any of the other commercially available plastic entrapment sacks as these sacks can be easily perforated with the morcellating forceps; indeed, in a decade the authors have had only two acute bowel injuries during laparoscopic renal surgery, both occurred when attempting morcellation with the kidney in a plastic sack.

The 8 x 10-inch LapSac is appropriately sized for the majority of renal specimens (i.e., </= 1700 g). On the back table, a guidewire (i.e., nitinol) is passed through the holes in the neck of the LapSac that also contain the

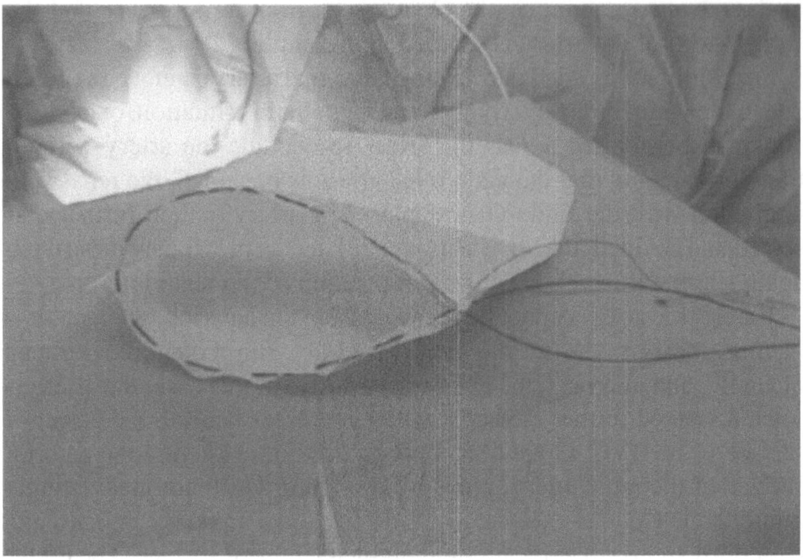

**Fig. 5.** Picture of guidewire inserted through the same holes through which the nylon drawstring passes on a Lapsac; the guidewire facilitates opening the sack.

drawstring. The two free ends of the guidewire should exit the edge of the sack at the same point that the blue nylon drawstring exits the edge of the sack, thereby facilitating both the introduction and subsequent opening of the mouth of the sack (Fig. 5). The LapSac is then loaded on the two-tined introducer leaving the tines on the outer surface of the sack. Usually, the sack is rolled counterclockwise from the bottom upward; the handle of the introducer, the two ends of the guidewire, and the nylon drawstring should all be parallel to one another and on the same side of the sack. As the 8 x 10-inch LapSac will not pass through a 12-mm trocar, the uppermost 12-mm trocar is removed and the entrapment sack loaded on the two-tined introducer is passed through the 12-mm abdominal incision, deeply into the abdomen and pelvis and then unfurled by twirling the introducer clockwise. Following the removal of the introducer, the 12-mm trocar is replaced. Using two atraumatic grasping forceps, the LapSac is completely unfolded and flattened within the abdomen. The laparoscope can now be moved from the paramedian port to the uppermost 12-mm port. Now two traumatic, locking 5-mm grasping forceps are introduced and the upper and lower tabs on the mouth of the LapSac are grasped. The LapSac is opened broadly such that its inferior edge is pulled just beneath the edge of the liver with the traumatic grasper passed via the paramedian 12-mm port, while the apex of the sack is pulled anterior via the lower midclavicular line port. The laparoscope can be passed into the LapSac, and with circular motions the entrapment sack is further opened. The specimen is then rolled off of the liver into the mouth of the sack; the forceps on the ureter is directed at the forceps holding the upper tab of the sack. As the specimen enters the sack, the forceps on the inferior edge of the sack's mouth is moved cephalad and anterior to trap and push the specimen deeper into the sack.

If entrapment using a two-instrument approach is difficult, then a fifth right trocar (5 mm) is placed just above or at Petit's triangle (just above the iliac crest in the midaxillary line). Now the LapSac is opened using three points of fixation by placing a traumatic locking grasping forceps on each of the three tabs. When the sack is opened in this manner, the middle grasper pulls the lip of the sack upward against the underside of the abdominal wall forming the apex of a tent-like opening in the sack; the medial and lateral 5-mm graspers are used to pull the bottom of the sack in opposite directions (i.e., medial and lateral, respectively), while displacing the sack posterior, thereby pulling the neck of the sack between them taut and creating the base of the tent. As such, this triangular opening of the sack results in the base of the tent running parallel with the edge of the liver while the apex of the tent lies at the anterior portion of the underside of the abdominal wall. The base of the sack is then positioned further posterior and cephalad until it lies just under the lower edge of the liver. The surgeon now moves the ureteral grasper toward the grasper on the apex of the sack. In doing this, the specimen rolls off of the liver and into the sack; as this occurs, the assistant holding the medial and lateral graspers on the sack moves the base of the sack anterior thereby pushing the specimen deeper into the sack. Specimen entrapment in this manner requires three people: the surgeon who controls the ureteral grasper and thus guides the specimen into the sack, the camera operator who holds the laparoscope and the middle grasper on the sack (apex of the tent), and an assistant who holds the medial and lateral graspers (base of the tent) on the sack.

**7b: Entrapment for Intact Removal.** If intact removal is planned, then a 15-mm Endocatch II (U.S. Surgical Inc., Norwalk, CT) or Endopouch (Ethicon Inc., Cincinnati, OH) is introduced and opened just beneath the liver; the self-opening design of this entrapment sack facilitates the entrapment process; however, morcellation should not be performed with these bags as the posterior "unseen" section of the plastic sack can be perforated with even a ring forceps. The 15-mm entrapment sack cannot be passed through a 12-mm trocar. As such, the trocar is removed and the barrel of the 15-mm entrapment sack deployment mechanism is gently passed through the trocar incision site under direct endoscopic vision.

**Step 8: Morcellation vs Intact Removal.** If morcellation of the specimen is planned, then the neck of the LapSac is delivered through the upper midclavicular line port. The port incision is enlarged to 20 mm. The surgical field around the port site is further isolated by the sequential placement over the neck of the sack of a sterile adhesive "10,10" drape, a fenestrated absorbent towel, and a nephrostomy drape; the neck of the sack is passed through a hole in each of these drapes. These precautions are taken to help prevent possible wound contamination with any "spilled" tumor cells.

Mechanical morcellation with a ring forceps can then be performed. With the 2-cm opening, the tissue can be fragmented under the direct vision of the surgeon. It is important for the surgeon and the assistant to each use one hand to hold up either side of the LapSac and to pull it taut. This will help deliver the specimen to the morcellating clamps and will make it easier for the second assistant to keep the sack in view. It is essential for the camera operator to be ever vigilant of any loss of pneumoperitoneum implying puncture of the LapSac. If the LapSac is perforated, the port-site incision is immediately enlarged so the remainder of the specimen within the LapSac can be delivered immediately. To date, the author is unaware of any perforation of a LapSac when morcellation was performed with a ring forceps. After completion of morcellation, the surgeon and all other members of the surgical team who participated during morcellation should re-gown and re-glove. The port site used for the delivery of the sack is swabbed with betadine. Using this approach, over the past 12 years, the authors have not experienced a wound seed or peritoneal contamination in any of their more than 100 renal cell cancer patients.

For intact removal, it is recommended to make a lower midline abdominal or a Pfannenstiel incision. The specimen is then extracted intact within the entrapment sack. One should resist the temptation to connect the medial and lateral upper or lower port sites for extraction purposes. The former will result in a more cephalad and possibly more painful incision, while the latter is a "weaker" incision and may result in a delayed postoperative hernia.

**Step 9: Exiting the Abdomen.** Regardless of whether the specimen has been removed intact or morcellated, at the end of the procedure the abdomen is carefully inspected at 5 mm Hg pneumoperitoneum pressure. Once hemostasis has been assured, the operative extraction site can be closed in two layers of 0-Vicyrl; the security of this closure can be assessed both manually and endoscopically. If the specimen was morcellated, then the extraction site is closed using two passages of the Carter Thomason device thereby placing two full thickness sutures of

0-Vicryl. The other port sites, since they were placed with an atraumatic trocar, do not require fascial closure and thus can be removed under direct endoscopic control. The only exception to this approach is for a midline port (i.e., >/= 10 mm); in this case we routinely close the fascia as there is no overlying muscle. All skin sites are closed with a 4-0 subcuticular absorbable suture.

### Left Side

**Step 1: Peritoneal Incisions and Pararenal Dissection.** The template for anatomic dissection of the left kidney assumes the configuration of an inverted cone (i.e., a water scooper) (Fig. 6). The lateral side of the cone is formed by the line of Toldt that is incised from the pelvic brim, cephalad to the level of the diaphragm. There are often adhesions from the descending colon at the splenic flexure to the anterior abdominal wall that need to be sharply released in order to complete the incision alongside the spleen up to the diaphragm. This cephalad incision serves to release any splenophrenic attachments thereby mobilizing the spleen from the abdominal sidewall (Fig. 6).

The medial aspect of the cone is then formed by retracting the peritoneal reflection of the descending colon medially and developing the plane between Gerota's fascia and the colonic mesentery. This natural plane between the mesentery of the descending colon and Gerota's fascia is most easily identified and entered along the lower pole of the kidney or just inferior to the kidney. The colon is mobilized medially and cephalad up to the spleen. The anterior upper curve of the cone is formed by the spleno-colic ligament, which is incised in order to fully mobilize the descending colon medially. The posterior upper curve of the cone is formed by the spleno-renal ligament; the potential for tearing of the splenic capsule is prevented by incising these ligaments. The dissection then follows the plane between the spleen and the superior portion of Gerota's fascia. At this point, the en bloc area of dissection has been defined and incorporates all of Gerota's fascia, the pararenal and perirenal fat, and the adrenal gland.

**Step 2: The Gonadal Vein.** The left gonadal vein is the most important structure to identify during a left nephrectomy as it reliably leads the surgeon to the renal vein. The gonadal vein can most easily be exposed inferiorly and traced superiorly. In obese patients, the surgeon can expose the inguinal ring in order to reliably identify the gonadal vein and trace it cephalad. Anteriorly along the gonadal vein, there should be no tributaries thereby providing the surgeon with a safe plane of dissection all the way up to the insertion of the gonadal vein into the main renal vein.

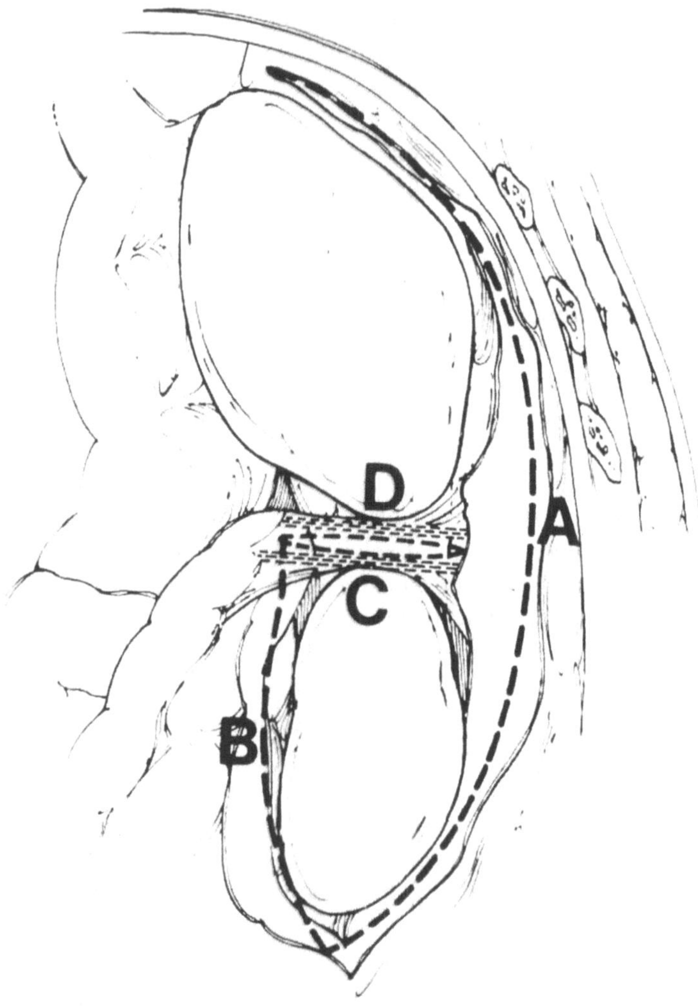


**Fig. 6.** Diagram demonstrating the inverted cone template for *en bloc* dissection during left radical nephrectomy. Unlike on the right side, the reflection of the colon comes to the lateral sidewall and thus an incision in the line of Toldt parallel to the kidney needs to be made; this incision is not carried deeply in an effort to hold the kidney lateral, which helps somewhat with the hilar dissection. (A: line of Toldt and splenophrenic attachments, B: plane between colonic mesentry and Gerota's fascia, C: spleno-colic ligament, D: spleno-renal ligament.)

**Step 3: Securing the Ureter.** The left ureter usually lies just posterior and lateral to the gonadal vein. It is carefully dissected from the retroperitoneal tissues and treated in the same manner as the right ureter was for a right nephrectomy.

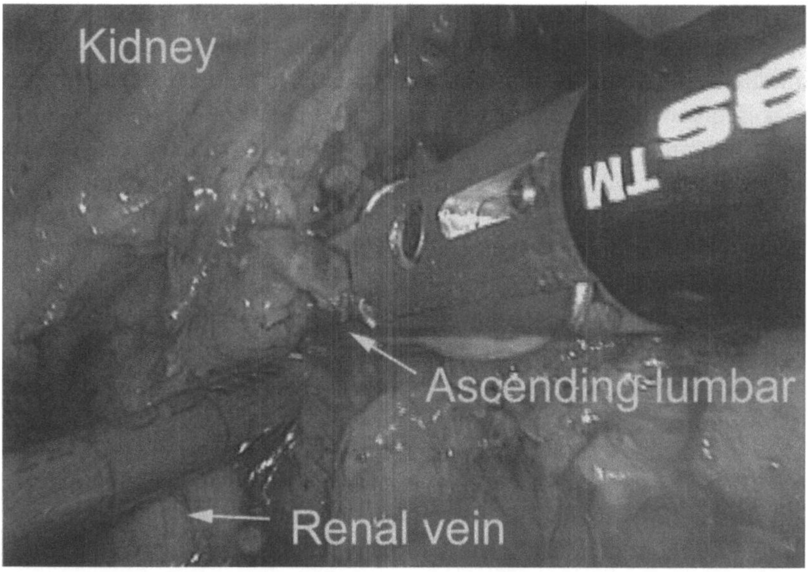


**Fig. 7.** Laparoscopic view of the Ligasure device on the left ascending lumbar vein. The 10-mm Ligasure device can be used in place of clips on the left renal vein tributaries preventing Endo-GIA failure secondary to clips.

**Step 4: Securing the Renal Hilum.** After tracing the gonadal vein to its junction with the main renal vein, it is secured and divided with four 9-mm vascular clips or the 10-mm Ligasure device. The ascending lumbar vein must also be carefully dissected and divided if present; it may enter either the renal vein posteriorly or the gonadal vein near its insertion into the renal vein (Fig. 7). The superior border of the renal vein is then freed by dissection of the adrenal vein; this vein usually lays parallel with or just medial to the insertion of the gonadal vein. It is similarly occluded with clips and divided or can be sequentially secured and incised with the Ligasure device. It is important to place the clips on these three renal vein tributaries such that they lie at least 1 cm from the main body of the renal vein; this will facilitate the subsequent safe placement of the Endo-GIA vascular stapler across the renal vein without risking interference of the stapler's function from any of the previously applied clips. If the surgeon inadvertently fires the stapler across a clip, the stapler may "freeze-up" and it cannot be properly released (3). In this situation, it may be necessary to convert to an open procedure or proceed to further dissect the renal vein medially in order to place a second Endo-GIA stapler across the vein; the decision of which way to proceed depends on the surgeon's experience.

If the surgeon tries to identify the left renal hilum by dissecting the area where it "should be," it is not uncommon for the dissection to drift medially. This can become quite problematic and indeed, one may even risk injury to the duodenum, which often lies at the bottom of this "medial hole." Again, the surest way to the renal vein is to trace the left gonadal vein cephalad. Vascular control, specimen dissection, entrapment, and morcellation or intact removal are all identical to the description for the right side. The only exception is that the left kidney specimen is displaced onto the anterior surface of the spleen just prior to entrapment. Exiting the abdomen is as described for a right nephrectomy.

## RETROPERITONEAL RADICAL NEPHRECTOMY

### *Access*

A 1.5–2.0-cm skin incision is created just below and posterior to the tip of the 12th rib (i.e., in the midaxillary line) with the scalpel and spread further open with a Kelly forceps. The underlying flank musculature is bluntly divided and the underlying thoracolumbar fascia is sharply incised to enter the pararenal fat of the retroperitoneum. It is helpful to use "S" type or "Army-Navy" retractors during this portion of the procedure so one can both see and feel the retroperitoneal fat. If the surgeon's index finger is in the retroperitoneal space, he or she should then be able to rotate the finger 180° and assuredly palpate the psoas muscle. Using the index finger, the fat can be further bluntly dissected following which a balloon dilator is introduced and inflated to 800 cc of air. A 10- or 12-mm blunt-tip cannula (U.S. Surgical Inc., Norwalk, CT) is inserted and the balloon on the distal portion of the cannula is inflated; the soft peritrocar outer ring of material is then snugged down onto the skin thereby sealing the body wall between the inner balloon and outer compression ring of the cannula; this tight seal will largely preclude gas leakage into the subcutaneous tissues. The pneumoretro-peritoneum is established and the 10 mm, 30° laparoscope is inserted to scan the operative field. Visualization of the working field is significantly different than the transperitoneal approach. On initial examination, it is usually easy to first identify the psoas muscle and at times, the genitofemoral nerve. If one follows the psoas muscle cephalad and medial in a thin patient, the visual pulsation of the renal artery should next be found. Gerota's fascia and the ureter are typically visible, although this may be difficult in the obese patient or in those patients with any degree of scarring or fibrosis in the retroperitoneal space. A small amount of venous blood overlying the tissues is normal, but there should be no active bleeding.

Accessory ports are placed under endoscopic control. Insertion of additional working ports is performed under endoscopic guidance. Alternatively, Gill has described the use of finger-guided "S" retractors to facilitate digital guidance for placement of additional working ports into the retroperitoneum that may be otherwise difficult to place under direct endoscopic vision. All ports placed into the retroperitoneum are of the blunt, not bladed, nature, thereby making it safer to use digital guidance. A 10- or 12-mm port is placed at the lower midaxillary line 2 cm cephalad to the iliac crest; a 5- or 12-mm port is placed at the level of the 12th rib in the posterior axillary line; and a 5-mm port is placed at the level of the 11th rib on the anterior axillary line. The placement of the ports should form a "T." Alternatively, ports can be placed only in a subcostal array (three-port "I" approach, as described by Gill) or a fifth port can be added anterior to the lower midaxillary line port, thereby creating a "W" array *(4)*.

## SURGICAL TECHNIQUE

The psoas muscle is cleared of any overlying tissue. This muscle can be followed medially, thereby moving the dissection well under the posterior surface of the kidney. This is a key concept because if one fails to create this depth of dissection, one runs the possibility of dissecting anterior to the kidney, thereby obscuring the hilum completely. The medial most upper 5-mm port is used for passage of a retractor (e.g., diamond flex "snake" or PEER); the retractor is opened and positioned on the posterior surface of the kidney. The retractor is then used to elevate and pull the kidney medially; the retractor can then be fixed to an Endoholder, thereby ensuring continued reliable retraction. Gerota's fascia must be incised to gain full access to the hilum; this incision should be created 1 to 2 cm anterior the medial edge of the psoas muscle. Dissection is initiated around the renal artery and then the renal vein with clip ligation and Endo-GIA stapling, respectively. However, it is perfectly acceptable to take the renal artery with the Endo-GIA. One caveat is that on the left side, the surgeon may encounter the posterior-directed ascending lumbar vein prior to seeing the renal artery; this vein should be dissected (four clips or Ligasure), secured, and then incised. Circumferential mobilization of the kidney is performed. The dissection is continued in a cephalad direction that will lead to the adrenal vein, which is secured and divided between four clips or with a Ligasure device. The ureter is transected between four clips and the remaining retroperitoneal attachments are divided.

Next, if the goal is intact removal, then the initial port site is extended, horizontally to 8–10 cm, and the entire specimen is retrieved intact after entrapment in a rapidly deployable plastic sack as previously described. Alternatively, if morcellation is desired the specimen can be secured in a LapSac. To do the latter, however, requires opening of the peritoneal cavity to provide sufficient space to maneuver the sack and the specimen.

Parenthetically, entering the peritoneal cavity at some point during the dissection does not require conversion to a transperitoneal technique. The peritoneal cavity is commonly entered during dissection of the anterior portion of Gerota's fascia.

As with the peritoneal approach to renal surgery, it is important to systematically exit the retroperitoneal space. Following completion of the surgical procedure, the $CO_2$ pressure in the retroperitoneum is reduced to 5 mm Hg and the operative and port sites are examined to ensure adequate hemostasis. The operative extraction site is closed in one or two layers of 0-Vicryl. Due to the retroperitoneal approach, the remaining port sites require no fascial closure. The ports are removed under direct visualization. The port sites are irrigated with saline and the skin is closed with a subcuticular 4-0 nonabsorbable suture.

## RESULTS

The advantages characteristic of minimally invasive procedures have been demonstrated for the laparoscopic radical nephrectomy (LRN). Operative results from the Nagoya experience of 60 patients in the laparoscopic arm and 40 patients in the open arm revealed that the mean operative time was longer than that of open surgery (5.2 vs 3.3 h, $p < 0.001$) *(5)*. However, the benefits of decreased blood loss (255 cc vs 512 cc, $p < 0.001$) and shorter time to full convalescence was statistically significant (23 vs 57 d, $p < 0.001$). Conversion to open surgery was only performed in one patient who had uncontrolled bleeding from an injury to the left renal artery. A transperitoneal approach was used in 45 patients and retroperitoneal in 15. Of note, the first 26 patients had intact extraction of the kidney, whereas the last 34 had their kidneys morcellated.

The mean weight of the laparoscopically dissected specimens was 279 g, whereas in the open group it was 339 g. The mean number of lymph nodes removed was seven from both the laparoscopic and open series; all lymph nodes were negative for tumor. The final tumor stage for the laparoscopic group was T1 in 15 patients, T2 in 43 patients, and T3 in 2 patients. In the open group, 11 patients had T1 disease, whereas the remainder had T2. All patients in the laparoscopic series were alive; two had metastatic disease without local recurrence or seeding of any port site. The calculated disease-free rate was 95.5% at 5 yr. Of the 40 patients who underwent ORN, 39 were alive with a median followup of 28.5 mo. The calculated disease-free survival in this group was 97.5% at 5 yr.

Of interest, was the postoperative recovery where 18 of the 60 laparoscopically treated patients did not receive any narcotics. The remaining 42 received a mean dose of 43 mg of pentazocine. In the open group, all patients required narcotics with an average dose of 68 mg of pentazocine ($p < 0.001$).

Chan summarized the Johns Hopkins experience where 67 LRNs were performed and compared to a contemporary cohort of 54 patients who underwent an ORN *(6)*. The mean operative time was 4.2 h for the LRN group and 3.2 h for the ORN group ($p < 0.001$). Notably, there was a significant decrease in the operative time between the first 15 and last 15 LRNs. The mean estimated blood loss (EBL) was 289 cc for laparoscopy and 309 cc for open surgery; there was no significant difference in this regard. Only one patient in the LRN group was converted to an open procedure; this patient had a renal vein that was visually suspicious for renal vein thrombus. The thrombus was successfully controlled through an ORN approach. The mean hospital stay for LRN and ORN groups was 3.8 and 7.2 d, respectively; this difference was statistically significant. Pain medication requirements and convalescence were not reported.

The kidney was approached via a transperitoneal approach in 66 out of 67 cases. The specimen was morcellated in 40 cases and thus routine pathologic staging was not available in these cases. Of the morcellated specimens, two were determined to be stage pT3 disease based on perinephric fat invasion in one case and renal vein invasion in the other patient. Of the intact specimens, 11 were determined to be pT3. One foreign patient was lost to followup. Eight patients in this group have died, including two with metastatic disease. Thus, 59 patients had no evidence of metastatic disease or recurrence; no patient had a port-site recurrence. Of the ORN population of 54, 40 patients had pathologic pT1 and 14 had pT2. Overall, 41 patients were alive at time of report and only two cancer-specific deaths were reported. Two other patients had lung metastasis appear and one patient with von Hippel-Lindau (VHL) disease recurred in the opposite kidney. Kaplan-Meier analysis revealed that the mean actuarial survival time was 6.9 yr in the LRN group and 5.9 yr in the ORN group; mean disease-free survival was 7.2 yr and 6.8 yr, respectively. There was no statistically significant difference in either comparison.

Table 1
Laparoscopic Radical Nephrectomy: Worldwide Experience, 2002

| *Author (Reference)* | *Cases* | *Operating Time (h)* | *EBL (cc)* | *Spec. Wt. (g)* | *Stage* | *Hosp. Stay (d)* | *Recovery (wk)* | *Followup (mo)* | *Comp (major/minor)* | *Seeding* |
|---|---|---|---|---|---|---|---|---|---|---|
| Janetschek et al. *(13)* | 31 | 2.4 | NS | NS | T1/T2 | 2.9 | NS | 18 | 0%/0% | None |
| Ono et al. *(5)* | 91 | 4.9 | 300 | 289 | T1/T2 | NS | 3.0 | 22 | 11% | None |
| Barrett et al. *(14)* | 72 | 2.9 | NS | 402 | T1/T2 | 4.4 | NS | 21 | 1 death 3%/8% | One |
| Dunn et al. *(11)* | 61 | 5.5 | 172 | 452 | T1/T2/T3b (r.v.) | 3.4 | 3.6 | 25 | 3%/34% | None |
| Gill *(7)* | 100 | 2.8 | 212 | 403 | T1/T2/T3 | 1.6 | 4.2 | 16 | 3%/11% | None |
| Chan *(6)* | 67 | 4.3 | 289 | NS | T1/T2/T3 | 3.8 | NS | 36 | 15% overall | None |
| Total | 422 | 3.8 | 243 | 387 | T1/T2/T3a/T3b | 3.2 | 3.6 | 23 | Mortality 0.3% | 0.3% |

EBL = estimated blood loss; NS = nonsignificant; r.v. = renal vein.

Gill recently reported the Cleveland Clinic experience of LRN making comparison of his first 100 cases with a retrospective cohort of 40 ORN *(7)*. All specimens were extracted intact and the retroperitoneal approach was used 73 times. A comparable operative time was achieved in this study with the LRN and ORN group with a mean of 2.9 h and 3.1 h, respectively. EBL was significantly lower in the LRN group (187 vs 670 mL). The LRN conversion rate was 2%, in both cases due to hemorrhage. The operative time in this series also decreased with increasing experience despite the observation that the specimen size increased over time.

Preoperative computed tomography (CT) scans for the LRN and ORN groups revealed a mean size of 5.1 and 5.4 cm, respectively. Staging in the LRN group consisted of 61 pT1 tumors, 6 pT2 tumors, 12 pT3 tumors, and 1 pT4 tumor. The ORN group's pathologic staging was as follows: 27 pT1 tumors, 4 pT2 tumors, and 9 pT3 tumors. Specimen weight was equivalent at 569 g for the laparoscopic group and 559 g for the open group. There were no positive surgical margins in either group. Over a mean followup period of 1.3 yr, no local or port-site recurrences were noted. Two patients with pT1 tumors developed metastatic disease.

Portis assembled a multi-institutional study with the longest followup after LRN reported to date *(8)*. This study compared the LRN group of 64 patients (median followup of 4.5 yr) vs a cohort of 69 patients (median follow-up of 5.8 yr) treated with ORN; all patients in this series were more than 3 yr out from their surgery. In this study, EBL was significantly less for laparoscopy (219 vs 354) and the operating room time was longer (4.8 hr vs 2.1 hr).

Preoperative CT in this study revealed that the ORN group had a significantly larger tumor size (6.2 cm vs 4.3 cm). Despite this, the specimen weight was not different between LRN and ORN at 425 g and 495 g, respectively. Local recurrence occurred in one patient in each of the ORN and LRN series. Distant metastasis was noted in 3 patients after LRN; in the ORN series, this occurred in 10 patients. The 5-yr Kaplan-Meier survival curves were calculated and no difference was noted in overall survival, disease-free survival, and cancer-specific survival.

## MORBIDITY

In series of laparoscopic transperitoneal standard nephrectomy, the complications have included transfusion, ileus, bowel obstruction, wound infection, medical complications, and other organ injuries. In the Nagoya experience, out of 60 patients, 2 required blood transfusion. There were intraoperative injuries to the left renal artery, spleen, duodenum, adrenal gland, and a periureteral artery. The duodenal and left renal artery injuries required conversion. Postoperatively, two patients suffered an ileus and another suffered a pulmonary embolus *(5)*. Two patients in the ORN group suffered intraoperative complications (one injury to the left renal vein and the spleen). Three patients received a blood transfusion. One patient suffered a postoperative ileus.

The group from Washington University also critically examined their series of 61 LRNs and found two major complications (ligation of the superior mesenteric artery and bleeding requiring conversion). There were 21 minor complications including congestive heart failure, atelectasis, various nerve palsies due to positioning, ileus, incisional hernia, LapSac leakage, and pleural effusion *(8)*. Complications were noted in the ORN cohort in this summary in 18 patients; the four major complications included injury to the superior mesenteric artery, colon injury, postoperative pulmonary embolus, and a 3000 cc EBL requiring transfusion. Three patients required intraoperative transfusions and two required postoperative transfusions. Fourteen minor complications included fever, pneumothorax, cardiac arrhythmias, and wound infection. The incidences of major and minor complications were both higher in the open group.

Abbou and his group summarized an experience of 50 retroperitoneal laparoscopic nephrectomies. Two patients had minor complications of atelectasis and local inflammation. Two major complications were encountered: one colon injury requiring temporary diversion and one conversion due to bleeding *(4)*. Gill reported on his series of 53 retroperitoneal nephrectomies and had two major complications including splenectomy and renal arterial injury requiring conversion. Eight minor complications occurred including infection, hematoma, ileus, atelectasis, skin rash, and cutaneous hyperesthesia *(9)*.

In a recent study at the Cleveland Clinic, Gill and colleagues prospectively randomized patients to transperitoneal (43 cases) or retroperitoneal (45 cases) laparoscopic nephrectomy. There was no statistically significant difference in hospital stay, analgesics, or blood loss. However, the retroperitoneal approach, in their hands, resulted in shorter operative time, 2.6 h vs 3.4 h and there was a trend toward fewer complications *(10)*.

## COSTS

The major drawback of LRN in the past has been one of cost effectiveness. The increased expense of the laparoscopic equipment and the increased operative time, plus the premium charged for the laparoscopic approach, resulted in most cases in a situation in which the LRN cost upward of $2000 more than a standard ORN approach *(11)*. However, with increasing operator experience and with a decrease in the amount of disposable equipment used during the laparoscopic procedure, the costs have come down signi¡ficantly. In a recent review of this topic, Cadeddu and associates showed that once the operative time for LRN fell below 4.7 h, combined with a hospital stay of less than 5.8 d and intraoperative costs of less than $5500, the savings incurred by a laparoscopic approach were $1200. Currently, at most centers, the time for the procedure has dropped to 4 h and the hospital stay is routinely less than 3 d. As such, the LRN in many centers is now more cost effective than an ORN *(12)*.

## CONCLUSIONS

In summary, in regard to efficiency, complications, oncologic results, and cost effectiveness, the LRN has truly evolved into a standard of care for treating T1–2 lesions of the kidney for which a radical nephrectomy is indicated. In many centers, it has now completely replaced open surgery for these lesions.

## REFERENCES

1. Clayman RV, Kavoussi LR, Soper NJ, et al. Laparoscopic nephrectomy: initial case report. J Urol 1991; 146: 278–282.
2. Chan DY, Su LM, Kavoussi LR. Rapid ligation of renal hilum during transperitoneal laparoscopic nephrectomy. Urology 2001; 57: 360–362.
3. Chan D, Bishoff JT, Ratner L, et al. Endovascular gastrointestinal stapler device malfunction during laparoscopic nephrectomy: early recognition and management. J Urol 2000; 164: 319–321.
4. Cicco A, Salomon L, Hoznek A, et al. Results of retroperitoneal laparoscopic radical nephrectomy. J Endourol 2001; 15: 355–359.
5. Ono Y, Kinukawa T, Hattori R, et al. Laparoscopic radical nephrectomy for renal cell carcinoma: a five-year experience. Urology 1999; 53: 280–286.
6. Chan DY, Cadeddu JA, Jarrett TW, et al.: Laparoscopic radical nephrectomy: cancer control for renal cell carcinoma. J Urol 2001; 166: 2095–2099.
7. Gill IS, Meraney AM, Schweizer DK, et al. Laparoscopic radical nephrectomy in 100 patients: a single center experience from the United States. Cancer 2001; 92: 1843–1855.
8. Portis AJ, Yan Y, Landman J, et al. Long-term followup after laparoscopic radical nephrectomy. J Urol 2002; 167: 1257–1262.
9. Gill IS. Laparoscopic radical nephrectomy for cancer. Urologic Clinics of North America 2000; 27: 707–719.
10. Gill IS, Strzempkowski B, Kaouk J, et al. Prospective randomized comparison: transperitoneal versus retroperitoneal laparoscopic radical nephrectomy. J Urol 2002; 167(suppl): 19.
11. Dunn MD, Portis AJ, Shalhav AL, et al. Laparoscopic versus open radical nephrectomy: a 9-year experience. J Urol 2000; 164: 1153–1159.
12. Lotan Y, Gettman MT, Roehrborn CG, et al. Cost comparison for laproscopic nephrectomy and open nephrectomy: analysis of individual parameters. Urology 2002; 59: 821–825.

13. Janetschek G, Jeschke K, Peschel R, et al. Laparoscopic surgery for stage T1 renal cell carcinoma: radical nephrectomy and wedge resection. Eur Urol 2000; 38: 131–138.
14. Barrett PH, Fentie DD, Tarager LA. Laparoscopic radical nephrectomy with morcellation for renal cell carcinoma: the Saskatoon experience. Urology 1998; 52: 23–28.

# 2 Role of Laparoscopic Nephrectomy in Metastatic Renal Cell Carcinoma

*Stephen E. Pautler,* MD, FRCSC
*and McClellan M. Walther,* MD, FACS

*CONTENTS*

INTRODUCTION
INDICATIONS
CONTRAINDICATIONS
OVERVIEW OF SURGICAL TECHNIQUE
RESULTS
CONTROVERSIAL ISSUES
SHORTCOMINGS OF LAPAROSCOPIC TECHNIQUE
REFERENCES

## INTRODUCTION

Renal cell carcinoma (RCC) is a life-threatening disease with a significant health burden to society. In 2001, there were an estimated 12,100 deaths from RCC in the United States *(1)*. Presentation with advanced kidney cancer occurs in approximately one-third of patients *(2)* leading to significant morbidity and mortality. The use of systemic immunotherapy affords this patient population the best chance at survival, although various trials have demonstrated suboptimal response rates *(3,4)*. Results of recent studies from single institutions and two multicenter randomized trials suggest a survival benefit for patients who underwent cytoreductive nephrectomy followed by some form of systemic immunotherapy *(5–7)*. Unfortunately, many patients are not

From: *Laparoscopic Urologic Oncology*
Edited by: J. A. Cadeddu © Humana Press Inc., Totowa, NJ

fit to receive systemic immunotherapy following surgery. In an effort to decrease morbidity from the procedure and to increase the number of patients fit for systemic treatment, the National Cancer Institute (NCI) group began performing cytoreductive laparoscopic radical nephrectomies (LRNs) in appropriate candidates. Herein, we describe the procedure and the early outcomes.

## INDICATIONS

The most broadly accepted indications for surgery in the patient with metastatic kidney cancer are symptoms attributed to the primary tumor. These symptoms include intractable gross hematuria, significant pain due to pressure effects or local invasion, and various debilitating paraneoplastic syndromes in selected patients. Furthermore, in the small population of patients who present with an isolated metastasis, nephrectomy in conjunction with metastasectomy can be curative *(8,9)*. Currently, cytoreductive nephrectomy is considered relative indication for patients with a good performance status despite multiple metastases and who are eligible for inclusion in a clinical trial of systemic therapy for treatment of their metastases. It has been extremely rare to observe a response to systemic immunotherapy in the primary tumor *(10)*. Other rationales for cytoreduction include the reduction in tumor burden and the source of future metastases, for harvesting of tumor-infiltrating leukocytes, and for identification of tumor-specific antigens for trials involving tumor vaccines.

## CONTRAINDICATIONS

Resectability of the primary tumor must be assessed on a case-by-case basis. A specific size criterion does not exist to preclude a laparoscopic approach, although the surgeon must be cognizant of adjacent organ involvement, working space limitations, and surgeon experience. Several contraindications do exist including poor performance status of the patient, a level III or greater vena cava tumor thrombus, uncorrectable coagulopathy, and massive intraperitoneal tumor metastases. Relative contraindications to cytoreductive LRN include the patient's unwillingness to participate in a clinical trial of systemic therapy, pregnancy, metastases to the central nervous system, and abnormal body habitus impeding positioning. With respect to adjacent organ involvement, techniques have been developed for laparoscopic resection of the diaphragm *(11)*, tail of the pancreas, and spleen if necessary. Recent reports of advanced laparoscopic management of level I–II vena caval thrombi have been reported *(12–14)*.

## OVERVIEW OF SURGICAL TECHNIQUE

Preoperatively, patients undergo a mechanical/antibiotic bowel prep and aggressive hydration through a large intravenous (iv) cannula. Subcutaneous heparin and pneumatic stockings are used for deep vein thrombosis prophylaxis. Additionally, patients receive a single dose of iv first generation cephalosporin prophylaxis. A urethral catheter and an orogastric tube are placed. Nitrous oxide anesthetic is avoided to prevent bowel distension. To maximize the working space between the lower costal margin and the anterior superior iliac spine, the patient is positioned with the affected side up and table flexion is used without the use of a beanbag or kidney rest. Generous padding is required; including an axillary roll and support for the ipsilateral arm (Fig. 1)

The preferred approach is transperitoneal due to the increased working space and the ability to survey the abdominal organs for metastases. We prefer an open access rather than a Veress technique because often times the primary tumors are quite large and there can be distortion of the intra-abdominal anatomy leading to an access-related injury if the Veress needle is employed. The camera port is placed in the ipsilateral paramedian line and two working ports are placed in a triangular fashion to facilitate an ergonomic approach to the kidney (Fig. 2). On the right side, an additional subxiphoid port is required for cephalad retraction of the liver using a fan or snake-type retractor. A retractor holder eliminates the need for an assistant to hold the retractor throughout the case *(15)*. Routine use of the AESOP robotic arm for control of the camera is a useful adjunct to reduce surgical assistant fatigue.

The basic steps of dissection follow those pioneered by Clayman and colleagues *(16)*. Several important considerations deserve attention. The key to the procedure is identification and control of the renal hilum. In cytoreductive LRN, there is a higher risk of renal vein and/or vena cava involvement due to the advanced nature of disease. Once the ureter is identified on the right or the gonadal vein on the left, then cephalad dissection following these structures will lead to the hilum. We recommend isolation of the artery and vein separately using meticulous dissection. A right-angled dissector is useful for separation of the vessels. Counter-traction on the kidney aids in identification of the hilar structures. If the primary tumor is large, standard laparoscopic instruments do not provide enough strength for retraction. A gynecological instrument called the spoon/cup biopsy forceps has a solid shaft that allows even very large tumors to be retracted. During left-sided dissections, the surgeon should ligate the gonadal vein prior to dissecting out the renal vein. The lumbar vein can be in close proximity to the renal artery and requires

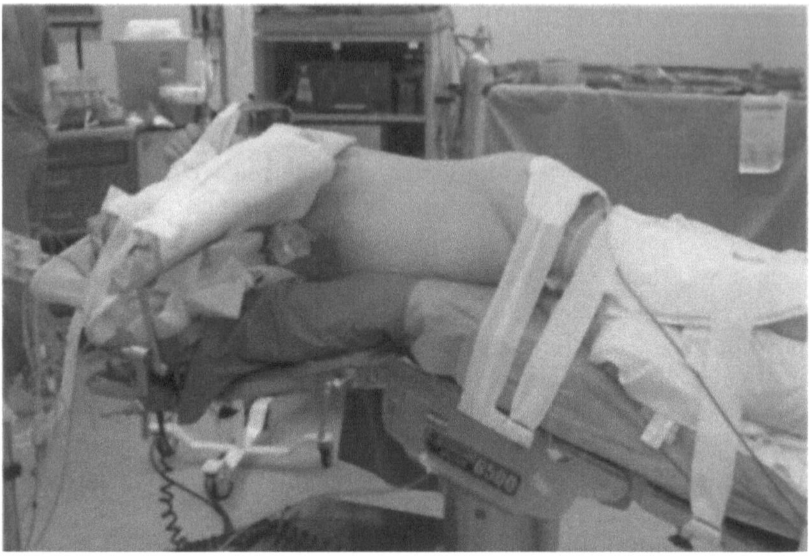

**Fig. 1.** Patient positioning for cytoreductive laparoscopic radical nephrectomy. Patient is in the flank position with the table flexed and adequate padding of all pressure points.

careful attention. Once the hilum is fully dissected, the artery is ligated using clips or an endovascular-stapling device. Inspection of the renal vein is mandatory to ensure it has collapsed. An instrument can be passed behind the vein to tent it up to ensure the absence of a tumor thrombus or additional arteries. Doppler ultrasound performed using a laparoscopic probe is required if there is any question of tumor thrombus or multiple arteries. The vein is secured using an endovascular stapler.

If adjacent organ resection is required, then the approach should be considered in detail preoperatively. The endovascular staplers are very useful for isolation of the tail of the pancreas and for ligation of the splenic hilum and short gastric arteries if splenectomy is required. Diaphragm resection is occasionally indicated *(11,17)*. A harmonic scalpel or shears provide sufficient vascular control in the majority of cases. During resection, care must be taken not to injure the lung parenchyma or the phrenic nerve. Attention must be paid to the patient's ventilatory status and if hypercarbia or respiratory compromise occurs, then immediate chest tube placement or conversion to open is required *(11)*.

Specimen removal following LRN for localized disease remains somewhat controversial. In the cytoreduction setting, morcellation of the specimen is an attractive option. The data that exists directly com-

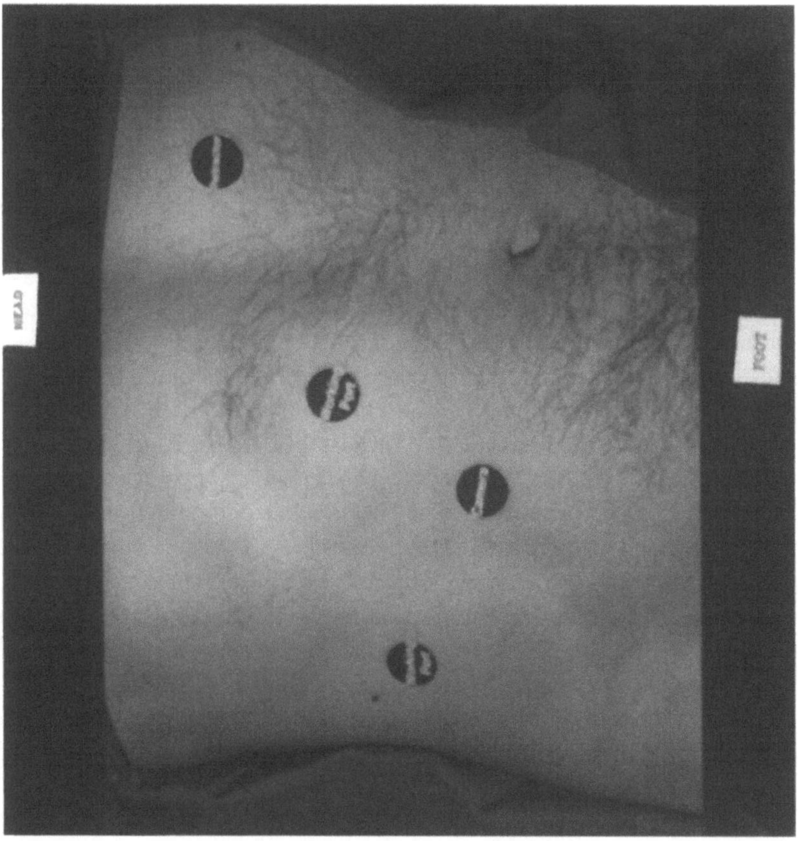

**Fig. 2.** Port placement for a right-sided cytoreductive laparoscopic radical nephrectomy.

paring intact removal and morcellation in patients undergoing cytoreduction demonstrated an advantage for the morcellation group in terms of postoperative narcotic requirement and time to receive systemic immunotherapy *(18)*. Concern of port-site tumor implantation is less ominous in this population because these patients have documented metastases elsewhere and will be receiving adjuvant therapy. Morcellation requires use of the impermeable LapSac (Cook Urological, Spencer, IN) to prevent tumor spillage. The size limitation of this sack is a specimen diameter of 15 cm. The specimen should freely spin 360° prior to attempting to place it in the sack. Generally, three graspers are used to hold the sack open mandating placement of an additional port in most cases. Recently, a device to hold open the sack has been described *(19)*. Alternatively, a guidewire can be placed through the mouth of the sack to open it *(20)*. Extra drapes and a skin barrier are used to protect the operative field from tumor spillage.

## RESULTS

In the initial NCI pilot series, operative results of cytoreductive LRN revealed significantly longer operative times in comparison to open cytoreduction. Blood loss was not significantly improved via the laparoscopic approach likely reflecting the advanced nature of the disease and difficulty of dissection. Benefits of the pure laparoscopic approach (with specimen morcellation) included less postoperative narcotics, a shorter hospital stay, and a shorter time to the administration of adjuvant high-dose Interleukin (IL)-2 therapy. Previously, up to 38% of patients who underwent open cytoreductive LRN at the NCI were unfit to receive systemic high dose IL-2 due to poor performance status or progressive disease *(7,21,22)*. Mortality associated with open cytoreduction LRN has been reported to be up to 4% in some series *(23)*. To date, no deaths have occurred in hospital following cytoreductive LRN in our series.

Oncologic outcomes are somewhat more difficult to assess. Cytoreductive LRN has been performed in the setting of a large randomized phase III trial of systemic IL-2 therapy, thus limiting the ability to draw any conclusions about the efficacy of LRN in these patients. Clearly, adjuvant therapy is required for these patients and the current standard of care in the United States is systemic IL-2 therapy. With respect to laparoscopy-specific oncology outcomes, no port-site recurrences have occurred.

Cytoreductive LRN is comparable to open cytoreductive nephrectomy with significant complication rates ranging from 13 to 50% *(21,22,24–26)*. The type and severity of complications are similar for the two approaches including blood loss and postoperative ileus. The blood loss seen with laparoscopic cytoreduction is greater than that during LRN for localized disease likely due to the abundant tumor vessels, adjacent organ involvement, and the bulky hilar lymphadenopathy found with advanced disease. We have observed a disproportionate number of cases of skin blistering and even cases of contralateral psoas necrosis due to the prolonged operating times with the patients in the flank position during cytoreductive LRN.

## CONTROVERSIAL ISSUES

Experience with cytoreductive LRN is limited. Walther et al. published the largest series to date. There was a statistically significant improvement in morbidity measures such as postoperative narcotic use and time to treatment with immunotherapy. To date, these results have yet to be validated at other institutions. For cytoreductive LRN to be fairly assessed, a multicenter prospective trial involving experienced laparoscopic urologic oncologists will have to be completed to prove benefit.

Further information has been published suggesting that the presence of retroperitoneal lymphadenopathy portends a poor prognosis in patients with metastatic kidney cancer *(27)*. Additionally, the UCLA group has found that patients with lymphadenopathy at the time of cytoreductive nephrectomy who do not undergo debulking lymphadenectomy have a poorer survival. Thus, if lymphadenopathy is present at the time of cytoreduction, the surgeon should endeavor to perform a lymphadenectomy. Using the laparoscopic approach, retroperitoneal lymphadenectomy can be performed, although no data currently exists regarding the completeness of the dissection or outcomes for metastatic kidney cancer. Clearly, further study is required.

The last subject of controversy remains specimen morcellation. As mentioned earlier, morcellation is an attractive option for patients with metastatic kidney cancer because these patients are able to receive systemic immunotherapy sooner and require less postoperative analgesia *(18)*. Some authors have argued that intact removal and morcellation lead to the same analgesia requirement in the localized kidney cancer setting *(28)*, but these tumors were all small relative to those found at the time of cytoreduction where the incision for intact removal can be quite large. Obtaining an accurate pathological diagnosis is critical prior to the administration of systemic therapy and morcellation in the cytoreductive setting does provide sufficient material for diagnosis *(29)*.

## SHORTCOMINGS OF LAPAROSCOPIC TECHNIQUE

Cytoreductive LRN remains a new technique with few centers performing the procedure. To date, the results of an initial pilot series are encouraging although further study must be done to determine the suitability of this procedure in the management of patients with metastatic kidney cancer. The laparoscopic technique is not recommended for patients with large tumor thrombi or extensive adjacent organ involvement in which massive reconstructive procedures will be required. The feasibility and thoroughness of lymphadenectomy for enlarged nodes remains to be proven.

## REFERENCES

1. American Cancer Society. Cancer Facts and Figures; 2001.
2. Hock LM, Lynch J, Balaji KC. Increasing incidence of kidney cancer in the last 2 decades in the United States: An analysis of surveillance, epidemiology and end results program data. J Urol 2002; 167: 57–60.

3. Fyfe G, Fisher RI, Rosenberg SA, et al. Results of treatment of 255 patients with metastastic renal cell carcinoma who received high-dose recombinant interleukin-2 therapy. J Clin Oncol 1995; 13: 688–696
4. Figlin RA. Renal cell carcinoma: Management of advanced disease. J Urol 1999; 161: 381–387.
5. Flanigan RC, Salmon SE, Blumenstein BA, et al. Nephrectomy followed by interferon alfa-2b compared with interferon alfa-2b alone for metastatic renal-cell cancer. N Engl J Med 2001; 345: 1655–1659.
6. Mickisch GHJ, Garin A, van Poppel H, et al. Radical nephrectomy plus interferon-alfa-based immunotherapy compared with interferon alfa alone in metastatic renal-cell carcinoma: a randomized trial. Lancet 2001; 358: 966–970.
7. Walther MM, Yang JC, Pass HI, et al. Cytoreductive surgery before high dose interleukin-2 based therapy in patients with metastatic renal cell carcinoma. J Urol 1997; 158: 1675–1678.
8. Cerfolio RJ, Allen MS, Deschamps C, et al. Pulmonary resection of metastatic renal cell carcinoma. Ann Thorac Surg 1994; 57: 339–344.
9. Friedel G, Hürtgen M, Penzenstadler M, Kyriss T, Toomes H. Resection of pulmonary metastases from renal cell carcinoma. Anticancer Res 1999; 19: 1593–1596.
10. Wagner JR, Walther MM, Linehan WM, et al. Interleukin-2 based immunotherapy for metastatic renal cell carcinoma with the kidney in place. J Urol 1999; 162: 43–45.
11. Pautler SE, Richards C, Libutti SK, Linehan WM, Walther MM. Intentional resection of the diaphragm during cytoreductive laparoscopic radical nephrectomy. J Urol 2002; 167: 48–50.
12. Dunn MD, Portis AJ, Shalhav AL, et al. Laparoscopic versus open radical nephrectomy: A 9-year experience. J Urol 2000; 164: 1153–1159.
13. Savage SJ, Gill IS: Laparoscopic radical nephrectomy for renal cell carcinoma in a patient with level I renal vein thrombus. J Urol 2000; 163: 1243–1244.
14. Sundaram CP, Rehman J, Landman J, Oh J. Hand assisted laparoscopic radical nephrectomy for renal cell carcinoma with inferior vena caval thrombus. J Urol 2002; 168: 176–179.
15. Pautler SE, McWilliams GW, Harrington FS, Walther MM. An articulating retractor holder to facilitate laparoscopic adrenalectomy and nephrectomy. J Urol 2001; 166:198–199.
16. Dunn MD, McDougall EM, Clayman RV. Laparoscopic radical nephrectomy. J Endourol 2000; 14: 849–855.
17. Rehman J, Landman J, Kerbl K, Clayman RV. Laparoscopic repair of diaphragmatic defect by total intracorporeal suturing: Clinical and technical considerations. J Soc Lap Surg 2001; 5: 287–291.
18. Walther MM, Lyne JC, Libutti SK, Linehan WM. Laparoscopic cytoreductive nephrectomy as preparation for administration of systemic interleukin-2 in the treatment of metastatic renal cell carcinoma: A pilot study. Urology 1999; 53: 496–501.
19. Pautler SE, Harrington FS, McWilliams GW, Walther MM. A novel laparoscopic specimen entrapment device to facilitate morcellation of large renal tumors. Urology 2002; 59: 591–593.
20. Sundaram CP, Ono Y, Landman J, Rehman J, Clayman RV. Hydrophilic guide wire technique to facilitate organ entrapment using a laparoscopic sack during laparoscopy. J Urol 2002; 167: 1376–1377.
21. Levy DA, Swanson DA, Slaton JW, Ellerhorst J, Dinney CPN. Timely delivery of biological therapy after cytoreductive nephrectomy in carefully selected patients with metastatic renal cell carcinoma. J Urol 1998; 159:1168–1173.

22. Walther MM, Alexander RB, Wiess GH, et al. Cytoreductive surgery prior to interleukin-2-based therapy in patients with metastatic renal cell carcinoma. Urology 1993; 42: 250–257.
23. Flanigan RC, Yonover PM. The role of radical nephrectomy in metastatic renal cell carcinoma. Sem Urol Oncol 2001; 19: 98–102.
24. Rackley R, Novick A, Klein E, Bukowski R, McLain D, Goldfarb D. The impact of adjuvant nephrectomy on multimodality treatment of metastatic renal cell carcinoma. J Urol 1994; 152: 1399–1403.
25. Bennett RT, Lerner SE, Taub HC, Dutcher JP, Fleischmann J. Cytoreductive surgery for stage IV renal cell carcinoma. J Urol 1995; 154: 32–34.
26. Franklin JR, Figlin R, Rauch J, Gitlitz B, Belldegrun A. Cytoreductive surgery in the management of metastatic renal cell carcinoma: the UCLA experience. Sem Urol Oncol 1996; 14: 230–236.
27. Vasselli JR, Yang JC, Linehan WM, et al. Lack of retroperitoneal lymphadenopathy predicts survival of patients with metastatic renal cell carcinoma. J Urol 2001; 166: 68–72.
28. Savage SJ, Gill IS. Intact specimen extraction during renal laparoscopy: muscle-splitting versus muscle-cutting incision. J Endourol 2001;15: 165–169.
29. Pautler SE, Hewitt SM, Linehan WM, Walther MM. Specimen morcellation after laparoscopic radical nephrectomy: Confirmation of histological diagnosis using needle biopsy. J Endourol 2002; 16: 89–92.

# 3 Morcellation vs Intact Specimen Removal

## *Clinical Implications and Risk of Tumor Recurrences*

*Steve Y. Chung,* MD
*and Timothy D. Averch,* MD

*CONTENTS*

INTRODUCTION
DEVICES
MORCELLATION VS INTACT SPECIMEN
FUTURE
REFERENCES

## INTRODUCTION

Morcellation is the fragmentation of whole tissue performed either manually or by high-speed electrical motor. This was initially described in the gynecologic literature in 1970 in 109 successful vaginal hysterectomies *(1)*. It has now taken a role in laparoscopic nephrectomy but its use is a subject of controversy and ongoing debate.

Laparoscopy has gained popularity in the field of urology, but it is only recently that the first laparoscopic total nephrectomy was performed and the use of morcellation was described *(2)*. This took place in June 1990 at Washington University in an 85-yr-old woman for a right-sided 3-cm renal mass. Upon complete dissection, the specimen was placed into a nylon organ sack and fragmented using a newly developed laparoscopic tissue morcellator. The morcellation took only 7 min and made it possible to deliver the 190 g fragmented kidney through an 11-mm port site.

From: *Laparoscopic Urologic Oncology*
Edited by: J. A. Cadeddu © Humana Press Inc., Totowa, NJ

Since the initial report, numerous studies have established the use of laparoscopy as an acceptable alternative for the removal of benign renal disease. Successful outcomes have been reported for the extirpation of renal malignancy using minimally invasive techniques as well *(3,4)*. Long-term followup has suggested that laparoscopy has an overall 5-yr recurrence-free and cancer-specific survival statistically equivalent to that of the traditional open approach *(5)*. The advantages of using laparoscopy are decreased perioperative morbidity, length of hospital stay, postoperative narcotic requirement, and complete convalescence *(6)*.

Although not an issue with benign disease, laparoscopic applications in cancer have raised debate over specimen retrieval. To preserve information on staging and to reduce the risk for seeding, patients have been subjected to incisions up to 7 cm for intact specimen removal. This has been achieved by extending a midline trocar incision or by creating a separate Pfannenstiel incision. In select female patients, Gill and colleagues described intact specimen removal through the vagina *(7)*. Although intact specimen incisions are smaller and carefully placed to limit patient discomfort, they somewhat detract from the cosmetic affect of minimally invasive surgery. Morcellation allows for the removal of a specimen through a port site while maintaining the cosmetic benefits of a laparoscopic approach and possibly reducing the risk of incisional hernia formation.

At the expense of preserving cosmesis, morcellation is not without risks and many questions remain. Prolonged operative time, complications, problems with staging, risks of port-site recurrence, efficacy of long-term tumor control, and costs are issues that need to be addressed.

## DEVICES

Morcellation requires two main instruments: durable organ sack and morcellator. Over the past decade, these devices have not strayed too far from their original design. This has allowed consistency among numerous institutional studies but has potentially averted the introduction of newer and possibly more improved devices.

### *Organ Sacks*

In 1990, the LapSac (Cook Urological, Spencer, IN) and introducer were introduced (Figs. 1, 2). The LapSac is made of a reinforced double-layered plastic and nylon pouch with the inner coating made of impermeable polyurethane. Presently, it is the only sack that has been shown to be strong enough for high-speed electrical morcellation in

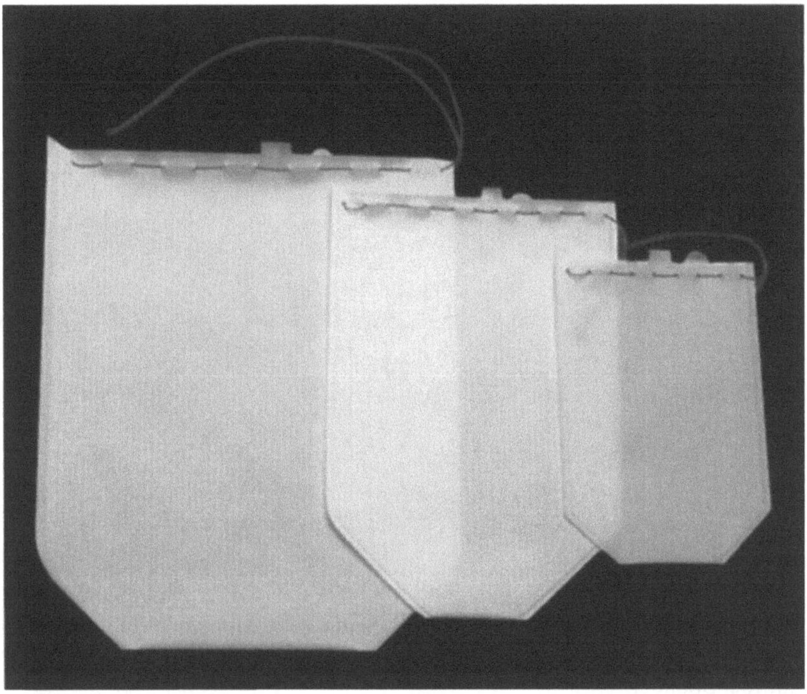

**Fig. 1.** LapSacs, in three various sizes, are the only acceptable sacks durable enough for high-energy morcellation. (Reprinted with permission from Cook Urological Inc. Spencer, IN.)

laparoscopic nephrectomy *(8–11)*. One drawback to the LapSac is the lack of an integral deployment mechanism. Entrapping the kidney in the sack can be very time consuming and awkward, especially for inexperienced laparoscopists. Novel methods in deployment have been described to ease the burden for the surgeon, such as the use of a guidewire inserted parallel to the drawstring *(4,12)*.

The Endocatch (Auto Suture Company, The United States Surgical Corporation, Norwalk, CT) has also been shown to successfully entrap organs. The 15-mm outer sheath easily retracts releasing the transparent entrapment bag, and the 10-cm opening is maintained by two thin pieces of metal. Although the device is simpler to use and the organ can be visualized, the Endocatch is not durable enough for high-speed electrical morcellation *(11)*. On mechanical testing, the Endocatch system has been found to resist breakage during specimen retrieval and require less force for withdrawal *(13)*. This was attributable to its stretching and molding capabilities.

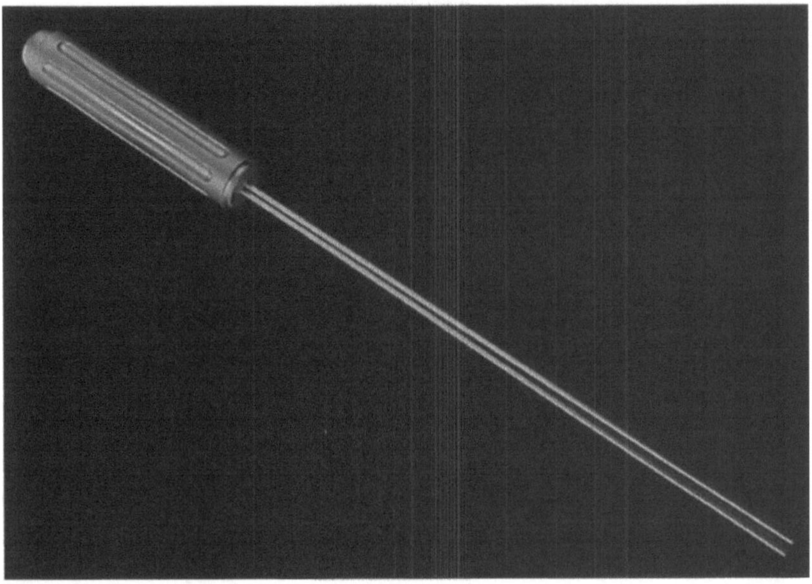

**Fig. 2.** The LapSac is rolled around the introducer and placed through ports to eliminate risks of perforation. (Reprinted with permission from Cook Urological, Inc. Spencer, IN.)

## *Morcellators*

Most studies on morcellation in the urologic literature have commented on the safety and clinical efficacy of the high-speed electrical morcellator (Cook Urological, Spencer, IN); however it is no longer available for clinical use. The Steiner electromechanical morcellator (Karl Storz, Culver City, CA), which is often used in gynecological cases *(14)*, and the electrical prostate morcellator (EPM, Coherent, Sturbridge, MA), which was made for intravesical morcellation of prostate tissue after holmium laser prostatectomy, have been applied to porcine kidney morcellation *(11)*. The Steiner has been shown to morcellate kidneys two to four times quicker than the conventional morcellator. Renal fragments were also significantly larger, which allowed for better histological examination *(11,14)*. The EPM, although not as fast, morcellated tissue into smaller fragments allowing for easy extraction *(11)*. Other morcellators available for clinical use, although mostly reported in gynecological literature, are the battery operated Serrated Edged Macro Morcellator (SEMM, Wisap America, Lenexa, KS), X-tract morcellator (Gynecare, Piscataway, NJ), and Morce-power (Richard Wolf Medical Instruments,Vernon Hills, IL) (Fig. 3). These may serve a role in laparoscopic nephrectomies in the near future due to their availability and ease of use.

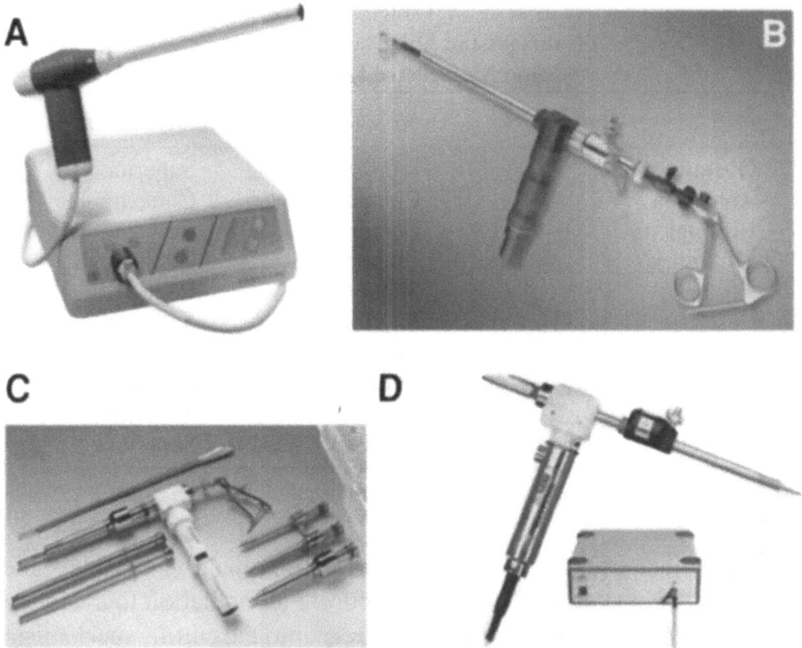


**Fig. 3.** Morcellators used in laparoscopic surgery. (**A**) X-tract morcellator; (**B**) Steiner (image courtesy of Karl Storz Endoscopy); (**C**) Serrated Edged Macro Morcellator (image courtesy of WISAP America); (**D**) Morce-power (image courtesy of Richard Wolf Medical Instruments Corp.)

## *Method of Morcellation*

The primary goals throughout tissue morcellation are to maintain clinical safety, uphold tenets of oncological surgery, and judiciously apply these principles throughout morcellation. Before an organ sack is introduced to the surgical field, all sharp instruments should be removed to lessen the risk of sack perforation. The sack should then be filled with normal saline to check for possible leakage. Once integrity is confirmed, the sack may be placed into a port using blunt-tip trocars or Cook's introducer (Fig. 2). Intra-abdominally, the sack should be handled with care, and instruments used for morcellation should not be reused. Frequent glove changes may also reduce the risk of tumor spread. Detailed steps for intra-abdominal passage of entrapment sacks are thoroughly outlined by Nakada and colleagues *(15)*.

During morcellation, the surgeon should be cognizant of certain principles. Firm and gentle rotational strokes should be applied while the morcellator is in direct contact with tissue. The surgeon should also avoid prolonged morcellation contact along the sack. Failure of both

Table 1
Advantages and Disadvantages in Intact and Morcellated Specimens

| | *Morcellation* | *Intact speciman* |
|---|---|---|
| Operative time | Inferior | Superior |
| Analgesia | Comparable | Comparable |
| Hospital stay | Comparable | Comparable |
| Morbidity | Comparable | Comparable |
| Cosmesis | Superior | Inferior |
| Cost-effectiveness | Inferior | Superior |
| Pathologic staging | Inferior | Superior |
| Surgical margins | Inferior | Superior |
| Followup prognostication | Inferior | Superior |
| Port-site recurrence | Inferior | Superior |

Used with permission of Med Reviews (from ref. *16*).

principles increases the risk of sack perforation. Finally, it is advisable to maintain constant pull on the sack during morcellation to avoid the creation of folds in the sack that may creep into the cutting mechanism during suctioning *(10)*.

## MORCELLATION VS INTACT SPECIMEN

The topic of morcellation is a controversial issue in laparoscopic nephrectomies. Several well-designed studies in literature have been published to address particular aspects of this subject matter. These are summarized in Table 1 *(16)*. However, as new data continue to be reported the debate will continue regarding postoperative quality of life, costs, complications, staging, port-site tumor seeding, and tumor control.

### *Postoperative Assessment*

Several studies comparing intact extraction after transperitoneal or retroperitoneal laparoscopic nephrectomies vs traditional open techniques demonstrated significant improvement in decreased analgesia requirements, complications, and hospital stay *(3,4,6,17)*. When comparing laparoscopic nephrectomies with and without tissue morcellation, Walther and co-workers showed a significant decrease in hospital stay and postoperative analgesic usage *(18)*. However, most studies reveal no significant difference in analgesia, hospital stay, or convalescence (Table 2). Dunn and colleagues noted an insignificant trend toward less narcotic requirements and hospital stay, and time to complete convalescence was shorter for the intact specimen group *(6)*. Likewise, others have noted insignificant differences in hospitalization or conva-

## Table 2
**Operative Time, Analgesia Requirements, Hospital Stay, and Convalescence in Intact vs Morcellated Kidney Specimens[a]**

| | *Ono et al. (20)* | | | *Dunn et al. (6)* | | | *Chan et al. (19)* | | | *Gettman et al. (21)* | | |
|---|---|---|---|---|---|---|---|---|---|---|---|---|
| | *Intact* | *Morcellate* | *p* | *Intact* | *Morcellate* | *p* | *Intact* | *Morcellate* | *p* | *Intact* | *Morcellate* | *p* |
| Patients | 26 | 34 | | 21 | 39 | | 27 | 40 | | 5 | 7 | |
| Operative time (min) | 318 | 306 | NS | 381 | 299 | S | n/a | n/a | n/a | 209 | 184 | NS |
| Specimen (g) | 276 | 281 | NS | 5.4 cm | 5.3 cm | NS | n/a | n/a | n/a | n/a | n/a | n/a |
| Postop analgesia (mg) | 34 | 29 | NS | 36 | 24 | NS | n/a | n/a | n/a | 15 | 34 | NS |
| Hospital stay (d) | n/a | n/a | n/a | 3.8 | 3.2 | NS | 3.9 | 3.6 | NS | 2.6 | 2.6 | NS |
| Convalescence (d) | 23.6 | 23.3 | NS | 19.6 | 28.7 | NS | n/a | n/a | n/a | 16 | 22 | NS |

[a]Single studies reveal no significant differences.
NS = nonsignificant; n/a = not applicable.

lescence between the two groups *(19,20)*. A preliminary prospective study evaluating subjective pain and activity assessments at time intervals of up to 2 wk noted similar findings *(21)*. The study, however, is limited because of the small cohort of patients. Larger randomized clinical studies will be necessary before conclusive statements can be made.

### *Operative Time and Costs*

The time required for tissue entrapment and morcellation is variable and operative times can increase by up to 1 h *(8)*. With familiarity with the morcellation technique, laparoscopic nephrectomies now take generally less than 3 h, with or without tissue morcellation *(9,21)*. When the extraction site is lengthened from 12 mm to 2 cm, Landman and co-workers have publicized a total morcellation and average extraction time of only 13.6 min (6–20 min) in in vitro studies of renal tumors averaging 4.9 cm in diameter *(8)*. Furthermore, with increasing surgeon experience, total operative time with morcellation and extraction should continue to improve.

The additional costs associated with morcellation cannot be overlooked. The traditional morcellator (least expensive) costs $1975, whereas the Steiner and EPM morcellators have an overhead cost of $9995 and $18,000, respectively. Additionally, the disposable blade and organ sack costs a combined $175.25 *(8)*. Prolonged operative time for novice surgeons may add additional operating room expenses.

### *Complications*

Urban and colleagues initially evaluated the integrity of organ sacks in 1993 *(10)*. They tested 24 LapSacs after in vivo use with the high-speed electrical tissue morcellator and noted 4 sacks to have pinhole perforations. The authors were unable to determine the exact time point of puncture. The remaining 20 LapSacs underwent permeability testing with serum albumin, indigo carmine (American Regent, Shirley, NY), and mouse bladder tumor cells. They were found to be impermeable to bacteria and tumor cells after the morcellation process. In a different study of 15 tested LapSacs, only 1 had gross perforation after ex vivo morcellation *(8)*. Although it occurred in a formalin-fixed specimen, thus possibly making the tissue harder to morcellate, an obvious perforation was noted. Tumor spillage was certainly possible and would violate principles of oncological surgery.

One report of bowel injury is reported in a series of 40 morcellated specimens *(19)*. It was promptly identified, and the trocar site was extended to allow for bowel resection and copious irrigation. This patient is reported to be tumor free at 2 yr followup. Presently, there are no other direct complications associated with the tissue morcellator.

An issue commonly discussed is the risk of incisional hernias after intact specimen removal. Elashry and co-workers reported five cases of incisional hernias after intact specimen removal through a transverse, lower flank, muscle-cutting incision after transperitoneal laparoscopic nephrectomies *(22)*. The authors now approach specimen removal through either a subcostal or midline incision. Two incisional hernias at intact specimen retrieval sites were also noted in a multicenter study *(23)*. In a single institutional study of 1311 various urological laparoscopic cases, three umbilical trocar site hernias, and three incisional hernias at the site of intact specimen removal were recognized *(24)*. Barrett and colleagues also reported a port-site hernia after 72 laparoscopic nephrectomies *(9)*. It appears the incidence of hernia formation will be equivalent whether a specimen is retrieved whole or morcellated.

## *Staging*

Proponents of intact specimen retrieval claim proper pathologic staging is lost after specimen morcellation. Additionally, although information on pathologic staging currently does not affect treatment in most cases of low-stage renal cancer, it may be used as a prognosticator when obtaining careful, long-term followup.

Advocates of morcellation acknowledge the potential loss of traditional pathologic staging after morcellation. In the current era of fine cut computed tomography (CT) scanning and three-dimensional reconstruction, clinical tumor staging is becoming more accurate and almost equivalent to pathologic staging, especially for low-stage tumors *(25,26)*. Shalhav and colleagues found no clinical understaging in 22 patients undergoing laparoscopic nephrectomy with intact specimen removal for stage T3a or lower tumors using the current tumor-node-metastasis (TNM) staging guidelines *(26)*. This is notwithstanding reports of clinically over or understaging of renal tumors occurring in 5–35% *(27–29)*. This includes a series by Gill and colleagues of 125 patients undergoing laparoscopic nephrectomy with intact specimen extraction. After histopathologic examination, CT scanning was found to understage 9% of tumors after invasion to perirenal fat, adrenal, and vein were identified. The authors claim that pathologic detail would have been missed had morcellation been performed *(17)*. To further study the issue of pathological evaluation after morcellation, radical nephrectomy specimens were reviewed by pathologist before and after in vitro high-speed electrical tissue morcellation. In 13 of 14 specimens, morcellation did not alter the identification of histology, grade, or local invasiveness of tumor *(8)*. Similar findings were suggested in another published series *(30)*.

Table 3
Possibility of Pathologic Staging after Evaluation of Morcellated Kidney Specimens

| | *Morcellated specimen* |
|---|---|
| Tumor size | Not possible |
| Renal vein involvement | Not possible |
| Histology | Possible |
| Grade | Possible |
| Vascular invasion | Difficult |
| Fat invasion | Difficult |
| Capsular invasion | Difficult |
| Adrenal invasion | Difficult |
| Surgical margin | Not possible |
| Urothelial carcinoma invasion | Difficult |

A potential pitfall of morcellation is the loss of identification of surgical margins. Although cancer recurrence is ultimately dependent on the biology of the cancer and unique to each patient, status of surgical margins may impart a better or worse prognosis. Attempts have been made to maintain this fundamental aspect of oncological surgery with the use of morcellators. The use of methylene blue (Faulding, Aguadilla, Puerto Rico), India ink (Schaeffer, Fort Madison, IA), and indigo carmine to stain kidneys in an organ bag were performed at the University of California at San Francisco. Their technique showed undiluted India ink to be superior in grossly and microscopically staining the outer surface of the specimen, while leaving internal structures stain free after manual morcellation *(31)*. With larger and more aggressive renal and adrenal tumors being removed laparoscopically, the role of pathologic staging will become more paramount. Methods to facilitate staging after morcellation should continue to be addressed.

Currently, there are no guidelines for pathologists in sampling morcellated tissue. Morcellation also does not meet the guidelines of the American Joint Committee on Cancer. Pathologic TNM staging cannot be applied after fragmentation of kidney due to potential loss of identification of tumor size, surgical margins, and renal vein involvement (Table 3). For urothelial tumors, invasion of renal pelvis cannot be fully evaluated as well. To add clarity to this issue, a specimen-sampling algorithm was recently created based on preoperative imaging studies, specimen gross weight, and tumor-to-kidney volume ratio (TKR) *(32)*. Based on statistical modeling, it was found that for TKR greater than 0.1 15% sampling yielded 99% chance of tumor identification. This initial study may lead to further methods of analyzing morcellated specimens. Additionally, long-term studies are needed to determine if outcome is affected by lack of pTNM staging for morcellated renal tumors. Perhaps a new pTNM staging system for morcellated kidneys may be required.

### *Port-Site Recurrence*

Port-site and abdominal wall implantation of tumor in the gynecologic and surgical literature have been described in adenocarcinoma of ovary and colon, respectively *(33,34)*. The urologic literature reports three cases of port-site tumor implantation with transitional cell and prostatic carcinoma *(35,36)*. For renal tumors, one report of port-site seeding 25 mo postsurgery of an 862 g, Stage 3, grade IV tumor has been reported from Canada. This was at the 12-mm port site where morcellation was performed *(37)*. No evidence of recurrent tumor was found in the renal fossa, retroperitoneum, liver, or nodes. Castilho and colleagues also noted multiple abdominal masses at the port site 5 mo after nephrectomy and morcellation of a grade II renal mass *(38)*. It was unclear if carcinomatosis was present in the ascites noted at the time of nephrectomy. The incidence of port-site seeding appears to be a rare event after morcellation, especially with the use of an impermeable entrapment sack. However, until long-term results materialize, it is difficult to assume seeding after morcellation equates the 0.4% incidence associated with open radical nephrectomies *(39)*.

There has been no report of intraperitoneal seeding after morcellation with an impermeable sack. Caddedu and colleagues investigated 157 laparoscopic nephrectomy cases with 142 specimens removed after morcellation *(23)*. At mean 19 mo followup, no port-site or local tumor recurrence have been noted. Studies with longer followup have not encountered seeding as well *(9,19,20)*.

### *Tumor Control*

Long-term data is currently lacking investigating tumor control after morcellation. To date, Fentie and colleagues report the longest followup at mean 33.4 mo after all specimens were initially morcellated. In 57 patients, 3 (5%) were found to have metastatic disease after laparoscopic nephrectomy and morcellation *(37)*. The incidence of these metastases based on the characteristics of the original tumor does not deviate from the natural history of renal cell carcinoma *(40)*.

## FUTURE

The role of morcellation in cancer surgery continues to invite controversy and speculation. Although morcellation appears to be safe and efficacious for both clinical safety and oncological control, long-term data have not definitively established its role. More specifically, until we review long-term data on cancer control, we will not know whether intact specimen retrieval or morcellation is superior. It may turn out that both are equally efficacious.

Meanwhile, as both modalities pursue a common endpoint, other factors need to be addressed. Pathologic staging may ultimately need to include fragmented specimens. The patient and physician are not given the benefit of knowing pathologic tumor staging after morcellation with present pTNM guidelines. Furthermore, as larger and more invasive tumors are extirpated laparoscopically, there may be a potential need for tissue morcellation and thorough pathologic evaluation. Another factor that may ease the burden of pathologic staging is improved imaging studies. It is possible we may soon have the capabilities to precisely stage all renal tumors clinically.

As technology moves forward, studies to support or criticize inventive and useful laparoscopic techniques will inevitably be delayed. In the end, morcellation may be disregarded as "oncologically risky," but contemporary literature suggests otherwise. As minimally invasive technology continues to improve, so will new topics of controversy.

## ACKNOWLEDGMENTS

We would like to thank David Cuellar, MD and Benjamin J. Davies, MD for assistance in preparing this manuscript.

## REFERENCES

1. Pratt J H, Gunnlaugsson GH. Vaginal hysterectomy by morcellation. Mayo Clin Proc 1970; 45: 374–387.
2. Clayman RV, Kavoussi LR, Soper NJ, et al. Laparoscopic nephrectomy: initial case report. J Urol 1991; 146: 278–282.
3. McDougall EM, Clayman RV, Elashry OM. Laparoscopic radical nephrectomy for renal tumor: the Washington university experience. J Urol 1996; 155: 1180–1185.
4. Ono Y, Katoh N, Kinukawa T, Matsuuro O, Ohshima S. Laparoscopic radical nephrectomy: the Nagoya experience. J Urol 1997; 158: 719–723.
5. Portis A, Yan Y, Landman J, et al. Long-term followup after laparoscopic radical nephrectomy. J Urol 2002; 167: 1257–1262.
6. Dunn MD, Portis AJ, Shalhav AL, et al. Laparoscopic versus open radical nephrectomy: a 9-year experience. J Urol 2000; 164: 1153–1159.
7. Gill IS, Cherullo EE, Meraney AM, Borsuk F, Murphy DP, Falcone T. Vaginal extraction of the intact specimen following laparoscopic radical nephrectomy. J Urol 2002; 167: 238–241.
8. Landman J, Lento P, Hassen W, Unger P, Waterhouse R. Feasibility of pathological evaluation of morcellated kidneys after radical nephrectomy. J Urol 2000; 164: 2086–2089.

9. Barrett PH, Fentie DD, Taranger LA. Laparoscopic radical nephrectomy with morcellation for renal cell carcinoma: the Saskatoon experience. Urology 1998; 52: 23–28.
10. Urban DA, Kerbl K, McDougall EM, Stone AM, Fadden PT, Clayman RV. Organ entrapment and renal morcellation: permeability studies. J Urol 1993; 150: 1792–1794.
11. Landman J, Collyer WC, Olweny E, Andreoni C, McDougall E, Clayman RV. Laparoscopic renal ablation: an in vitro comparison of currently available electrical tissue morcellators. Urology 2000; 56: 677–681.
12. Sundaram CP, Ono Y, Landman J, Rehman J, Clayman RV. Hydrophilic guide wire technique to facilitate organ entrapment using a laparoscopic sack during laparoscopy. J Urol 2002; 167: 1376–1377.
13. Singhvi SK, Allan W, Williams ED, Small PK. Assessment of the physical properties of endoscopic retrieval systems. Br J Surg 2002; 89: 1183–1187.
14. Steiner RA, Wight E, Tadir Y, Haller U. Electrical cutting device for laparoscopic removal of tissue from the abdominal cavity. Obstet Gynecol 1993; 81: 471–474.
15. Nakada SY, McDougall EM, Clayman RV. Laparoscopic extirpation of renal cell cancer: feasibility, questions, and concerns. Semin Surg Oncol 1996; 12: 100–112.
16. Kaouk JH, Gill I. Laparoscopic radical nephrectomy: morcellate or leave intact? Leave intact. Rev Urol 2002; 4: 38–42.
17. Gill IS, Meraney AM, Schweizer DK, et al. Laparoscopic radical nephrectomy in 100 patients: a single center experience from the United States. Cancer 2001; 92: 1843–1855.
18. Walther MM, Lyne JC, Libutti SK, Linehan WM. Laparoscopic cytoreductive nephrectomy as preparation for administration of systemic interleukin-2 in the treatment of metastatic renal cell carcinoma: a pilot study. Urology 1999; 53: 496–501.
19. Chan DY, Cadeddu JA, Jarrett TW, Marshall FF, Kavoussi LR. Laparoscopic radical nephrectomy: cancer control for renal cell carcinoma. J Urol 2001; 166: 2095–2099.
20. Ono Y, Kinukawa T, Hattori R, et al. Laparoscopic radical nephrectomy for renal cell carcinoma: a five-year experience. Urology 1999; 53: 280–286.
21. Gettman MT, Napper C, Corwin TS, Cadeddu JA. Laparoscopic radical nephrectomy: prospective assessment of impact of intact versus fragmented specimen removal on postoperative quality of life. J Endourol 2002; 16: 23–26.
22. Elashry OM, Giusti G, Nadler RB, McDougall EM, Clayman RV. Incisional hernia after laparoscopic nephrectomy with intact specimen removal: caveat emptor. J Urol 1997; 158: 363–369.
23. Cadeddu JA, Ono Y, Clayman RV, et al. Laparoscopic nephrectomy for renal cell cancer: evaluation of efficacy and safety: a multicenter experience. Urology 1998; 52: 773–777.
24. Vallancien G, Cathelineau X, Baumert H, Doublet JD, Guillonneau B. Complications of transperitoneal laparoscopic surgery in urology: review of 1,311 procedures at a single center. J Urol 2002; 168: 23–26.
25. Rassweiler J, Fornara P, Weber M, et al. Laparoscopic nephrectomy: the experience of the laparoscopy working group of the German Urologic Association. J Urol 1998; 160: 18–21.
26. Shalhav AL, Leibovitch I, Lev R, Hoenig DM, Ramon J. Is laparoscopic radical nephrectomy with specimen morcellation acceptable cancer surgery? J Endourol 1998; 12: 255–257.

27. McClennan B, Deyoe, L. The imaging evaluation of renal cell carcinoma: diagnosis and staging. Radiol Clin North Am 1994; 32: 55–69.
28. Myneni L, Hricak H, Carroll P. Magnetic resonance imaging of renal cell carcinoma with extension into the vena cava: staging accuracy and recent advances. Br J Urol 1991; 68: 571–578.
29. Newhouse J. the radiologic evaluation of the patient with renal cancer. Urol Clin North Am 1993; 20: 231–246.
30. Pautler SE, Hewitt SM, Linehan WM, Walther MM. Specimen morcellation after laparoscopic radical nephrectomy: confirmation of histologic diagnosis using needle biopsy. J Endourol 2002; 16: 89–92.
31. Meng MV, Koppie TM, Duh Q, Stoller M. Novel method of assessing surgical margin status in laparoscopic specimens. Urology 2001; 58: 677–681.
32. Rabban JT, Meng MV, Yeh B, Koppie T, Ferrell L, Stoller ML. Kidney morcellation in laparoscopic nephrectomy for tumor. Am J Surg Pathol 2001; 25: 1158–1166.
33. Childers JM, Aqua KA, Surwit EA, Hallum AV, Hatch KD. Abdominal-wall tumor implantation after laparoscopy for malignant conditions. Obstet Gynecol 1994; 84: 765–769.
34. Ramos JM, Gupta S, Anthone GJ, Ortega AE, Simons AJ, Beart RW. Laparoscopy and colon cancer. Is the port site at risk? A preliminary report. Arch Surg 1994; 129: 897–899.
35. Anderson JR, Steven K. Implantation metastasis after laparoscopic biopsy of bladder cancer. J Urol 1995; 153: 1047–1048.
36. Bangma CH, Kirkels WJ, Chadha S, Schroder FH. Cutaneous metastasis following laparoscopic pelvic lymphadenectomy for prostatic carcinoma. J Urol 1995; 153: 1635–1636.
37. Fentie DD, Barrett PH, Taranger LA. Metastatic renal cell cancer after lapa-roscopic radical nephrectomy: long-term follow-up. J Endourol 2000; 14: 407–411.
38. Castilho LN, Fugita OE, Mitre AI, Arap S. Port site tumor recurrences of renal cell carcinoma after videolaparoscopic radical nephrectomy. J Urol 2001; 165: 519.
39. Uson AC. Tumor recurrence in the renal fossa and/or abdominal wall after radical nephrectomy for renal cell cancer. Prog Clin Biol Res 1992; 100: 549–560.
40. Rafla S. Renal cell carcinoma: natural history and results of treatment. Cancer 1970; 25: 26–40.

# 4 Hand-Assisted Laparoscopic Radical Nephrectomy

*Patrick S. Lowry,* MD *and Stephen Y. Nakada,* MD

*CONTENTS*

INTRODUCTION
INDICATIONS
CONTRAIDICATIONS
PATIENT PREPARATION
ANESTHETIC CONSIDERATIONS
POSITIONING
ROOM SET-UP
PLACEMENT OF TROCARS AND HAND PORT
HAND-ACCESS DEVICES
STEPS OF PROCEDURE
POSTOPERATIVE CARE
DISCUSSION
SUMMARY
REFERENCES

## INTRODUCTION

Radical nephrectomy has been the mainstay for the treatment of localized renal cell carcinoma (RCC) since first described by Robson in 1969 *(1)*. The laparoscopic radical nephrectomy (LRN) has introduced a new standard of care to the field of urology. LRN is an advanced procedure requiring training in laparoscopic techniques. An intra-abdominal hand gives improved tactile feedback to the urologist, thereby

From: *Laparoscopic Urologic Oncology*
Edited by: J. A. Cadeddu © Humana Press Inc., Totowa, NJ

making LRN less daunting. Hand-assisted laparoscopy (HAL) also provides another tool to help urologists perform more complex and challenging radical nephrectomies.

## INDICATIONS

Radical nephrectomy is the procedure of choice for localized RCC. Hand-assisted laparoscopic radical nephrectomy (HALRN) may be performed on almost any patient who requires radical nephrectomy. There are no absolute size limitations as this depends on the expertise and comfort level of the individual surgeon. Removal of tumors larger than 10 cm, however, should probably be left to experienced laparoscopic surgeons. HALRN may also be performed on patients with metastatic disease either for the palliation of symptoms or for potential combination with adjuvant immunotherapy. Prior abdominal or renal surgery is not a contraindication to HALRN. In fact, an advantage of HALRN over traditional laparoscopic nephrectomy is the tactile feedback of the intra-abdominal hand for the taking down of adhesions from prior abdominal or renal surgery, perirenal inflammation, or infection. An alternative for patients with prior intra-abdominal surgery is the retroperitoneal laparoscopic approach.

## CONTRAINDICATIONS

Until recently, the only absolute contraindication to HALRN was the presence of inferior vena cava (IVC) tumor thrombi. However, a recent case report cited that the recent development of laparoscopic vascular instruments and the advantage of hand assistance allowed this limit to be extended for select cases with caval thrombi *(2)*. Patients with renal vein thrombi can also be treated effectively. This illustrates that the growth of laparoscopy and the benefits of the hand assistance have enabled urologists to progress to the point that with the exception of large caval thrombi, there are no absolute contraindications. Each surgeon must individually set limits according to his or her experience and comfort level.

There are circumstances that make HALRN more complex, with a higher potential for morbidity. These circumstances include a history of bowel obstruction, peritonitis, and abdominal wall infection. Specific conditions that may predispose a patient to increased risks with HALRN include large tumor size (>10 cm), prior inflammation (pyelonephritis, xanthogranulomatous pyelonephritis, history percutaneous renal access), and prior transabdominal or renal surgery. All factors should be considered by the surgeon prior to planning the operation.

## PATIENT PREPARATION

The standard workup of a renal mass should be complete before deciding the surgical approach. Therefore, the evaluation should be the same as for an open radical nephrectomy (ORN). Renal function should be evaluated with a serum creatinine. If the creatinine is elevated, or if the radiologic imaging reveals an abnormal contralateral kidney, a differential renal scan may be considered. Patients with renal insufficiency or compromised contralateral renal function may need further consideration for renal-sparing surgery.

A metastatic survey should include a posterolateral and lateral chest X-ray or chest computed tomography (CT), serum calcium, serum alkaline phosphatase, and an abdominal CT scan. The CT scan is also useful to assist in surgical planning. Bone scan is advised for patients with elevated calcium, elevated alkaline phosphatase, or bone pain *(3)*.

## ANESTHETIC CONSIDERATIONS

The insufflation pressure on the kidneys may produce a temporary oliguric state. Rather than increasing intravenous (iv) fluid, relatively low maintenance fluid rate of 5 cc/kg/h should be administered, and intraoperative blood loss should be replaced. A Foley catheter allows monitoring of urine output, as well as keeping the bladder decompressed. After the HALRN is completed, low urine output should resolve over the next day with conservative management as mobilization of fluid occurs.

Insufflation pressure causes diffusion of $CO_2$ into the blood, but is rarely a clinical problem. End tidal $CO_2$ should be monitored and kept between 30–40 mm Hg. Increased end tidal $CO_2$ values should prompt decreasing the insufflation pressure.

Nitrous oxide can support combustion when used with cautery or laser. It should be avoided both as an inhalant for anesthesia as well as an insufflant. It may lead to bowel dilation as well.

An orogastric or nasogastric tube should be in place during the case to keep the stomach deflated. This should be removed at the end of the case.

## POSITIONING

The patient is positioned in a modified flank position (Fig. 1). Although the table may be rotated to more of a flank during the case to allow the bowel to fall away and facilitate dissection, initial placement in a modified flank position with the abdomen aimed slightly more anteriorly simplifies placement of the hand-assist device. The kidney rest is raised minimally to avoid neurologic/pressure injuries, and the

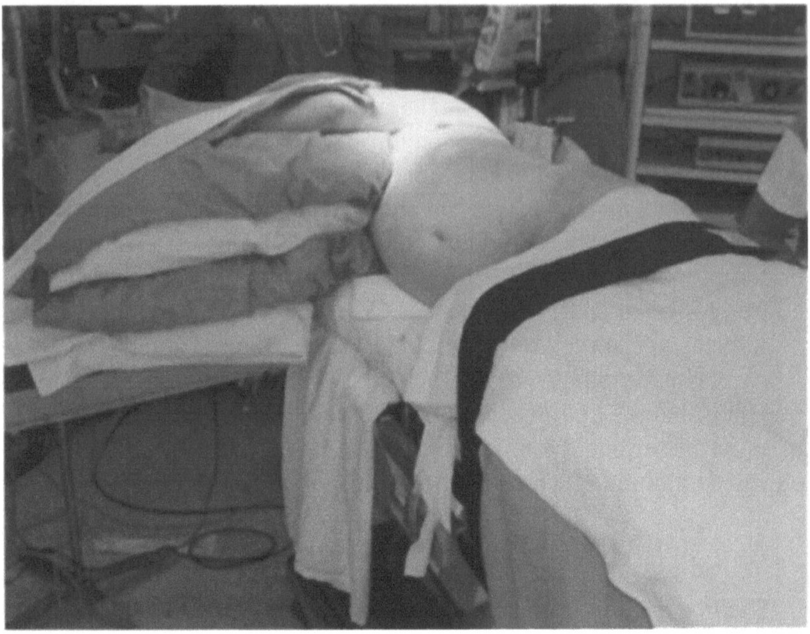

**Fig. 1.** Modified flank position for left HALRN. Note minimal use of the kidney rrest and pillows to support upper arm.

table is minimally flexed (15–20°). The downward leg is flexed, and the knee and ankle are well padded with foam or gel pads. The upward leg is straight and well supported with pillows. The lower arm is well padded at the elbow and wrist, and an axillary roll is placed. The upper arm may be suspended or placed on a padded Mayo stand (Fig. 1). The patient is carefully examined to ensure no points of excess pressure exist. Areas of concern should receive additional padding or change of position. Wide cloth tape affixed to the bed and placed over the shoulder and greater trochanter increase stability. Tape blisters are avoided by placing towels or tegaderm between the cloth tape and the skin. The patient's entire abdomen and flank is then prepped and draped.

## ROOM SET-UP

The surgeon and assistant stand together on the opposite side from the kidney to be removed (Fig. 2). The surgeon is closest to the head of the patient to facilitate hand port and working port access. The assistant stays closer to the feet to run the camera and, if necessary, an additional retractor. The surgical technician stays on the same side as the surgeons, closer toward the foot of the bed. The surgical instrument tables are on

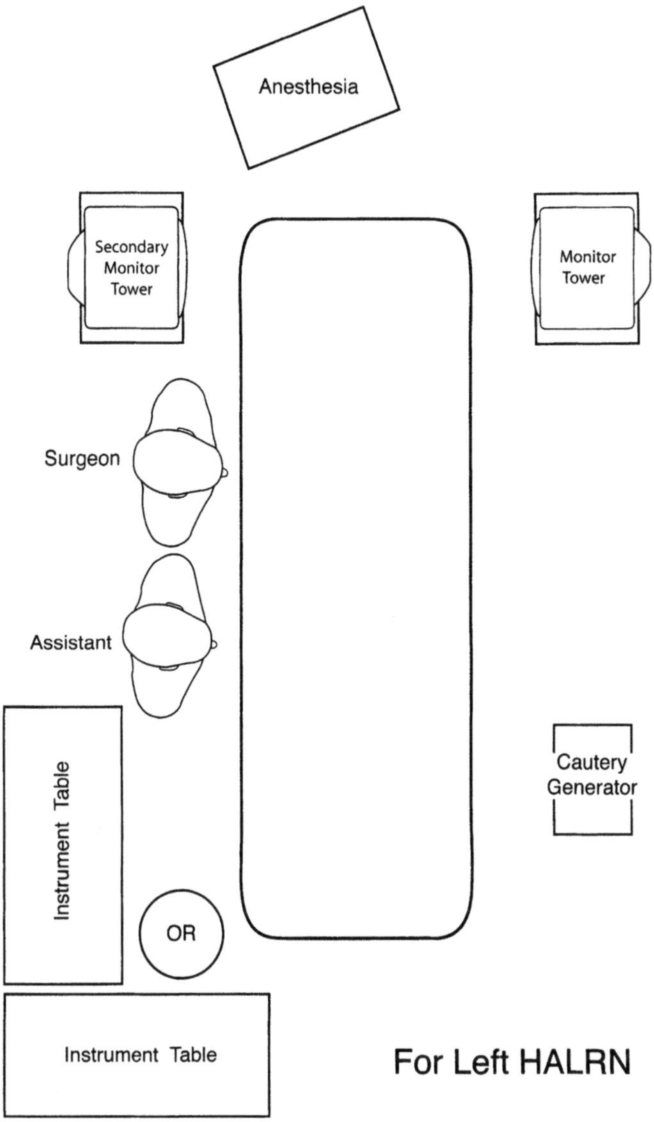


**Fig. 2.** Recommended room set-up for left HALRN.

the side of the surgeon at the feet and behind the surgeons, and the power generators (i.e., cautery, harmonic scalpel) are across the patient from the surgeons (see Table 1 for list of instruments). Monitors are placed at the level of the patients' shoulders on both sides of the patient.

An open instrument set should always be available should conversion to an open procedure be necessary.

**Table 1**
**HALRN Instrument List, the University of Wisconsin**

| |
|---|
| *Nondisposable* |
| Two monitors, flat screen (Stryker) |
| 5-mm or 10-mm (Stryker) 30° laparoscope |
| 5-mm or 10-mm (Stryker) 0° laparoscope |
| High-flow insufflator |
| Three-chip camera (Stryker) |
| 5-mm Maryland dissector |
| 5-mm Atraumatic grasper |
| 5-mm scissors, curved and straight blades |
| 5-mm suction/irrigation system (Nehzat) |
| Carter-Thomason closure device (Inlet Medical, Eden Prairie, MN) |
| 5-mm curved harmonic scalpel (Ethicon) |
| *Disposable* |
| Hand-access device (Gelport, Applied Medical) |
| Nonbladed trocars, one 5 mm, two 10 mm (Visiport, Ethicon) |
| Port reducers (Ethicon) |
| LapSac (Cook) |
| Endo-GIA stapler, vascular load (10 mm) (Ethicon) |
| Sutures, 1 PDS for fascial closure of hand port |
| 0 Vicryl for 10-mm ports |
| 4-0 Vicryl for skin closure |

## PLACEMENT OF TROCARS AND HAND PORT

For the right-handed surgeon performing a left HALRN, we recommend the hand port be placed in a midline incision just above the umbilicus (Fig. 3). For a right HALRN, a right-handed surgeon could place the hand port in the right lower quadrant (Fig. 4). This would allow the right-handed surgeon to use his or her dominant hand for the working port instruments. Alternatively, the right-handed surgeon could use the mirror-image set-up (Fig. 3) as on the left side, and work with his or her dominant hand in the abdomen. The hand device is typically placed prior to the trocars without the pneumoperitoneum. The length of the incision should correspond to the glove size of the surgeon. After being placed, the device is closed and the abdomen insufflated. The camera port can be placed through the inflated hand-access device. After inspecting the abdomen, the remaining ports can be placed under direct visualization. This facilitates better placement, and one can avoid the access-related complications that may occur with Veress needle placement.

In addition to the hand port, two or three trocars are required; one 5- or 10-mm camera, one 10-mm working port, and sometimes an addi-

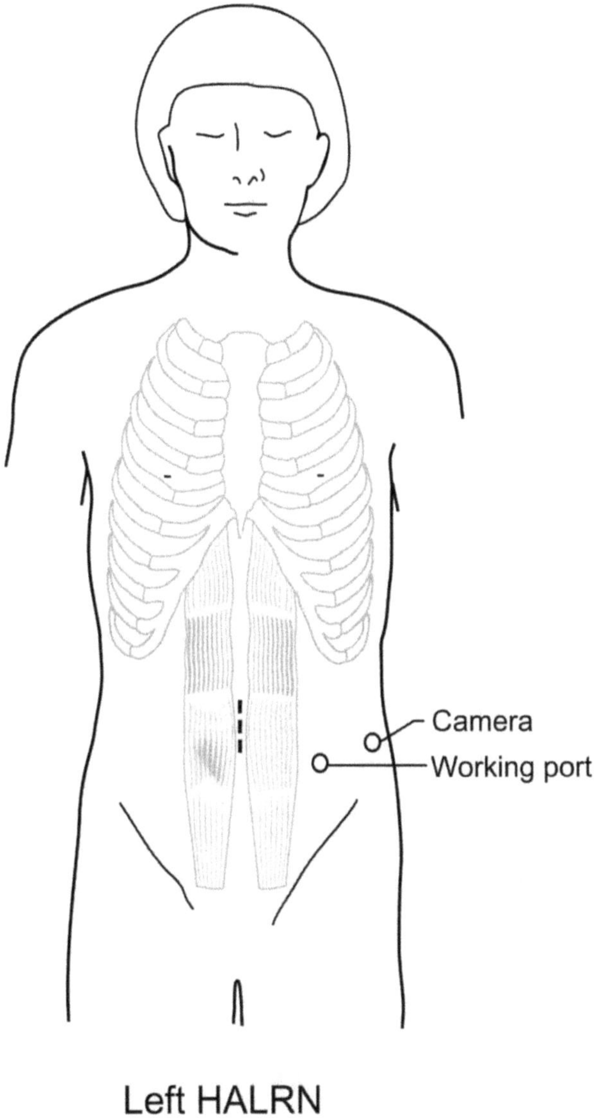


**Fig. 3.** Trocar and hand-access position for left HALRN for right-handed surgeon.

tional 5-mm working port for additional retraction, particularly on the liver for right-sided tumors. Location of the ports will vary depending on the size of the patient, surgeon preference, and surgeon experience. In general, the camera port should be placed lateral to the rectus muscle in the midclavicular line at or slightly above the level of the umbilicus. The 10-mm working port should be placed in the midaxillary line in a

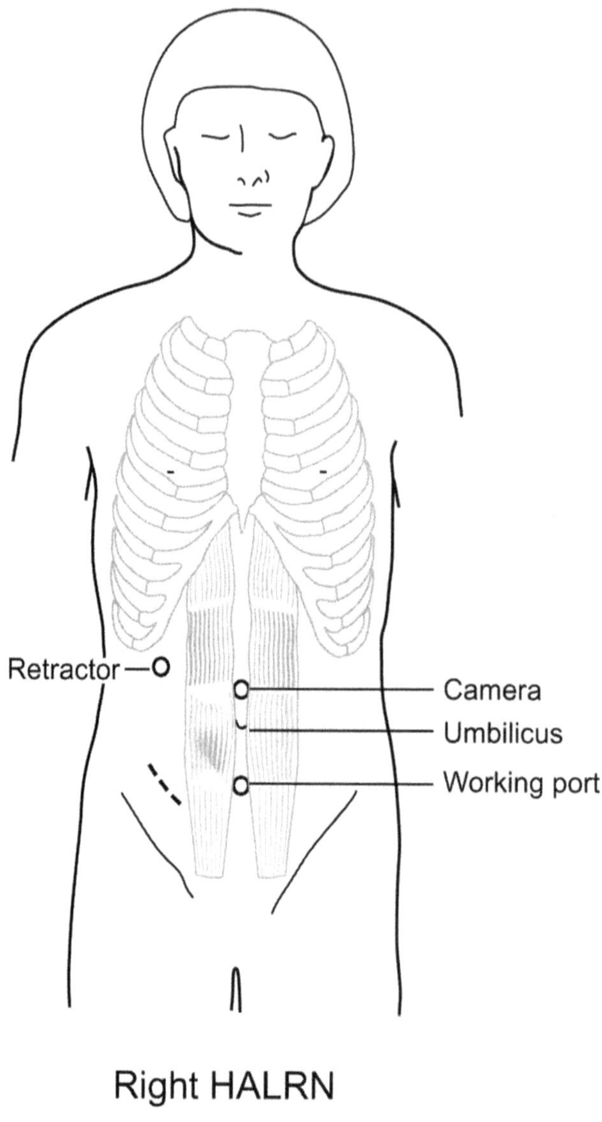


**Fig. 3.** Trocar and hand-access position for left HALRN for right-handed surgeon.

position more cranial than the camera port. If needed for retraction, an additional 5-mm working port may be placed laterally in the subcostal region, somewhere between the midaxillary line and the midclavicular line, or wherever the surgeon believes it will be of the best use. We prefer the Diamond flex triangle (Genzyme) or the PEER retractor (Jarit) for the spleen or liver.

If a port is so poorly placed that it is of no use, it should be left in place and another port placed in a more ideal location. An additional port (particularly 5 mm) adds minimal morbidity and is preferable to struggling with suboptimally located ports.

For obese patients, placement of the hand-access device in the usual location may put the hand port an uncomfortable distance from the kidney, making dissection difficult. We recommend placing the hand-access device lateral of the midline in order to stay closer to the kidney. Trocar positioning should be adjusted as well to allow for the more lateral location of the hand-access device.

## HAND-ACCESS DEVICES

Although different devices exist, each maintains the pneumoperitoneum while allowing the hand to stay in the abdomen. Three early devices include the HandPort (Smith and Nephew, Andover, MA), the Intromit (Applied Medical, Rancho Santa Margarita, CA), and the Pneumosleeve (Dexterity, Atlanta, GA) *(4)*. The HandPort and the Pneumosleeve are two-piece devices that use a template on the abdomen and a sleeve worn by the surgeon. The sleeve attaches in an airtight manner to both to the abdominal template and the wrist of the surgeon, preventing loss of air. The Intromit is a one-piece device that inflates around the surgeon's wrist, causing an airtight seal by the pressure of the inflation. Both the Intromit and the Handport will maintain the pneumoperitoneum with only an instrument or laparoscope in the device.

Later generation devices include the Gelport (Applied Medical, Rancho Santa Margarita, CA), Omniport (Weck, Research Triangle Park, NC), and LapDisc (Ethicon, Cincinatti, OH). The LapDisc prevents loss of air pressure by using an adjustable system that tightens around the wrist. The Omniport uses an inflatable collar to create an airtight seal around the wrist. The Gelport uses a soft gel-type cap with a small slit through which the surgeon places a hand (Fig. 5). The port stretches around the wrist, providing an airtight seal. The Gelport is unique in that it allows transfer of the hand in and out of the port without loss of the pneumoperitoneum.

## STEPS OF THE PROCEDURE

### *Step 1: Survey the Abdomen*

As with any surgery, an initial survey of the abdominal structures should be performed to evaluate for metastatic disease or adhesions. Liver and spleen should be visually examined and palpated for abnor-

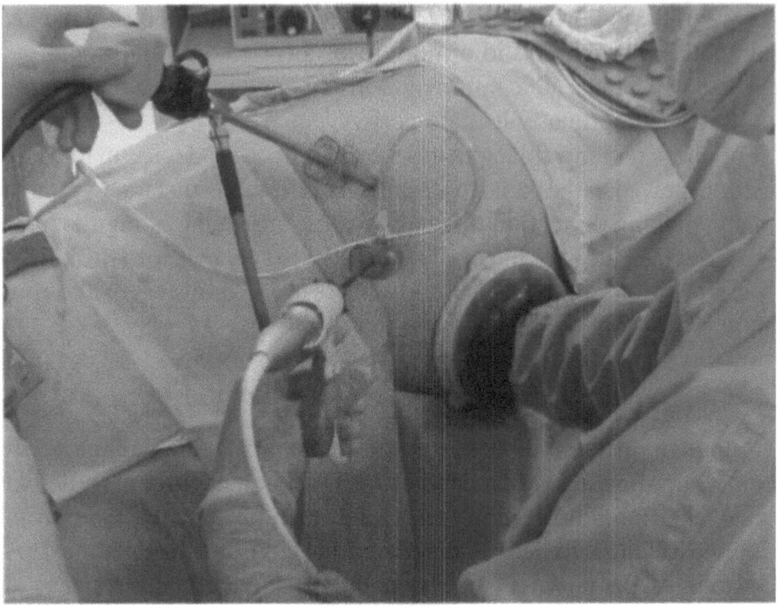

**Fig. 5.** Gelport hand-access device in use during right HALRN. Note part configuration inverted as surgeon is left-handed.

malities. Position of the caudal edge of the liver and spleen should be noted. A brief inspection of the pelvis can then be performed. The intra-abdominal hand allows palpation of major structures similar to that afforded in open surgery.

### *Step 2: Incise the Line of Toldt*

The intra-abdominal hand should be used to place medial traction on the colon to clearly delineate the line of Toldt. The 5-mm curved-tip Harmonic scalpel or electrocautery shears are used to incise a small area on the white line. Through this small defect, a finger can be inserted in the plane behind the fascia to push the colon away and expose a bloodless plane through the peritoneal attachments. These attachments are then incised to free the colon from the lateral abdominal wall.

### *Step 3: Mobilize the Colon*

Prior to mobilizing the colon, the entire line of Toldt should be detached from the iliac vessels to the hepatic or splenic flexure. Each step in the mobilization of the colon should occur at one level throughout the length of the colon before proceeding deeper. This keeps all of the mobilization in the same plane, rather than having areas of different depths of dissection.

Caudally, the colon should be mobilized to the level of the iliac vessels. Cranially, the colon to the level of should be freed from the liver or spleen. After the colon is liberated from the abdominal sidewall and liver/spleen, medial retraction with the hand reveals the anterior surface of Gerota's fascia.

For a right nephrectomy, the fascial attachments from the colon to the liver should be divided. The colon should then be swept medially, fulgurating small vessels, lymphatics, or strands of fascia as needed to expose Gerota's fascia. The liver is released from the sidewall by incising the triangular ligament to allow it to be retracted superiorly. Once the duodenum is identified, the Kocher maneuver should be performed to reflect the duodenum medially and expose the IVC.

In the case of left nephrectomy, the line of Toldt should be incised to the level of the spleen, and then over the upper pole of the kidney lateral to the spleen. Traction injuries to the spleen are by incising lateral attachments of the peritoneum from the spleen to the diaphragm, allowing the spleen to fall medially to expose the plane between the spleen and the upper pole of the kidney. Dissection should be superficial to include only the peritoneal layer, and should be performed close to the spleen in order to avoid perforation of the diaphragm. One should also keep in mind that the stomach can come around the lateral aspect of the spleen. The splenic flexure between the colon and the spleen is not taken down, but left intact so that after the spleen is released, the plane between the spleen and the upper pole of the kidney can be developed to allow the both spleen and colon to fall away medially. The colon may then be retracted medially across the midline to adequately provide access to the renal hilum.

### *Step 4: Free Lateral and Superior Attachments to the Kidney*

With the anterior surface of Gerota's fascia visible, attention is turned to mobilization of the lateral and superior attachments of the kidney. Conversely, in conventional laparoscopic technique (without hand assistance), these attachments are left in place until after the hilar vessels are secured so the kidney will remain more stable. The lateral aspect is freed up from the lower pole toward the upper pole. The upper pole attachments are liberated medially to the adrenal. The 30° lens facilitates dissection of the upper and upper lateral pole attachments. The posterior attachments should be left intact at this point in the case.

### *Step 5: Locate and Control the Ureter*

The ureter should be identified early in the case and divided between clips or with the vascular stapler. The ureter typically lies medial to the psoas, alongside the gonadal vein. During dissection of the ureter, care

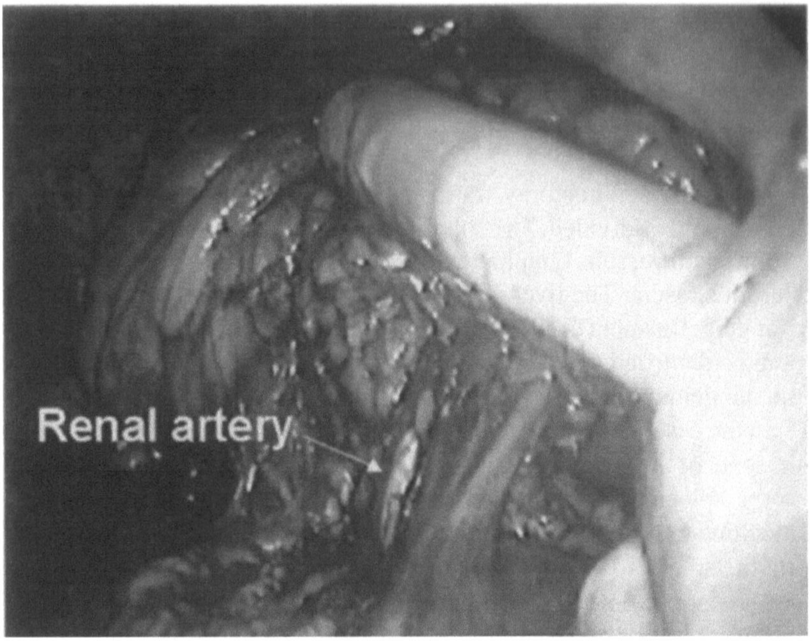


**Fig. 6.** Posterior control of the renal artery.

should be taken to avoid damaging the gonadal vein to avoid troublesome bleeding. During left nephrectomy, the gonadal vein can be followed cranially to the renal vein. On the right side, the gonadal vein comes off the vena cava, and the surgeon should be careful not to avulse the gonadal vein off the cava. After division, the proximal ureteral stump can be used to assist with retraction of the kidney.

### *Step 6: Free Attachments to the Lower Pole of the Kidney*

The lower pole should be now completely mobilized. Using fingertip dissection and the harmonic scalpel to expose and coagulate the attachments, the lower pole should be freed up in a lateral to medial direction. Care should be taken in the direction of the hilum to beware of unrecognized lower pole vessels.

### *Step 7: Identify and Mobilize the Renal Vein and Artery*

The anterior surface of the vein should be identified and carefully cleaned off. On the left side, the adrenal and gonadal vein branches should be located. The artery should be located by palpation. The renal vein and artery should be dissected free. If this is difficult, or if the vascular anatomy appears complex, the dissection may be facilitated by

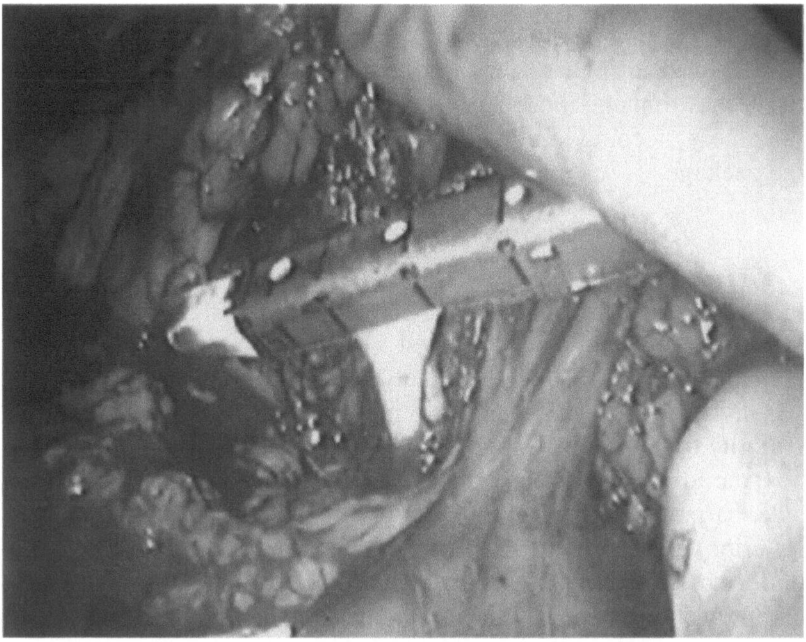

**Fig. 7.** Stapling the renal artery.

freeing the posterior attachments to the kidney and flipping the kidney anteriorly for a posterior approach to the renal artery (Fig. 6).

### *Step 8: Free the Posterior Attachments to the Kidney*

After the renal vein and artery have been identified, the posterior attachments to the kidney should be freed up. The only remaining attachments are at the hilum and superiorly at the adrenal gland.

### *Step 9: Divide the Renal Artery and Vein*

The renal artery is divided with a vascular stapler using posterior artery control (Fig. 7) *(13,19)*. This involves flipping the kidney medially to expose the renal artery. The renal vein can then be stapled with a vascular stapler. Prior to activating the stapler, the surgeon needs visual confirmation that the device extends across the entire vein. The surgeon can also palpate the tips of the stapler. If necessary, the 30° lens can be used. Stapling over clips can cause staple misfire, resulting in hemorrhage. If clips have been used prior to this point to control the adrenal vein, gonadal vein, or lumbar veins,then one must take great care to insure that no clips are between the jaws of the stapling device.

### *Step 10: Free the Remaining Medial Attachments*

After division of the artery and vein, medial lymphatics and adipose tissue may remain. These can be taken down with the harmonic scalpel or cautery, keeping in mind that an aberrant vessel may be hidden in the package.

### *Step 11: Spare or Remove the Adrenal*

If the adrenal is to be spared, the plane between the upper pole of the kidney and the adrenal, which may have been started during freeing of the upper pole, should be developed. Using the harmonic scalpel in this plane, the adrenal can be completely separated from the kidney. Care should be made to stay lateral and inferior to the adrenal to avoid the majority of the vessels supplying and draining the adrenal.

If the adrenal is to be taken, it should be removed en bloc. On the left side, harmonic scalpel or clips are used to free to posteromedial and superior vessels. The main adrenal vein coming from the renal vein is divided between clips. On the right side, dissection should proceed very carefully between the vena cava and the adrenal gland until the adrenal vein is found. Dissection should proceed in such a direction as to move fat and vessels away from the gland. The adrenal vein should be clipped twice on the cava side if possible and once on the gland side. One must take care when clipping the left adrenal, as clips on the renal vein can interfere with the stapler.

### *Step 12: Lower the Pneumoperitoneum and Assess for Bleeding*

Working insufflation pressures (usually 15 mm Hg) may tamponade venous bleeding. Lowering the pressure to the 5 and again surveying the hilar area, the upper pole area, and the area where the ureter was dissected and transected may find bleeding that was undetected at higher pressures.

### *Step 13: Removal of the Specimen*

Prior to removal, the specimen must be placed into a bag in order to protect the wound from potential tumor seeding. The Lapsac (Cook, Spencer, IN) is currently the only extraction bag that is impenetrable to tumor cells. To facilitate placement of the specimen into the bag, one side of the open end should be grasped with an instrument, and the other edge held open with a finger. After the tumor is carefully placed into the opening, the drawstring is pulled to close the bag, which may be extracted through the hand port site. For large tumors, the fascial incision may need to be slightly enlarged.

### *Step 14: Close the Port Sites and Hand-Access Site*

The hand should be removed, and the hand port device closed such that the camera may visualize the abdomen through the hand device. The Carter-Thomason device (Inlet Medical, Eden Prairie, MN) is then used to place a stitch in all 10-mm sites. Five-mm ports should be closed in children to prevent herniation of omentum. After sutures are placed, the laparoscope is used to visualize the removal of all ports, and the sutures are tied down. The fascia in the hand-site incision is closed with a running 1-0 PDS, and the skin is closed with a 4.0-Vicryl to avoid the need to remove skin staples.

## POSTOPERATIVE CARE

Patients wear sequential compression devices on the lower extremities until ambulating well. Ambulation is begun the night of surgery. Patients are offered clear liquids the morning of the first postoperative day. Diet is advanced as tolerated. Patients are generally discharged on postoperative d 3 or 4.

## DISCUSSION

Laparoscopic nephrectomy is not new to urology *(5)*. Despite being more than 11 years removed from the first laparoscopic nephrectomy, this procedure remains limited in the urologic community outside of academic centers *(6)*. Many factors have caused this lack of progress. Most practicing urologists received little training in laparoscopy in the early and mid-1990s. As of early 2003, not all residency programs were performing laparoscopy. Additionally, laparoscopic nephrectomy is perceived as a technically challenging, more time-consuming procedure. Fellowship training is often required to learn the techniques, and the learning curve can be steep. Cases with potential laparoscopic application may not be as prevalent for practicing urologists, leading to difficulty in retaining the skills to consistently perform the procedure. Finally, due to disposable instruments and increased operative time, laparoscopic nephrectomy is costly to perform. Although all of these concerns have merit, the use of HAL helps alleviate many of these concerns by providing distinct advantages for both the surgeon and the patient.

The ability to perform surgery despite the loss of tactile sensation during dissection is a primary challenge to mastering laparoscopic surgery. An attempt to circumvent this lack of feedback has been described by the insertion of a finger through a port site to help with identification of anatomy *(7)*. Since 1997, when the first HALRN using a commercial sleeve was performed *(8)*, hand assistance has been extended to donor nephrectomy (HALDN), nephroureterectomy (HALNU), pyeloplasty, and partial nephrectomy (HALPN) *(9–12)*. The insertion of a hand into the operative field provides a tool that today cannot be replaced with a laparoscopic instrument. Only the human hand provides tactile information, assists with dissection, retracts and protects nearby organs, and palpates unidentified structures to help with tissue recognition. Additionally, an intra-abdominal hand facilitates hemostasis, exposure, and suturing if necessary during HALRN. The hand-access site may also be used for the introduction of a sponge or even a small instrument. It is evident that hand assistance facilitates laparoscopic nephrectomy, particularly for larger renal lesions.

HAL enables advanced laparoscopists to perform more difficult cases including large renal tumors (10 cm), HALDN, HALNU, HALPN, or simple nephrectomy (HALN) for inflammatory conditions (XGP, pyelonephritis, prior surgery). Additionally, use of hand access might prevent conversion to an open procedure in a standard laparoscopic case *(13)*. If a specimen is to be removed intact via incision, little is lost by hand access, and the benefits can broaden the scope of a surgeon's practice.

Disadvantages of HALRN include cost of hand-access device, operative time to set up the hand device, restricted port placement, incisional morbidity, and a decrease of the operative space with the introduced hand. The newer devices often do not have a template, and interfere with port placement less. The operative space is decreased, but usually the advantages of HAL surgery (HALS) outweigh this. The incision used is 6.5–7.5 cm, depending on the surgeon's glove size. Unless one is morcellating the specimen, an incision will need to be made anyway.

In 2002, the laparoscopic approach became the standard of care for kidney removal. When compared to open surgery at Washington University, LRN was associated with less blood loss, fewer complications, and decreased analgesia requirements. Patients were able to take liquids earlier, return home sooner, and experience full recovery faster *(14)*. More importantly, long-term followup at 5 yr was equivalent with recurrence-free survival and cancer-specific survival over 90% for both ORN and LRN *(15)*. Outcomes of HALRN compare favorably to transperitoneal LRN with morcellated specimen removal, having been shown to have similar recovery and morbidity, yet with a shorter operative time *(16)*. Compared to retroperitoneal LRN with intact specimen removal, HALRN had no significant difference in operative time, blood loss, analgesia requirements, time until oral intake, length of stay, or activity level after 2 wk *(17)*. Laparoscopic donor nephrectomy (LDN) has also been compared to the hand-assisted approach, with HAL showing sig-

Table 2
HALRN vs ORN: The University of Wisconsin Experience

| | *HALRN* (*n = 50 in 48 patients*) | *ORN* (*n = 18*) |
|---|---|---|
| Tumor Size | 5.9 cm (2–12) | 6.4 cm (3–11) |
| Patient age | 58 (29–83) | 61 (44–92) |
| OR time | 233 (134–356) | 117 (34–120) |
| EBL | 170 cc | 210 cc |
| LOS (median days) | 4 d (2–22) | 5 d (4–7) |
| ASA | 2.6 | 2.5 |
| Complication (%) | 12% | 11% |

HALRN = hand-assisted laparoscopic radical nephrectomy; ORN = open radical nephrectormy; OR = operating room; EBL = estimated blood loss; LOS = length of stay; ASA = American Society of Anesthesiologists.

Table 3
HALRN vs ORN: Time from Surgery Until Patients Can Resume Normal Activity, Return to Work, and Feel 100% Recovered

| | *HALRN* | *ORN* | *p = value* |
|---|---|---|---|
| Normal activity (d) | 13 | 23 | $p = 0.01$ |
| Work (d) | 29 | 53 | $p = 0.03$ |
| 100% recovered (d) | 31 | 150 | $p = 0.0001$ |

HALRN = hand-assisted laparoscopic radical nephrectomy; ORN = open radical nephrectomy.

nificantly reduced operative time, significantly shorter warm ischemia time, and no difference in length of stay *(18)*.

Our early series at the University of Wisconsin compared HALRN to ORN performed over the same time period. Patients in the HALRN had a shorter duration of hospitalization (3.9 vs 4.7 d), a quicker return to work (26.8 vs 53 d), and an earlier time to 100% recovery (28 vs 150 d) *(19)*.

The updated experience at the University of Wisconsin includes 50 HALRN in 48 patients (2 with bilateral nephrectomies). We compared these to 18 ORN at our institution performed over a similar time period (see Table 2). Average tumor size was similar (5.9 vs 6.4 cm), operative time was longer for HALRN (233 min vs 117 min), and average patient age was comparable (58 vs 61). We found blood loss to be less in HALRN (171 cc vs 210 cc). Length of stay was less for HALRN patients; the median day of discharge for HALRN patients was d 4, and for ORN patients was d 5 (Table 2). Patients recovered faster in the HALRN

Table 4
HALRN: Cancer-Specific Survival

| | *Months of followup* | *Cancer-specific survival* |
|---|---|---|
| First 10 patients | 41 | 100% |
| First 15 patients | 36 | 100% |
| First 20 patients | 32 | 100% |
| Overall—46 patients (Palliative nephrectomy excluded) | 12.4 | 100% |

HALRN = hand-assisted radical nephrectomy.

group (Table 3). Ability to return to nonstrenuous activity was at 13 d in the HALRN group, compared to 23 d in the ORN group ($p = 0.01$). HALRN patients returned to work after 29 d, and the ORN patients returned after 53 d ($p = 0.03$). On average, HALRN patients felt 100% recovered at 31 d, yet ORN patients did not feel fully recovered until after 150 d ($p = 0.001$). Average followup on the first 42 HALRN patients is 12.4 mo, and the only cancer-specific death occurred in a patient who underwent palliative nephrectomy. Although overall followup is 12.4 mo, we have longer followup on the earlier patients (Table 4). For the first 10 HALRN patients, the average followup is 41 mo; for the first 15 HALRN patients, the average followup is 36 mo; and for the first 20 HALRN patients, the average followup is 32 mo. As mentioned, the only cancer-specific death was in the palliative nephrectomy.

With the cost of medical care increasing, pressure to provide cost-effective health care makes the incorporation of new technology into current practice difficult. Although it can be argued that the improved outcomes seen with laparoscopic nephrectomy justify the increased cost that comes from disposable equipment and increased time in the operating room, the overall cost of surgery and hospitalization can be less. Lotan et al. showed not only that laparoscopic nephrectomy could be more cost effective when the total cost is considered, but also how it could be more cost effective *(20)*. With statistical cost analysis, they showed that by decreasing laparoscopic operative time and equipment costs, and by decreasing the length of stay, laparoscopic nephrectomy could in fact be cost effective.

Hand assistance can lower costs further. In the HALDN, Lindstrom et al. showed HAL lowered cost compared to standard LDN by shortening the operative and anesthesia time. Additionally, they showed that

HALDN, despite the addition of the hand port, decreased operative cost by alleviating the need for a retrieval bag, laparoscopic retractor, and one trocar *(21)*.

## SUMMARY

LRN remains the new standard of care for the treatment of localized renal cancer. HALS represents a pragmatic development in urologic laparoscopy. For many urologists, HALS is the only approach they will have the time and resources to learn. HALRN shortens the learning curve for the surgeon learning laparoscopy due to the familiarity and confidence gained with the advantages of tactile sensation. When planning any radical nephrectomy, hand assistance with intact removal has proven benefits for the patient and the surgeon.

## REFERENCES


1. Robson CJ. The results of radical nephrectomy for renal cell carcinoma. J Urol 1969; 101: 297–301.
2. Sundaram CP, Rehman J, Landman J, et al. Hand assisted laparoscopic radical nephrectomy for renal cell carcinoma with inferior vena caval thrombus. J Urol 2002; 168(1): 176–179.
3. Novick AC. Surgery of the kidney. In Campbell's Urology, 8th ed., (WB Saunders, Philadelphia, ed.), 2002, p 3587
4. Stifelman M, Neider, AM. Prospective comparison of hand-assisted laparoscopic devices. Urology2002; 59(5): 668–672.
5. Clayman RV, Kavoussi LR, Soper NJ, et al. Laparoscopic nephrectomy: the initial case report. J Urol 1991; 146: 278–282.
6. Kaynan AM, Lee KL, Winfield HN. Survey of urological laparoscopic practices in the state of California. J Urol 2002; 167(6): 2380–2386.
7. Winfield HN, Chen RN, Donovan, JF. Laparoscopic tricks of the trade: how to overcome lack of tactile feedback (abstract 513). J Endourol 1996; 10: S189.
8. Nakada SY, Moon TD, Gist M, et al. Use of the Pneumosleeve as an adjunct during laparoscopic nephrectomy. Urology 1997; 49: 612–613.
9. Wolf JS Jr, Tchetgen MB, Merion RM. Hand-assisted laparoscopic live donor nephrectomy. Urology 1998; 52(5): 885–887.
10. Keeley FX, Sharma NK, Tolley, DA. Hand-assisted laparoscopic nephroureterectomy. BJU Int 1999; 83(4): 504–505.
11. Kim C, Shichman S. Hand-assisted laparoscopic utereropelvic junction obstruction repair. J Urol 2001; 165(5S) 371.
12. Kim C, Shichman S, Stifelman M, et al. Hand-assisted laparoscopic partial nephrectomy. J Urol 2001; 165(5S) 371.
13. Nakada SY. Techniques in endourology: hand-assisted laparoscopic nephrectomy. J Endourol 1999; 13(1): 9–15.
14. Dunn MD, Portis AJ, Shalhav AL, et al. Laparoscopic versus open radical nephrectomy: a 9-year experience. J Urol 2000; 164(4): 1153–1159.
15. Portis AJ, Yan Y, Landman J. Long-term followup after laparoscopic radical nephrectomy. J Urol 2002; 167(3):1257–1262.

16. Nelson CP, Wolf JS Jr. Comparison of hand assisted versus standard laparoscopic radical nephrectomy for suspected renal cell carcinoma. J Urol 2002; 167(5):1989–1994.
17. Batler RA, Campbell SC, Funk JT. Hand-assisted vs. retroperitoneal laparoscopic nephrectomy. J Endourol 2001; 15(9): 899–902.
18. Lindstrom P, Haggman M, Wadstrom J. Hand-assisted laparoscopic surgery (HALS) for live donor nephrectomy is more time- and cost-effective than standard laparoscopic nephrectomy. Surg Endosc 2002; 16(3): 422–425.
19. Nakada SY, Fadden P, Jarrard DF, et al. Hand-assisted laparoscopic radical nephrectomy: comparison to open radical nephrectomy. Urology 2001; 58: 517–520.
20. Lotan Y, Gettman MT, Roehrborn CG, et al. Cost comparison for laparoscopic nephrectomy and open nephrectomy: analysis of individual parameters. Urology 2002; 59(6):821–825.
21. Lindstrom P, Haggman M, Wadstrom J. Hand-assisted laparoscopic surgery (HALS) for live donor nephrectomy is more time- and cost-effective than standard laparoscopic nephrectomy. Surg Endosc 2002; 16(3): 422–425.

# 5 Laparoscopic Management of the Complex Renal Cyst

*Ryan F. Paterson,* MD, *Tibério M. Siqueira, Jr.,* MD, *and Arieh L. Shalhav,* MD

*Contents*

Introduction
Management of Intermediately Complex Renal Cysts
Techniques
Conclusion
References

## INTRODUCTION

Renal cysts are present radiologically in approx 50% of adults over the age of 50 and the incidence rises with advancing age *(1,2)*. The majority of renal cysts are benign simple cysts and require no surgical intervention when asymptomatic. However, a minority of renal cysts can result in pain, hematuria, obstruction to renal drainage, infection, hypertension, and even compression of other intra-abdominal structures that necessitate radiologic or operative treatment. Additionally, cysts may have radiologic features that correlate with a higher likelihood of malignancy that necessitates definitive treatment (Table 1) *(3,4)*.

Traditional therapies for simple renal cysts include aspiration with or without sclerotherapy (the most common treatment) *(5,6)*, percutaneous or ureteronephroscopic marsupialization *(7–9)*, and open cyst decortication. Simple aspiration without sclerotherapy is primarily a diagnostic procedure in which the fluid can be sent for cytology to help

From: *Laparoscopic Urologic Oncology*
Edited by: J. A. Cadeddu © Humana Press Inc., Totowa, NJ

**Table 1**
**Bosniak Classification of Renal Cysts**

| *Type* | *Wall* | *Septations* | *Calcifications* | *Precontrast density (HU)* | *Enhancement* |
|---|---|---|---|---|---|
| I | Thin | None | None | 0–20 | None |
| II | Thin | None–few | Minimal | 0–20 | None |
| III | Increasing thickness | Multiple | Moderate | 0–20 | None |
| IV | Thick | Many | Coarse | > 20 | present |

From ref. *3*

exclude malignancy and the cessation of symptoms with decompression of the cyst can predict an improved result with later definitive treatment. However, aspiration in isolation is associated with recurrence rates of up to 81–96% after a single treatment *(10)*. Percutaneous cyst unroofing or ureteronephroscopic marsupialization remain commonly employed treatments for symptomatic cysts in the patient who has failed aspiration and sclerotherapy. In contrast, open cyst unroofing in the laparoscopic era is rarely required and is associated with significant morbidity (complications in 33% of patients in one study) *(11)*.

After confirming a diagnosis of a symptomatic simple renal cyst, the most commonly utilized therapy remains aspiration and sclerotherapy (e.g., ethanol, bismuth phosphate, tetracycline, povidone-iodine, lipidol, iophenylate) with an overall complete radiological resolution rate of approx 70% *(12,13)*. However, recurrence of the cyst(s) after aspiration and sclerosis is not uncommon and symptomatic patients who have failed this minimally invasive option are ideal candidates for laparoscopic management *(4,14,15)*, thereby avoiding the significant morbidity of an open surgical cyst decortication. Additionally, a laparoscopic approach is reasonable in those patients with a contraindication to sclerotherapy such as a peripelvic cyst. Peripelvic cysts are located in close proximity to the renal vasculature and collecting system, which commonly results in these cysts being associated with symptoms of obstruction, pain, infection, and stone formation *(16,17)*. Sclerotherapy in these cases has a significant risk of inducing peripelvic fibrosis and is rarely used today *(18)*. Likewise, anteriorly located renal cysts may also be poor candidates for sclerotherapy as the potential for bowel injury from the inflammatory reaction to the sclerosant may persuade the urologist to choose a laparoscopic approach as the first line of therapy *(19)*. Additional indications for choosing a laparoscopic approach initially include patients with very large renal cysts or multiple cysts, as in the authors' experience these cases may have an improved outcome with laparoscopic cyst unroofing.

In contrast to the surgical treatment of simple renal cysts, the laparoscopic treatment of complex or indeterminate renal cysts remains an area of controversy. The Bosniak radiologic classification of renal cysts (Table 1) has greatly improved the management of patients with renal cystic disease and has demonstrated that the more complex the radiologic appearance of a renal cyst, the greater the chance of finding malignancy on pathologic review *(3)*. Category I renal cysts are considered simple benign cysts and do not require further evaluation, whereas category IV renal cysts are malignant until proven otherwise and should be managed similarly to a solid renal mass. However, multiple options are currently advocated in the literature for the management of the indeterminate renal cyst (Bosniak category II and III cysts) including observation with serial imaging studies, laparoscopic unroofing with selective biopsy of the cyst wall, enucleation, laparoscopic partial nephrectomy (LPN), and laparoscopic radical nephrectomy (LRN). The results of multiple series evaluating the laparoscopic and open surgical management of simple and complex renal cysts are summarized in Tables 2 and 3 *(4,15,19–37)*.

## MANAGEMENT OF INTERMEDIATELY COMPLEX RENAL CYSTS

The Bosniak classification of renal cysts (Table 1) has allowed standardization of the management of renal cystic disease with the vast majority of asymptomatic Bosniak category II renal cysts followed radiologically, whereas Bosniak category III renal cysts undergo surgical exploration as there is an increased incidence of malignancy in these cases *(3)*. However, radiological followup as the sole treatment of category II renal cysts may result in a missed diagnosis of malignancy in a significant number of cases, and this has prompted investigators to re-evaluate the management of Bosniak category II renal cysts. Recently, Gary Bellman's group at the Kaiser Permanente Medical Center in Los Angeles reported the cumulative results from multiple studies evaluating the pathological findings of Bosniak category II and III renal cysts with the authors suggesting that up to 24% of Bosniak category II cysts and up to 33% of category III renal cysts are found to harbor renal cell carcinoma (RCC) *(24)*. A laparoscopic approach for treatment of an indeterminate renal cyst has multiple advantages including establishing a definitive diagnosis, minimizing intraoperative blood loss, improving patient comfort and cosmetic results, rapid convalescence, and reducing length of hospital stay *(24)*. These authors have the largest experience reported in the literature on the laparoscopic treatment of indeterminate renal cysts, consisting of 57 patients with indeterminate renal cysts (Bosniak category II and III renal cysts) who underwent transperitoneal laparoscopic localization, aspiration of the cyst, cytologic analysis, unroofing of the cyst wall, and biopsy of the cyst base. Pathologic evaluation of these specimens was performed intraoperatievely, and further management was based on the findings. The results are summarized in Tables 2 and 3. In patients undergoing laparoscopic cyst evaluation only with no further surgery (partial or total nephrectomy), no cases of renal functional deterioration occurred.

Of the 57 patients, 11 were found to have cystic RCC (19%), with the majority of tumors low grade (grade I or II clear cell or granular cell RCC) and low stage (9 cases T1; 2 cases T2). Importantly, the size of the cyst was not found to correlate with the presence of malignancy and only one patient had a positive cytology result (false-negative rate of 91%). Open partial nephrectomy was performed on five patients, open radical nephrectomy (ORN) was performed on four patients and two patients underwent laparoscopic nephrectomy. Of the 11 nephrectomies, 10 were performed immediately after the laparoscopic evaluation under the same anesthetic. After a mean followup of 40 mo (range 6–70 mo), no cases of local recurrence, port-site or peritoneal seeding, or distant metastatic disease have been encountered. This study suggests that laparoscopic evaluation of the indeterminate renal cyst is safe and effective for the treatment of both Bosniak category II and III renal cysts. Additionally, the results suggest that a large number of cystic RCCs would be missed if the surgeon over-relied on the results of the cytology obtained pre- or intraoperatively. In a similar study, Rubenstein et al. *(4)* reported two cases of RCC in 10 patients with symptomatic renal cysts undergoing laparoscopic renal cyst decortication. Both of these patients had negative aspiration cytology results preoperatively and the preoperative computed tomography (CT) images were consistent with Bosniak category I renal cysts. No tumor recurrence has been noted after ORN in either of these cases. Likewise, Roberts et al. *(15)* reported a single case of RCC in their series of 32 patients with peripelvic and parenchymal renal cysts undergoing laparoscopic cyst decortication. The isolated case of cystic RCC occurred in a patient with a 10-cm Bosniak category II renal cyst (minimally thickened wall) with both negative pre- and intraoperative cytology and a negative frozen section of the excised cyst wall. However, permanent pathological analysis of the specimen revealed a 0.8-cm focus of diffuse papillary RCC within the cyst wall adjacent to the base. The patient underwent an ORN with excision of the trocar site used for specimen removal and at 60 mo followup, no evidence of recurrence has been found. Along the same lines, Lifson et al. *(21)* reported one of nine patients with nonpolycystic kidney disease who was found to have RCC on pathologic review. Preoperatively, multiple large Bosniak category I cysts were noted with the preoperative cyst fluid cytology negative for malignancy. Under the same anesthetic, the patient underwent an ORN with the final pathological study revealing papillary RCC with negative surgical margins. No evidence of recurrence has been noted after 5 yr of followup. In summary, these studies suggest that cystic RCC found at the time of laparoscopic cyst decortication can be successfully treated with immediate partial or radical

Table 2
**Intraoperative and Postoperative Data for Laparoscopic Treatment of Renal Cysts**

| *Series* | *No. of pts* | *Previous perc. aspiration* | *TP/RP approach* | *Average OR time (hr)* | *Mean hospital stay (d)* | *Average narcotic require-ment* | *% pain relief* | *Duration of follow-up (mo)* | *Serum creatinine postop* | *Complications* |
|---|---|---|---|---|---|---|---|---|---|---|
| Rubenstein et al. *(4)* | 10 | 6 | 9/1 | 2.5 | 2.2 | 5.3 mg morphine equivalent | 80 | 10 | NA | Hematoma, ileus; flank parasthesia |
| Brown et al. *(20)* | 5 | 3 | TP | 2.4 | 2 | NA | 74 | 24 | NA | Umbilical/anterior abdominal hernia |
| Lifson et al. *(21)* | 9 | NA | TP | 2.3 | 2.2 | NA | 100 | 33 | Stable | Ileus, hemorrhage |
| Hoenig et al. *(23)* | 3 | 3 | 2/1 | 1.4 | 5.0 | NA | 100 | 3.5 | NA | Ileus |
| Hoenig et al. *(22)*[a] | 4 | 3 | 3/1 | 5.6 | 2.75 | 385 mg meperidine | 75 | 2–22 | NA | 1 renal pelvic laceration |
| Limb et al. *(24)* | 57 | NA | TP | 3.1 | 0.6 | NA | NA | NA | Stable[b] | 3/57 |
| Guazzoni et al. *(19)* | 20 | 20 | TP | 1.25 | 2.2 | No parenteral narcotics | 100 | 3–6 | stable | None |
| Denis et al. *(25)* | 10 | NA | 8/2 | 1.5 | 5.4 | NA | 100 | 8.3 | NA | 1 conversion 2° bleeding |
| Roberts et al. *(15)*[c] | 11 | 1 | 7/4 | 3.9 | 2.7 | NA 6.8 | 100 | 22.4 ± 6.8 | NA | 1 (9%) urinary fistula with ileus |
| Roberts et al. *(15)*[d] | 21 | 7 | 13/8 | 2.7 | 1.9 | NA | 100 | 15.8 ± 4.4 | NA | 3 (14%) mid ureteric stricture, diaphragmatic injury, peroneal |

| | | | | | | | | | | |
|---|---|---|---|---|---|---|---|---|---|---|
| Hemal et al. (26) | 5 | 5 | RP | 1.15 | 2.3 | 300 mg pethidine | 100% | 15-39 mo. | NA | Nerve palsy |
| Hemal et al. (26) | 2 | 0 | RP | 3.1 | 2.3 | 300 pethidine | 100% | 15-39 mo. | NA | None |
| Stanley et al. (27) | 4 | NA | TP | 2.5 | 1-2 | NA | 75% | NA | NA | NA |
| Austoni et al. (28) | 6 | NA | TP | 2.0 | NA | NA | 100% | NA | NA | 0% |
| Valdivia Uria et al. (29)[a] | 13 | NA | TP | NA | NA | NA | NA | 0–12 | NA | NA |
| Wada et al. (30) | 13 | NA | TP | NA | NA | NA | 83% | 3 | NA | NA |
| Ou et al. (31) | 4 | 4 | 7GRP/7RP | 0.87/1.73 | 4.6/3.7 | 71.4/2.21.4 mg meperidine | 100% | 7/9 | NA | 14.3/0% |
| Helal et al. (32) | 10 | 10 | TP | 2.92 | 2.5 | NA | 90% | NA | NA | 0% |
| Zuluaga Gomez[c] et al. (36) | 5 | NA | NA | NA | NA | NA | 100% | NA | NA | 1 case fretroperitoneal hematoma |
| Zanetti et al. (37)[d] | 18 | NA | NA | NA | NA | NA | 94% | 6 | NA | 11% |

[a]Laparoscopic treatment of peripelvic cysts.
[b]Forty-six of 57 patients who were not found to have RCC on laparoscopic evaluation.
[c]Laparoscopic treatment of 11 peripelvic renal cysts.
[d]Laparoscopic treatment of 21 parenchymal renal cysts.
[e]Retroperitoneal approach to renal cysts.
[f]Gasless retroperitoneoscopic approach (GRP) vs gaseous retroperitoneoscopic approach (RP).
TP = transperitoneal; RP = retroperitoneal; OR = operating room; NA = not applicable

Table 3
**Laparoscopic Treatment of Complex Renal Cysts**

| *Series* | *No. of pts* | *Mean cyst size (cm)* | *No. Bosniak Category II cyst* | *No. RCC (%)* | *No. Bosniak Category III cyst* | *No. RCC (%)* | *Grade of RCC* | *Stage of RCC* | *Duration of F/U pts with RCC (mo)* | *% Local recurrence or metastatic disease* |
|---|---|---|---|---|---|---|---|---|---|---|
| Limb et al. *(24)* | 57 | 5.3 ± 2.3 (1.5-10) | 28 | 3 (11%) | 29 | 8 (28%) | I or II | T1 (9) (T2 (2) | 40 (range 6-70) | 0% |
| Lifson et al. *(21)* | 9 | NA | Tumor in Bosniak I cyst | | | 1 (11%) | NA | T1 | 60 | 0% |
| Rubenstein et al. *(4)* | 10 | 11.4 (6–20) | Tumor in simple renal cysts | | | 2 (20%) | NA | NA | NA | NA |
| Roberts et al. *(15)* | 32 | NA | 8/32 Bosniak II/III cysts | | | 1 (3%) | NA | T1 | 60 | 0% |
| Aronson et al. *(34)*[a,b] | 15 | NA | 4 | 0 (0%) | 7 | 4 (57%) | NA | NA | NA | NA |
| Wilson et al. *(35)*[a,b] | 20 | NA | 5 | 4 (80%) | 4 | 4 (100%) | I or II | NA | NA | NA |
| Cloix et al. *(33)*[a] | 30 | NA | 7 | 1 (14%) | 13 | 4 (31%) | NA | NA | NA | 8% |

[a]Open surgical series.
[b]Retrospective series of patients with pathologically proven cystic renal masses.
RCC = renal cell carcinoma; F/U = followup.

nephrectomy with long-term followup confirming an absence of local recurrence or distant metastases. Additionally, these studies indicate a low yield of cyst fluid cytology in excluding renal malignancy, a finding supported by the study of Hayakawa et al., who reported that only 14% of 37 patients with cystic RCC had a preoperative positive cytology for malignancy *(38)*. The absence of local, regional, or metastatic disease in these cases may be a reflection of the improved prognosis related with cystic RCC compared to other subtypes of RCC *(39–41)*. Indeed, the majority of tumors in Bellman's study *(24)* were of a low grade and stage.

Despite promising results of laparoscopic treatment of Bosniak category I renal cysts in the literature, a recent case report of an RCC recurrence after laparoscopic cyst decortication of a Bosniak category I renal cyst is alarming and suggests continued caution in approaching renal cystic disease with only laparoscopic cyst decortication *(42)*. In this unfortunate case, Meng et al. reported a 60-yr-old patient with a left simple renal cyst who underwent an uncomplicated transperitoneal laparoscopic cyst decortication. No cytology was reported and no suspicious lesions were noted visually or on pathological review of the excised cyst wall. Seven months postoperatively, the patient presented with an enhancing left solid renal mass, lymphadenopathy, lung and liver metastases, and subcutaneous nodules at his port sites. The patient underwent immunotherapy and removal of his left kidney, spleen, and left colon with the final pathology report revealing chromophil and sarcomatoid RCC (Fuhrman grade 4) in all specimens with a stage of pT4N2M1.

The laparoscopic treatment of peripelvic cysts can also be difficult and must be approached with caution. Hoenig et al. *(22)* reported a success rate of 75% in their series of four patients treated with laparoscopic cyst unroofing. The authors recommended that a transperitoneal rather than retroperitoneal approach may be preferable due to the improved cyst exposure, intraperitoneal drainage of cyst fluid, more complete hilar dissection, and enhanced room to both repair inadvertent injuries of the collecting system, and to access the omentum for use as a "wick." Recently, Roberts and Kavoussi *(15)* reported the largest series to date on the laparoscopic treatment of peripelvic cysts (Tables 2 and 3). Eleven patients were treated, with 7 undergoing a transperitoneal approach and 4 a retroperitoneal approach. The authors compared their results to the laparoscopic treatment of parenchymal renal cysts and reported a longer mean operative time (233 min vs 164 min; $p = 0.003$) and larger mean operative blood loss (182 mL vs 98 mL; $p = 0.04$) with treatment of peripelvic cysts. Although all patients in both groups were symptom-free postoperatively, a single cyst recurrence was noted radiologically in the peripelvic group.

Our decision-making algorithm for asymptomatic and symptomatic Bosniak category I, II, and III renal cysts are outlined in Figs. 1, 2, 3 and 4. The laparoscopic technique used at our institution for cyst evaluation and ablation (lap cyst E&A) is detailed here.

For Bosniak category I and II cysts, if asymptomatic, our strategy is imaging followup unless significant change occurs; either rapid growth or increase in complex cyst features. Symptomatic Bosniak category I cysts are percutaneously treated, whereas symptomatic Bosniak category II cysts are managed with lap cyst E&A.

Our management strategy for the Bosniak category III renal cyst (Fig. 4) differs from those authors *(24)* who advocate laparoscopic cyst unroofing, as we have tended to approach these lesions in a similar manner to Bosniak category IV cysts (malignant renal tumors until proven otherwise) and if feasible, perform an LPN or LRN with no attempt at cyst aspiration or unroofing. However, if the size or location of the lesion does not permit a laparoscopic enucleation or LPN and there is a low clinical suspicion for malignancy, then we will proceed with a lap cyst E&A. In contrast, if the clinical suspicion of malignancy is high or the patient is found during cyst E&A to have either positive cyst cytology or a positive frozen section (or permanent section) for malignancy, then immediate partial or radical nephrectomy according to the size and location of the tumor should be performed. In those rare cases of a negative frozen section and a positive permanent section for malignancy, open partial or ORN should be performed within 1 wk of surgery. Bosniak category IV renal cysts are treated the same as a solid renal mass with the patient undergoing a LPN or LRN according to the tumor size, location and number, as well as any indications for nephron-sparing surgery.

## TECHNIQUES

### *Preoperative Evaluation*

Routine preoperative laboratory studies are obtained including electrolytes, complete blood count, urinalysis, and urine culture. The patient is routinely typed and screened as a more extensive surgery (LPN or LRN) may be required depending on the operative findings. Patients are informed of the risks inherent to laparoscopic exploration of a complex renal cyst especially the theoretical risk of cancer cell migration if a tumor-bearing cyst is opened. In addition, informed consent is obtained for both open and laparoscopic partial or radical nephrectomy if malig-

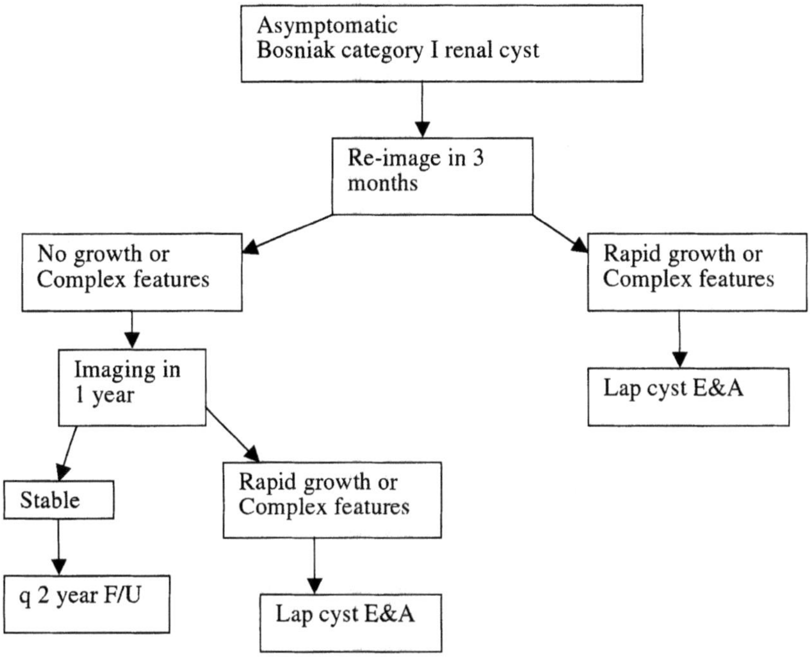


**Fig. 1.** Management of the asymptomatic Bosniak category I renal cyst. q = every ; F/U = followup; Lap cyst E&A = laparoscopic cyst evaluation and ablation.

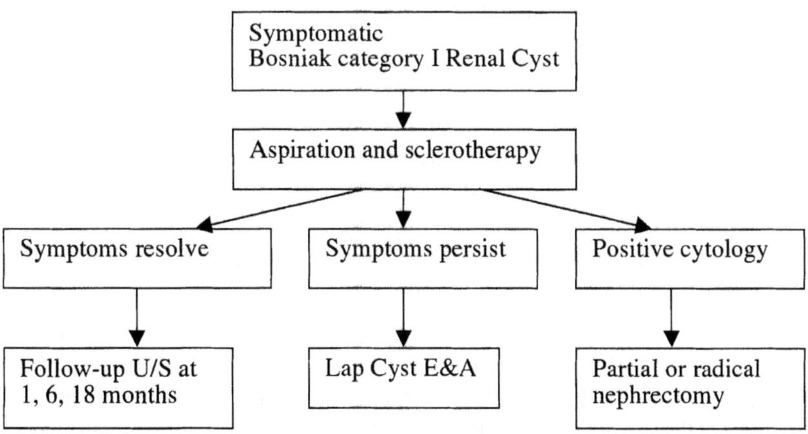


**Fig. 2.** Management of the symptomatic Bosniak category I renal cyst. U/S = ultrasound; Lap cyst E&A = laparoscopic cyst evaluation and ablation.

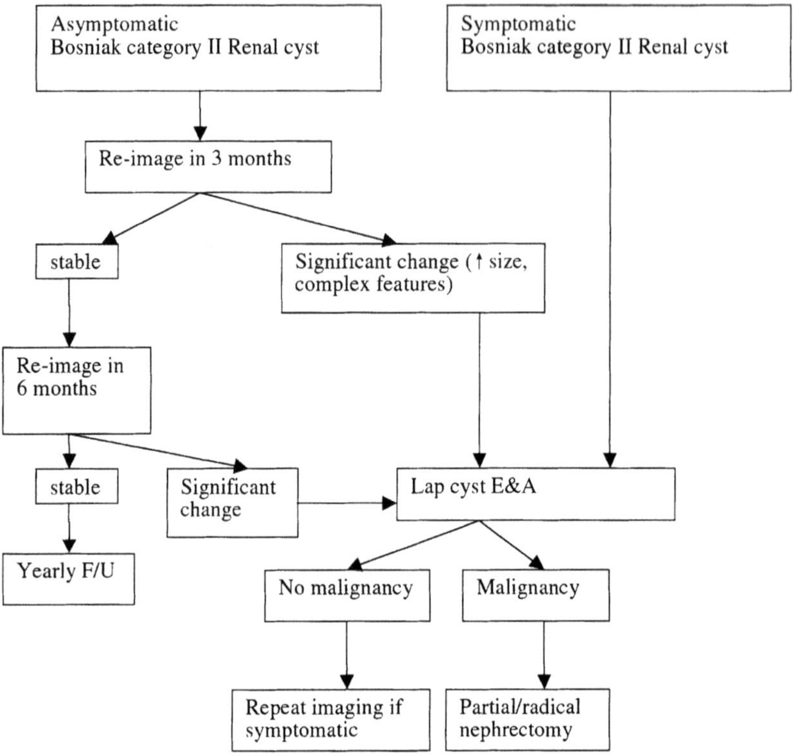


**Fig. 3.** Management of syptomatic and asymptomatic Bosniak category II renal cysts. F/U = followup; lap cyst E&A = laparascopic cyst evaluation and ablation.

nancy is detected at the time of cyst unroofing. Additionally, some researchers recommend that patients with indeterminate renal cysts warrant a preoperative metastatic workup that includes a chest X-ray and liver function tests *(24)*.

In patients with normal renal function, a renal protocol contrast CT scan (with and without intravenous [iv] contrast administration) is mandatory prior to consideration for surgical exploration. The appearance of the cyst on thin section (2.5–3 mm slice width) CT scans is the best guide to identify patients for laparoscopic exploration of renal cysts. In contrast, in those patients with impaired renal function, contrast allergy, or a hyperdense renal cyst, a magnetic resonance imaging (MRI) scan with the administration of contrast (gadolinium) is performed with reliance primarily on the T2 images *(12)*. However, in most of our patients, an ultrasound (US) study was part of their evaluation and furnished valuable information regarding the cyst grading.

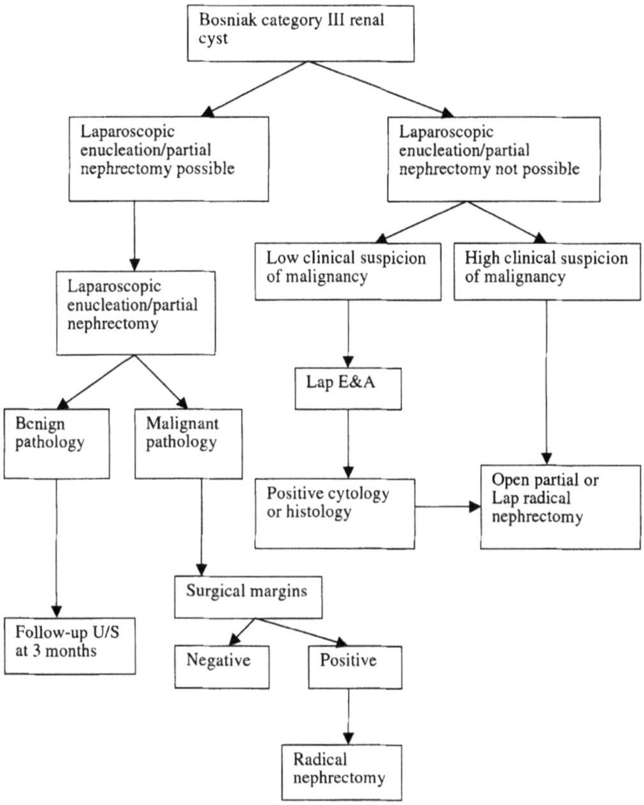


**Fig. 4.** Management of the Bosniak category III renal cyst. U/S = ultrasound; lap E&A = laparoscopic cyst evaluation and ablation.

## *Surgical Technique at Indiana University Hospital*

The choice of a retroperitoneal or transperitoneal approach to the renal cyst depends on multiple factors including the size, number, and location of the renal cyst(s); the suspicion of malignancy; the experience of the surgeon; and the presence of co-existent intra-abdominal pathology. As a general rule, cysts located on the anterior surface of the kidney are best approached via a transperitoneal approach, whereas cysts on the posterior surface can be more easily accessed via a retroperitoneal approach. However, many authors, including ourselves, advocate a retroperitoneal approach for the majority of renal cysts in order to prevent intraperitoneal spillage of cyst contents, to reduce postoperative ileus, and to avoid later intraperitoneal adhesion formation *(26)*.

Caution must be exercised when intraparenchymal renal cysts are being considered for laparoscopic management. Cysts deep in the kidney may be visible on intraoperative US but intact removal of the cyst can be very difficult and the dissection can result in significant bleeding and risk of injury to the renal-collecting system. An open approach in this setting may be more appropriate for the less experienced laparoscopist.

### Transperitoneal Approach

A light preoperative bowel preparation is not routinely required. Antibiotic prophylaxis with a single iv dose of a cephalosporin is adequate in the majority of cases and sequential pneumatic compression devices are placed on all patients. After induction of general anesthesia and endotracheal intubation, a Foley catheter and orogastric tube are inserted. The patient is placed in a 45° modified flank position with the kidney bar raised and the patient secured on a bean bag. The exposed flank is then prepared with povidone-iodine solution and drapes applied. Abdominal landmarks are noted and the position of the laparoscopic ports selected. The number and location of laparoscopic ports will vary with the body habitus of the patient, the presence or absence of prior abdominal surgery; the kidney affected; the preference of the surgeon; and the size, number, and location of the renal cyst(s). In general, in patients without previous upper abdominal incisions, we begin with a 12-mm port placed at the lateral border of the rectus muscle 5–10 cm cephalad to the umbilicus. However, in patients with large palpable cysts, we choose to place our initial port away from the mass in a location where the abdominal wall is not be compressed by the cyst. The initial port is placed with the aid of a 10-mm 0° lens and 12-mm Optiview visual obturator (Ethicon, Cincinnati, OH). Alternatives include the use of a Veress needle to enter the peritoneal cavity or an open direct insertion of the initial port using the Hasson technique.

Once the peritoneum is entered, pneumoperitoneum is established with a pressure limit of 14 mm Hg and the abdomen is inspected for injury to the solid and hollow viscera. The 10-mm 30° telescope is then inserted and additional ports are placed under direct vision. Usually, a 5-mm blunt port (Ethicon, Cincinnati, OH) is placed 5 cm below the rib cage at the lateral border of the rectus muscle, while in the lower quadrant midclavicular line, a 5- or 12-mm port is placed (approx 10 cm below the rib cage). Later, after reflection of the colon, an additional 5 mm port may be placed halfway between the 12th rib and the iliac crest in the midaxillary line to provide lateral retraction of the kidney when dissecting anteromedial cysts. For right-sided upper pole cysts, the presence of a 3- or 5-mm laparoscopic port in a midline subxiphoid location allows for retraction of the liver edge cephalad by anchoring a 3- or 5-mm locking toothed grasper to the body wall inferolateral to the liver.

In occasional cases, anteriorly located simple renal cysts can be safely approached by careful dissection through the mesocolon, minimizing colonic manipulation *(23)*.

Previous intra-abdominal surgery or prior inflammatory processes can result in significant adhesions that are divided as close to the abdominal wall as possible using the 5-mm harmonic endoshears. When minimal distance separates the bowel from the abdominal wall, sharp dissection with the 5-mm scissors without electrocautery is safest. Once all adhesions are divided, the colon is reflected medially by incising the peritoneum at the white line of Toldt. Wide mobilization of the colon from below the iliac vessels to the hepatic or splenic flexure is helpful and facilitates later dissection of the renal cyst. For access to upper pole renal cysts, the spleen or liver must be mobilized by dividing the peritoneal attachments to allow the spleen or liver to be retracted cephalad and medially. On the left this involves division of the phrenocolic, lienorenal, and splenocolic ligaments. For right-sided medial cysts, the duodenum must be carefully mobilized medially (Kocher maneuver) using sharp and blunt dissection and avoiding the use of electrocautery.

Further dissection of the kidney depends on the location, size, and number of renal cysts. In most cases, dissection of the renal hilum is not required except in cases of peripelvic cysts (see below). Gerota's fascia is incised and the perinephric fat is mobilized off of the renal capsule and surface of the renal cyst with the cyst dissected to its junction with the adjacent renal parenchyma. Large renal cysts are often visible through Gerota's fascia and appear as a well-delineated blue dome protruding from the surface of the kidney. When identification of the cyst remains difficult, intraoperative ultrasound can be performed to locate it. Complete dissection of the cyst is performed until 1 cm of normal kidney tissue is identified around the cyst. This portion of the dissection is performed while the cyst is preserved intact to facilitate the plane of dissection off the cyst wall.

The majority of symptomatic Bosniak category I and II renal cysts can be managed with laparoscopic unroofing of the renal cyst (Figs. 1–3). Using a laparoscopic 5-mm, 18-gauge needle aspirator, the cyst is aspirated and the color of the fluid noted (clear yellow in most cases). The cyst fluid is routinely sent for cytological analysis and in cases of suspected infection, a gram stain and culture is obtained. We do not routinely send the fluid from simple renal cysts for determination of protein, fat, and creatinine. Subsequently, the cyst is filled with sterile water for about 5 min to lyse any potential cancer cells. After the cyst is evacuated, the outer wall is grasped and, using the harmonic scalpel (Ethicon, Cincinnati, OH), the cyst wall is excised close to the junction of the cyst with the normal renal parenchyma using the coagulating energy level. An increase in bleeding is often encountered when the cyst is excised flush with the renal parenchyma and this should be avoided. Additional hemostasis is achieved by using bipolar cautery during and after excision of the cyst wall. Next, the base of the cyst is carefully inspected with the aid of the magnification offered with the 30° laparoscope and any suspicious areas undergo excisional biopsy using the endoshears and submitted for frozen section. Hemostasis is achieved using bipolar cautery avoiding damage to the collecting system or adjacent vessels. The excised cyst wall is placed into a 10-mm endocatch bag (Ethicon, Cincinnati, OH) and sent for frozen section and permanent pathological analysis. If malignancy is noted on frozen section, an immediate partial or radical nephrectomy is performed. If the final pathological report detects malignancy and a nephrectomy is indicated, then surgery is best performed within 1 wk of the initial procedure to facilitate dissection *(24)*.

If no suspicious areas are noted endoscopically and no malignancy is detected from frozen section analysis of the cyst wall, the base of the cyst is fulgurated using the argon beam coagulator (Birtcher Medical System, Allenwood, NJ) at a setting of 80 watts. A pedicle of perinephric fat or omentum is then placed into the cavity and anchored in place with freehand placed sutures of 3-0 Vicryl (SH needle) to act as a wick to prevent recurrence. Sterile water is used as the irrigant in all cases and at the end of the case, a thorough lavage of the peritoneal cavity is performed.

In occasional cases where the kidney must be extensively mobilized, a nephropexy is required to prevent postoperative torsion on the renal pedicle. The nephropexy is performed by affixing the kidney capsule to the posterolateral abdominal wall fascia with two or three 0-Vicryl sutures placed using an intracorporeal suturing technique. We do not reapproximate the colon to the body wall as we feel that the intraperitonealization of the cyst helps prevent recurrence. No drains are needed in the majority of cases. The pneumoperitoneum is reduced to 4 mm Hg and the surgical site inspected for hemostasis or collecting system injury. (If needed Methylen Blue and lasix are given iv to better asses for urine leak.) If needed, free-hand suturing is used to achieve hemostasis or to repair any collecting system injury. Should a drain be required due to questionable hemostasis or collecting system injury, a 5-mm Blake drain (Ethicon, Cincinnati, OH) can be placed exiting through a lateral 5-mm port site and anchored to the skin using a 2-0 nonabsorbable suture. Port sites larger than 5 mm are closed with 0-Vicryl with the aid of a fascial closure device by the majority of laparoscopic surgeons.

However, our short-term results with the use of the blunt-tipped visual obturator (Optiview, Ethicon, Cincinnati, OH) suggest that in adults, fascial closure of the 10- or 12-mm ports may be unnecessary *(43)*. The 5-mm port sites are then removed under direct vision followed by removal of the 12-mm camera port by back loading the 12-mm port and withdrawing the laparoscope, inspecting for bleeding on exiting the abdominal wall. A subcuticular 4-0 Vicryl is then used to close the port site skin followed by adhesive strips.

### Peripelvic Cysts

Peripelvic cysts represent a unique challenge to the laparoscopic surgeon based on their close proximity to the renal vessels and renal pelvis. In these cases, we begin with the patient positioned supine where flexible cystoscopy is performed to place a 5 French ureteral catheter to aid identification of the proximal ureter and renal pelvis and allow the instillation of Methylene blue to detect inadvertent collecting system injury. The open-ended ureteral catheter is secured to the Foley catheter and the patient is repositioned with the desired flank elevated. Dissection of the kidney proceeds as above with the addition of meticulous hilar dissection to dissect the ureter, renal pelvis, and renal vasculature off the cyst wall. In these cases, the peripelvic cyst is often draped by segmental vascular branches that can easily be injured resulting in significant blood loss. After cyst aspiration and irrigation with sterile water, the central portion of the renal cyst wall away from the vessels is grasped and incised with the endoshears or harmonic scalpel allowing further dissection of the cyst wall. The cyst wall is safely excised away from vital structures even if some cyst wall is left adjacent to this structures. The interior of the cyst and the remaining cyst wall vigilantly examined and suspicious areas are carefully biopsied as described above. No fulguration of the interior cyst surface is performed as fulguration is a risk factor for injury to the collecting system. Methylene blue is administered through the ureteral catheter to assess for collecting system injury. If no collecting system injury is noted, a tongue of perinephric fat or mobilized omentum is placed into the cyst cavity to prevent accumulation of cyst fluid and anchored in place with 4-0 or 5-0 Vicryl sutures (using a free-hand technique) to the exposed renal parenchymal edge. In cases of collecting system injury, the communication can be closed with figure-of-8, 4-0 Vicryl suture and a drain placed. The ureteral catheter is then internalized at the end of the procedure and the bladder drained for 24 h. The internal ureteral stent remains for up to 6 wk and a contrast study is recommended prior to stent removal to rule out ongoing urinary extravasation *(44)*. Patients are discharged home at 24–48 h if they are passing flatus, tolerating a regular diet, and their pain is controlled with oral pain medications.

### Retroperitoneal Approach

Posterior or lower pole Bosniak category I and II renal cysts can be optimally approached directly via the retroperitoneal approach. Indeed, as a general rule, we find that the retroperitoneal approach can be used for the majority of simple renal cyst decortications. The patient is placed in the 90° full flank position on a bean bag with the kidney rest elevated. The flank is prepared and draped and the bony landmarks of the 12th rib, paraspinal muscles, and iliac crest are noted. A 15-mm incision that will easily allow the insertion of the index finger is made 2 cm below the tip of the 12th rib. The 12-mm Optiview visual obturator (Ethicon, Cincinnati, OH) with a 10-mm 0° telescope is then used to enter the retroperitoneal space under vision. Once entered, the visual obturator is removed and the retroperitoneal space is dissected bluntly with a lubricated index finger. The underside of the 12th rib, psoas muscle, and lower pole of the kidney are key internal landmarks to palpate to allow for a successful retroperitoneal dissection. Gentle finger dissection allows the peritoneum to be mobilized medially by peeling the peritoneum off of the anterior abdominal wall. Wide peritoneal mobilization is necessary to prevent later peritoneal puncture during placement of the most anterior laparoscopic port. The retroperitoneum is then balloon dissected under direct vision with the aid of a pre-peritoneal balloon dissector (US Surgical, Norwalk, CT) or blindly with a Gaur balloon (finger cot of a size 8 glove tied over a 16 French red rubber catheter). Balloon dissection requires the balloon to be carefully placed in the space between the psoas muscle posteriorly and the kidney anteriorly. A common mistake during the retroperitoneal approach is to place the balloon anterior to the kidney. Once the retroperitoneal space is dissected, additional ports are placed under digital guidance. A 5-mm blunt port (Ethicon, Cincinnati, OH) is placed posteriorly at the junction of the 12th rib and the paraspinal muscle (avoiding the subcostal neurovascular bundle) and an additional 5-mm port is placed at the anterior axillary line 5 cm cranial to the anterior superior iliac spine. A 12-mm blunt-tipped balloon trocar (US Surgical, Norwalk, CT) is inserted at the camera port site inferior to the tip of the 12th rib. Pneumoretroperitoneum is then established (14 mm Hg) and the retroperitoneum examined for landmarks and to exclude perforation of the peritoneum. Gerota's fascia overlying the posterior surface of the kidney is incised in a cephalocaudad direction and the perinephric fat and Gerota's fascia mobilized off of the renal capsule and cyst. The cyst is than managed as in the transperitoneal approach.

The retroperitoneal approach is also conducive to partial and radical nephrectomy, however, at our center our preference is to approach potentially malignant lesions via the transperitoneal approach.

## CONCLUSION

Review of the literature and our own experience suggest that the majority of symptomatic Bosniak category I and II renal cysts can be safely managed laparoscopically with multiple treatment options available including lap cyst E&A. Additionally, laparoscopy is increasingly being chosen to both evaluate and definitely treat Bosniak category III renal cysts. Continued caution is warranted due to the isolated reports of RCCs found in association with both simple and complex renal cysts managed laparoscopically. However, the majority of studies report no excellent long-term outcomes when cystic RCC found at the time of laparoscopic cyst unroofing is definitely managed with LPN or LRN.

## REFERENCES

1. Terada N, Ichioka K, Matsuta Y, et al. The natural history of simple renal cysts. J Urol 2002; 167: 21–23.
2. Laucks SPJ, McLachlan MSF. Aging and simple cysts of the kidney. Br J Radiol1981; 54: 12–14.
3. Bosniak M. The current radiological approach to renal cysts. Radiology 1986; 158: 1–10.
4. Rubenstein S, Hulbert J, Pharand D, et al. Laparoscopic ablation of symptomatic renal cysts. J Urol 1993; 150: 1103–1106.
5. Delakis D, Karyotis I, Loumbakis P, et al. Long-term results after percutaneous minimally invasive procedure treatment of symptomatic renal cysts. International Urology and Nephrology 2001; 32: 321–326.
6. Chung B, Kim J, Hong C, et al. Comparison of single and multiple sessions of percutaneous sclerotherapy for simple renal cyst. BJU International 2000; 85: 626–627.
7. Kang Y, Noble C, Gupta M. Percutaneous resection of renal cysts. J Endourol 2001; 15: 735–738.
8. Liatsikos E, Siablis D, Karnabatidis D, et al. Percutaneous treatment of large symptomatic renal cysts. J Endourol 2000; 14: 257–261.
9. Weichert-Jacobsen K, Loch T, Kuppers F, et al. Clinical experience with percutaneous renal cyst resection. BJU International 1999; 84: 164–166.
10. Clayman RV, Kavoussi LR. Endosurgical techniques of noncalculus disease. In: Campbell's Urology, 6th ed. (Walsh PC, Stamey TA, Vaughan EDJ, eds.), WB Saunders, Philadelphia, 1992, pp. 2259–2261.
11. Kropp K, Grayhack J, Wendel R, et al. Morbidity and mortality of renal exploration for cysts. Surg Gynecol Obstet 1967; 125: 803–806.
12. Wolf JSJ. Evaluation and management of solid and cystic renal masses. J Urol 1998; 159: 1120–1133.
13. Pearle M, Traxer O, Cadeddu J. Renal cystic disease:laparoscopic management. Urol Clin North Am 2000; 27: 661–673.

14. Nieh PT, Bihrle WI. Laparoscopic marsupialization of massive renal cyst. J. Urol 1993; 150: 171–173.
15. Roberts W, Bluebond-Langner R, Boyle K, et al. Laparoscopic ablation of symptomatic parenchymal and peripelvic renal cysts. Urology 2001; 58: 165–169.
16. Holmberg, G., Hietala, S. O.: Treatment of simple renal cysts by percutaneous puncture and instillation of bismuth-phosphate. Scand J Urol Nephrol 1989; 23: 207–212.
17. Hinman FJ. Obstructive renal cysts. J Urol 1978; 119: 681–683.
18. Lang EK. Renal cyst puncture and aspiration: A survey of complications. Am J Roentgenol 1977; 18: 723–727.
19. Guazzoni G, Montorsi F, Bergamaschi F, et al. Laparoscopic unroofing of simple renal cysts. Urology 1994; 43: 154–159.
20. Brown JA, Torres VE, King BF, et al.: Laparoscopic marsupialization of symptomatic polycystic kidney disease. J Urol 1996; 156: 22–27.
21. Lifson BJ, Teichman JMH, Hulbert J. Role and long-term results of laparoscopic decortication in solitary cystic and autosomal dominant polycystic kidney disease. J Urol 1998; 159: 705–706.
22. Hoenig D, McDougall EM, Shalhav A, et al. Laparoscopic ablation of peripelvic renal cysts. J Urol 1997; 158: 1345–1348.
23. Hoenig DM, Leveillee RJ, Amaral JF, et al. Laparoscopic Unroofing of Symptomatic Renal Cysts: Three Distinct Surgical Approaches. J Endourol 1994; 9: 55–58.
24. Limb J, Santiago L, Kaswick J, et al. Laparoscopic Evaluation of Indeterminate Renal Cysts: Long-Term Follow-Up. J Endourol 2002; 16: 79–82.
25. Denis E, Nicolas F, Ben Rais N, et al. Laparoscopic surgical treatment of simple cysts of the kidney. Prog Urol 1998; 8: 195–200.
26. Hemal AK, Aron M, Gupta NP, et al. The role of retroperitoneoscopy in the management of renal and adrenal pathology. BJU International 1999; 83: 929–936.
27. Stanley KH, Winfield HN, Donovan JF. Laparoscopic marsupialization of renal cysts. J. Urol 1993; 149: 452A.
28. Austoni E, Trinchieri A, Zanetti G, et al. Renal cyst: Laparoscopic resection. Arch Ital Urol Androl 1993; 65: 235–237.
29. Valdivia Uria JG, Abril Baquero G, Monzon Alebesque F, et al. Laparoscopic ablation of renal cysts. Arch Esp Urol 1994; 47: 246–252.
30. Wada T, Kamiryo Y, Tsuchido M, et al. Laparoscopic unroofing of a renal cyst. Hinyokika Kiyo 1995; 41: 861–865.
31. Ou S, Yang CR, Chang YY, et al. The clinical experience of gasless retroperitoneoscopic and gasless retroperitoneoscopy-assisted unroofing of renal cyst. Chin Med J (Taipei) 1997; 59: 232–239.
32. Helal MA, Albertini JJ, Albrink M, et al. Laparoscopic renal cyst excision: An alternative treatment for patients failing percutaneous management. J. Endourol 1999; 13: A125.
33. Cloix P, Martin X, Pangaud C, et al. Surgical management of complex renal cysts: A series of 32 cases. J Urol 1996; 156: 28–30.
34. Aronson S, Frazier H, Baluch J, et al. Cystic renal masses: Usefulness of the Bosniak classification. Urologic Radiology 1991; 13: 83–90.
35. Wilson T, Doelle E, Cohan R, et al. Cystic renal masses: a recalculation of the usefulness of the Bosniak classification system. Academic Radiology 1996; 3: 564–570.
36. Zuluaga Gomez A, Arrabal Martin M, de la Fuente Serrano A, et al. Laparoscopic treatment of the symptomatic renal cyst. Arch Esp Urol 1995; 48: 284–290.

37. Zanetti G, Trinchieri A, Montanari E, et al. Laparoscopic renal cyst excision. Min Invas Ther Allied Tech 1996; 5: 567–570.
38. Hayakawa M, Hatano T, Tsuji A, et al. Patients with renal cysts associated with renal cell carcinoma and the clinical implications of cyst puncture: A study of 223 cases. Urology 1996; 47: 643–646.
39. Koga S, Nishikido M, Hayashi T, et al. Outcome of surgery in cystic renal cell carcinoma. Urology 2000; 56: 67–70.
40. Bielsa O, Lloreta J, Gelabert-Mas A. Cystic renal cell carcinoma: pathological features, survival and implications for treatment. Br J Urol 1998; 82: 16–20.
41. Onishi T, Oishi Y, Goto H, et al. Cyst-associated renal cell carcinoma: Clinicopathologic characteristics and evaluation of prognosis in 27 cases. Int J Urol 2001; 8: 268–274.
42. Meng M, Grossfeld G, Stoller M. Renal cell carcinoma after laparoscopic cyst decortication. J Urol 2002; 167: 1396.
43. Shalhav AL, Barret E, Lifshitz DA, et al. Transperitoneal laparoscopic renal surgery using blunt 12-mm trocar without fascial closure. J Endourol 2002; 16: 43–46.
44. Fabrizio M. Laparoscopic Evaluation and Treatment of Symptomatic and Indeterminate Renal Cysts. In: Atlas of Laparoscopic Retroperitoneal Surgery. (Bischoff J, Kavoussi L, eds.), WB Saunders, Philadelphia, 2000, pp. 135–150.

# 6 Laparoscopic Partial Nephrectomy

*D. Brooke Johnson,* MD
*and Jeffrey A. Cadeddu,* MD

*CONTENTS*

INTRODUCTION
INDICATIONS
OVERVIEW OF SURGICAL TECHNIQUE
MORBIDITY
ONCOLOGIC RESULTS
CONTROVERSIAL ISSUES
SUMMARY
REFERENCES

## INTRODUCTION

Throughout the 1990s, two surgical advances significantly changed the approach to treating renal masses. One of these was the progression of minimally invasive surgery. Clayman et al. accomplished the first laparoscopic nephrectomy in 1990 *(1)* and since then a number of investigators have reported their experience with laparoscopic nephrectomy using a variety of different approaches *(2–4)*. The other advancement was the acceptance of nephron-sparing surgery (NSS) as a treatment alternative for small renal tumors in patients with a normal contralateral kidney. Partial nephrectomy was initially shown to be effective in the treatment of renal tumors when preservation of renal function was essential *(5,6)*. Excellent local control was attainable for small renal tumors treated with partial nephrectomy. With further investigation, the role of partial nephrectomy in cases with a normal contralateral kidney has become widespread *(7)*.

From: *Laparoscopic Urologic Oncology*
Edited by: J. A. Cadeddu © Humana Press Inc., Totowa, NJ

Laparoscopic partial nephrectomy (LPN) combines these two advances to offer the benefits of decreased morbidity inherent to laparoscopy while preserving renal function afforded by partial nephrectomy. The purpose of this chapter is to evaluate the role of LPN in current renal surgical oncology.

## INDICATIONS

Partial nephrectomy for a malignant renal tumor is indicated in situations where radical nephrectomy would leave the patient anephric. This includes patients with bilateral renal tumors or tumors involving a solitary functioning kidney. Partial nephrectomy should also be considered in a patient with a unilateral renal tumor and a functioning contralateral kidney that is affected by a such conditions as calculous disease, chronic pyelonephritis, renal artery stenosis, and unilateral reflux or systemic diseases such as diabetes, hypertension, and nephrosclerosis *(8)*. Studies have also defined the role of elective partial nephrectomy in patients with unilateral renal tumors and normal contralateral kidneys *(7)*. For patients with localized, single tumors less than 4 cm in diameter, partial nephrectomy provides disease-free outcomes that are comparable to radical nephrectomy *(9,10)*.

The indications for LPN for malignant disease are generally more restricted due to technical limitations of the laparoscopic approach. However, advancements in laparoscopic instrumentation and technique have led to more aggressive application of LPN. Nevertheless, most investigators continue to limit LPN to patients with small (usually <3–4 cm) predominantly exophytic tumors *(11)*. Patient-dependent variables such as tumor location, previous renal surgery, a history of multiple abdominal surgeries, and the need for cold ischemia all must be weighed when considering LPN as a possible treatment option. Patients with large or intrarenal tumors that would require extensive reconstruction are best resected via an open surgical approach. Ultimately, each surgeon should evaluate the feasibility of LPN for a given patient based on tumor characteristics and his or her experience and skill with this and other laparoscopic procedures.

## OVERVIEW OF SURGICAL TECHNIQUE

The authors prefer to employ the transperitoneal approach to LPN. The creation of a pneumoperitoneum generally establishes ample working space and operative visualization. The transperitoneal approach also reveals familiar anatomic landmarks that aid in localization, identification, and resection of the tumor. The retroperitoneal approach has also been described *(11)*, and some tumors, namely those on the posterior surface of the kidney, are particularly suited to this approach.

### *Preoperative Preparation*

The day before the operation, the patient is placed on a clear liquid diet. A mechanical bowel prep of one bottle of magnesium citrate is given the evening before surgery. In the operating room, a 5 French open ureteral catheter may be placed into the renal pelvis and connected to a syringe of dilute indigo carmine solution. This can be used for evaluating collecting system injury after excising the lesion. Foley catheter and nasogastric tubes are also placed prior to patient positioning. Prophylactic intravenous antibiotics are given before making the first incision.

### *Positioning, Access, and Tumor Exposure*

The patient is placed in the modified lateral decubitus position as for laparoscopic nephrectomy *(12)*. Three or four laparoscopic ports are then placed depending on the position of the tumor and the need for a laparoscopic retractor. The mesocolon is reflected along the line of Toldt, leaving Gerota's fascia intact. The kidney is mobilized within Gerota's fascia and the renal hilum dissected. The tumor is localized and dissected, preferably leaving the perinephric fat overlying the tumor.

### *Resection, Hemostasis, and Closure of the Collecting System*

Currently, there is no consensus as to the optimal method for hemostasis and closure of the resection defect. Duplication of open surgery with hand suturing presents a difficult technical challenge *(11)*. As a result, hand-assisted laparoscopy (HAL) has been used in an attempt to bridge the gap and reduce this technical difficulty *(13)*. Similarly, advances in instrumentation and technology including parenchymal compression *(14,15)*, electrosurgical snare resection *(16)*, ultrasonic shears resection *(17)*, hydro-jet dissection *(18)*, microwave hemostasis *(19)*, and radiofrequency coagulation *(20,21)* have each been applied to LPN. Laparoscopic ultrasound, another technological advance, is routinely used in most studies to evaluate the depth and extent of the tumor being treated. The various approaches, along with their advantages and disadvantages, are discussed below.

#### Duplication of Open Surgery

One of the standards by which all laparoscopic procedures are judged is their ability to replicate the open surgical alternative. Gill et al. reported their single institutional experience in 50 patients with a mean tumor size of 3 cm undergoing LPN using a technique that aims to

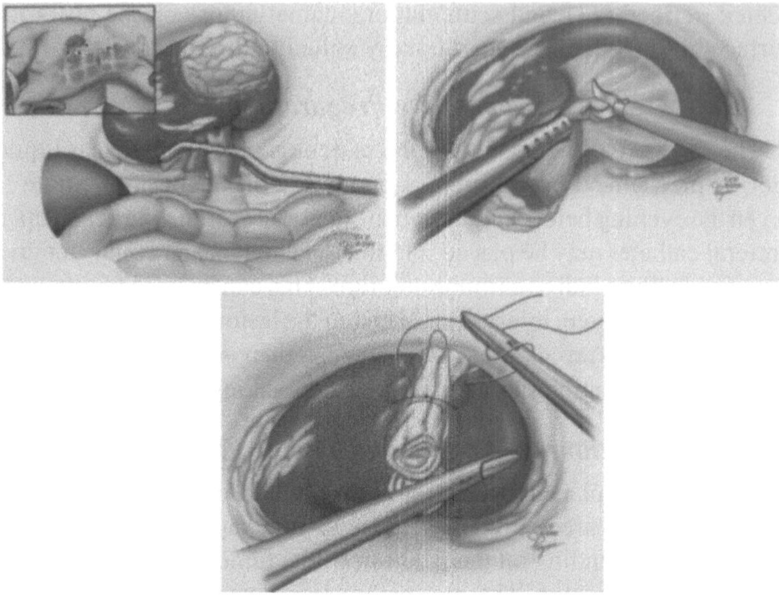

**Fig. 1.** Laparoscopic duplication of the open technique for partial nephrectomy. (Reproduced with permission from ref. *11*.)

duplicate the established principles of open partial nephrectomy *(11)*. They utilized either a transperitoneal or retroperitoneal approach depending on the location of the tumor. In each case, the renal hilum was controlled using a laparoscopic Satinsky or bulldog clamp, and in general, renal hypothermia was not induced. Perinephric fat and Gerota's fascia were left intact over the tumor. Using electrocautery and sharp dissection, care was taken to excise a 0.5-cm margin of healthy tissue with the tumor. Defects in the collecting system were closed with absorbable suture, and major vessels were closed with figure-of-8 sutures. Parenchymal defects were then closed over bolsters using figure-of-8 sutures (Fig. 1). Each of these steps was accomplished using intra-corporeal free-hand suturing. Mean warm ischemia time was 23 min and mean operative time was 3 h. Major and minor complications occurred in three (6%) and three (6%) patients, respectively.

Replicating the open technique offers the advantages of formal closure of parenchymal, vascular and collecting system defects, and the investigators felt this could be accomplished in an efficient and time-sensitive manner *(11)*. They must be commended for their results. However, the technical requirements of the procedure limit its widespread application. In an editorial comment following the article, Wolf stated

"Clamping the renal hilum and then operating 'under the gun' with the intention of completing tumor excision and closure of the collecting system and parenchyma in less than 30 minutes is a daunting task. [T]his challenge probably should be deferred by most urologists . . . [but] should be performed only by urologists with considerable laparoscopic experience" *(22)*.

### Hand-Assisted Laparoscopic Partial Nephrectomy (HALPN)

HAL has been developed in an attempt to improve the safety and speed of laparoscopic procedures without sacrificing the advantages of minimally invasive surgery. Wolf et al. demonstrated the increased efficiency of HAL nephrectomy without sacrificing convalescence as compared to standard laparoscopic nephrectomy *(23)*. This same approach has been applied to LPN.

In a multi-institutional study involving 11 patients (9 with presumed cancerous lesions), Stifelman et al. reported their experience with HALPN *(13)*. Utilizing a transperitoneal approach, the kidney was mobilized to provide posterior access to the renal hilum and the renal artery identified and controlled with a vessel loop as necessary. The intra-abdominal hand was used to compress the kidney just proximal to the resection site during tumor resection using ultrasonic shears and the argon beam coagulator. Surgical hemostasis was achieved using oxidized cellulose gauze pressed manually into the defect, and the renal capsule re-approximated using chromic pledget sutures. Gerota's fascia was then re-approximated over a second oxidized cellulose gauze bolster. Mean operative time was 273.6 min and estimated blood loss (EBL) was 319 mL. There were no major complications and only two (18%) minor complications reported.

HALPN offers the advantages of tactile sensation, proprioception, and improved three-dimensional orientation over purely laparoscopic techniques. An intra-abdominal hand also allows for direct manipulation of the kidney and compression of the parenchymal defect thereby facilitating hemostasis. The intent of this approach is to provide a safer, more widely accessible, and reproducible minimally invasive technique, although there have been no large or prospective studies to evaluate this assertion. However, hand-assistance does not overcome the surgical challenge of laparoscopic intercorporeal suturing. Furthermore, HALPN may be considered a compromise of minimally invasive principles, utilizing an incision large enough to introduce the surgeon's hand. This results in inferior cosmesis and a marginally lengthened convalescence, two characteristics typically considered advantages of the laparoscopic approach.

### Bipolar Electrocautery

A common surgical tool in both open and laparoscopic surgery, bipolar cautery has been used for resection and hemostasis in LPN. Janetschek et al. employed bipolar electrocautery to remove tumors less than 2 cm in size in five of the seven patients in their series *(24)*. The kidney was dissected laparoscopically, Gerota's fascia removed, and the tumor exposed. The renal artery was dissected and controlled in the first patient, but after that they did not feel renal artery dissection was necessary. A dissecting sponge and bipolar coagulation were used for dissection and hemostasis. Following excision, the tumor bed was cauterized with the argon beam coagulator and fibrin glue. The surface was then covered with oxidized cellulose and the fatty tissue of Gerota's fascia pulled over the defect and sutured into place. Operative time ranged from 2.5 to 5 h. Blood loss was between 190 mL and 280 mL for the patients in whom bipolar coagulation was employed.

Hoznek et al. also reported using bipolar coagulation in 5 of 13 patients *(25)*. Using a retroperitoneal approach, Gerota's fascia was incised and the perirenal fat removed to expose the tumor. Bipolar coagulation was used in cases where a large resection of parenchyma was planned. The renal pedicle was also entirely dissected for these cases to allow temporary arrest of renal circulation. An atraumatic vascular clamp was applied when bleeding could not be controlled with bipolar coagulation alone. After resection, the cut surface was covered with oxidized cellulose mesh impregnated with resorcinol formaldehyde glue. Mean operating time was 113 min. Mean blood loss was 72 mL. Warm ischemia time was less than 10 min in all cases. Two urinomas were reported, and in one of these patients, a subsequent open radical nephrectomy was necessary for cancer control.

Bipolar coagulation has the advantage of familiarity to all surgeons and ready availability. This provides simplicity and shortens the learning curve inherent to many laparoscopic techniques. However, hemostasis of larger vessels can be tenuous and requires that the surgeon be prepared with adjunctive hemostatic measures including renal pedicle occlusion.

### Cable Tie

As hemostasis is a major issue in LPN, investigators have focused on possible technical improvements to address it. Several tourniquet-like techniques have been evaluated as a way to control bleeding from the resection site. One such technique employs a cable tie and another uses a knitted double loop for parenchymal compression to create reversible, regional hypoperfusion.

McDougall et al. first described the use of a plastic hemostatic renal cable tie for LPN in a pig model *(26)*. Cadeddu et al. improved this technique in an animal model *(27)* and have since reported its use in treating a patient with a 3-cm upper pole renal tumor *(20)*. The tumor was exposed and a ¼-inch wide by 10-inch long gas sterilized cable tie was engaged in a loose loop (Fig. 2) and positioned around the upper pole below the tumor and above the renal hilum. The cable tie was tightened to render the entire upper pole ischemic and the tumor excised. The defect was coagulated and sealed with fibrin glue and oxidized cellulose. Operative time was 3.5 h. Warm ischemia time was 12 min each with two separate applications of the cable tie. EBL was 100 mL. Recovery was uncomplicated and the patient resumed normal activity 3 wk later. This approach has since been employed with good results in two additional patients.

### Double Loop Tourniquet

Gill et al. described a different type of hemostatic tourniquet consisting of 2 U-loop strips of knitted tape ⅛-inch wide extending from a 17 F plastic sheath *(15)*. This device was designed for use in both open partial nephrectomy and LPN to eliminate the need for renal artery occlusion and minimize ischemic renal damage. The double loop tourniquet was used in one LPN in their published report, as well as in six open partial nephrectomies.

In the laparoscopic approach, the kidney was first mobilized and the double loop tourniquet was positioned around the each pole. The tape around the pole containing the tumor was double looped and tightly cinched leading to circumferential compression and obstruction of blood flow. The other tape was left loosely positioned. The tumor was excised, and hemostasis was achieved using clips, the argon beam coagulator, electrocautery, or suture ligatures. In the series of both open partial nephrectomies and LPN there was no instance when the double loop tourniquet cut into the renal parenchyma, nor were there any occurrences of slippage of the device. Operative time, blood loss, and hospital stay were not reported.

The cable tie and double loop methods offer the advantages of reliable hemostasis, short warm ischemia time, and maintenance of perfusion to the uninvolved portions of the kidney. The minimal bleeding facilitates the ligation of larger vessels, closure of collecting system defects, and cautery of bleeding surfaces and simplifies the application of hemostatic agents. Parencymal compression devices also avoid global renal hypoperfusion that can lead to ischemic acute renal failure in patients undergoing partial nephrectomy *(28)*. However, these devices

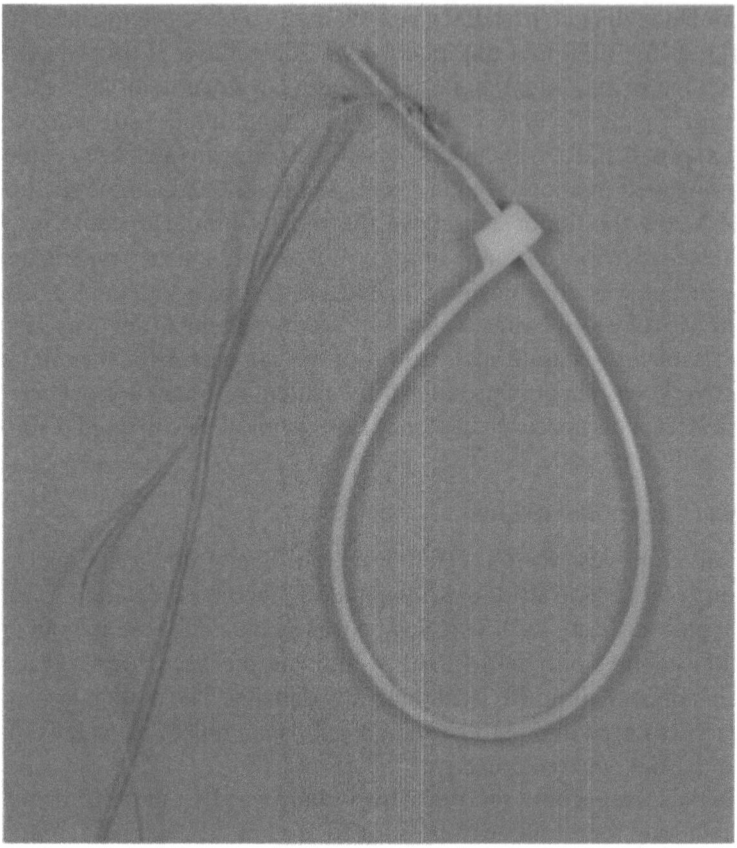

**Fig. 2.** Gas sterilized cable tie used for hemostatsis.

must be positioned between the renal hilum and the lesion, thus limiting their application to polar lesions. Another concern with compressive devices is that they have the possibility of slippage or cutting into the renal parenchyma.

### Ultrasonic Shears

Ultrasonic shears simultaneously divide and coagulate tissue using a titanium blade vibrating at 55,000 Hz. This creates temperatures in the range of 50–100°C, forming a denatured protein coagulum. Harmon et al. reported the use of ultrasonic shears during LPN in 15 patients with small (mean tumor size of 2.3 cm), predominantly solid renal masses *(17)*. Both the transperitoneal and retroperitoneal approaches were used depending on the position of the tumor, patient surgical history, and surgeon preference. No parenchymal compression or renal artery occlusion was employed. The laparoscopic ultrasonic shears were used to completely excise the tumor and the argon beam coagulator was used as necessary during resection to aid in hemostasis. Defects in the collecting system were closed using intracorporeally tied interrupted sutures. The exposed cut surface was again coagulated and oxidized cellulose gauze was welded into place using the argon beam coagulator. Mean operative time was 170 min and mean blood loss was 368 mL. There were no complications in the series. Harmon et al. determined the ultrasonic shears to be the safest method for dividing renal parenchyma without prior vascular control, and the argon beam coagulator the best method of renal surface coagulation after tumor excision.

Janetschek et al. also reported the use of ultrasonic shears in one of seven patients undergoing LPN *(24)*. Blood loss was "exceedingly high" when the ultrasonic shears were used and the investigators felt this tool to be unsatisfactory. They did admit that this was their initial experience with the device and that lack of experience may have contributed to the poor result.

Ultrasonic shears offer the advantage of tumor excision without vascular occlusion, thereby reducing the possibility of ischemic damage. However, the ultrasonic shears clearly do not provide complete hemostasis with large resections, and adjunct methods of coagulation are required.

### Water-Jet Dissection

Water-jet dissection uses a thin, ultra-coherent stream of fluid forced at high velocity through a small nozzle. The water pressure can be adjusted with the goal of cutting through renal parenchyma while preserving vessels and the collecting system. This technology has been applied in hepatic, corneal, and neurological surgery. Shekarriz et al. described the use of this tool in the porcine model for LPN *(18)*. They used the water-jet for parenchymal cutting at a setting of 30 atm and reported a virtually bloodless field with the vessels and collecting system preserved. Although the use of water-jet dissection has been reported in human patients for open partial nephrectomy *(29)*, use in humans for LPN has not been described.

### Microwave Coagulation

Microwave coagulation uses needle-type monopolar electrodes to apply microwave energy to the tissue surrounding the electrode. Microwaves, which comprise the 300 to 3000 MHz range of the electromagnetic spectrum, generate heat at the tip of the electrode, leading to the formation of a conical-shaped wedge of coagulated tissue *(30)*. Microwave cautery can coagulate vessels up to 3 mm in diameter *(31)*, allowing relatively bloodless resection through the area of coagulation.

Yoshimura et al. reported using microwave coagulation for LPN in six patients with small (11–25 mm diameter) exophytic renal tumors *(19)*. Once the kidney was exposed, the perirenal fat was dissected off the renal capsule overlying the tumor. Electrocautery was used to mark a circumferential line of incision 1 cm from the tumor edge in the renal capsule. Microwave coagulation at 2450 MHz was then applied around the circumferential line of incision using needle-type electrodes punctured into the renal parenchyma. Depending on the size of the lesion, 5 to 23 puncture sites were used 5–8 mm apart around the tumor to form a contiguous zone of coagulated tissue. The mass was excised without pedicle occlusion using scissors to cut within the midportion of the coagulated zone. No collecting system leaks were identified. Argon beam coagulation and oxidized cellulose were then applied to achieve complete hemostasis. Mean operative time was 186 min and blood loss was less than 50 mL. Two complications, a postoperative hematoma and transient gross hematuria, were reported. Both of these were managed conservatively.

This study demonstrated excellent hemostasis when using microwave coagulation for LPN. The small area of coagulation produced by each puncture allows for precise control of the area of tissue treated, but the probes must be placed at close intervals allowing for overlap, otherwise bleeding can occur. However, the authors warned of possible collateral thermal damage when using the microwave coagulator and recommended frequent port venting to prevent high intraperitoneal temperatures and pressures. They also expressed concern about the effect of microwave coagulation on the collecting system and the healing of microwave induced collecting system injury. They treated only peripherally located, exophytic tumors 3 cm or less in diameter to avoid injury to the collecting system.

### Radiofrequency Coagulation

Radiofrequency (RF) energy applied by electrodes placed into a grounded patient produces an electric current. Impedance within the tissue leads to the production of heat resulting in temperatures sufficient to cause tissue coagulation.

Originally applied as an ablative treatment for small renal masses, Corwin and Cadeddu reported encouraging results using RF coagulation as a hemostatic technique during LPN for a 1.5 cm partially exophytic mass *(20)*. More recently, Gettman et al. published their experience using

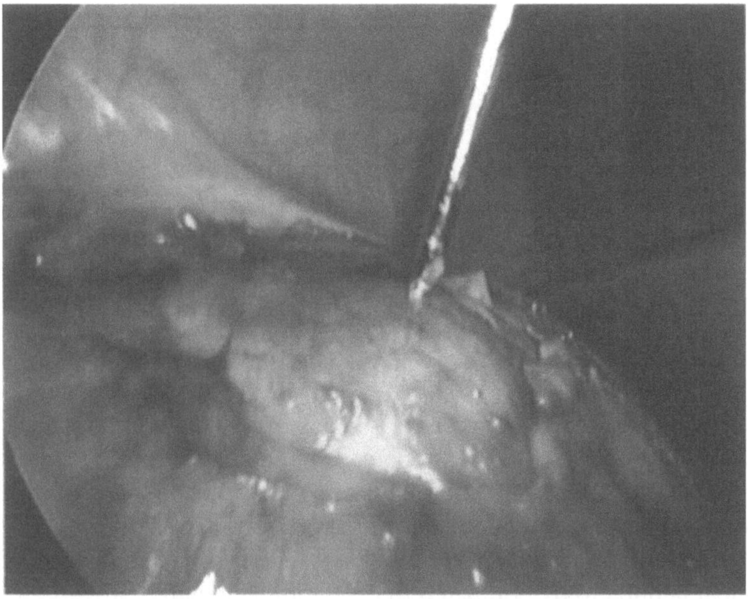

**Fig. 3.** Radiofrequency probe positioned to coagulate tumor.

RF coagulation in 10 patients with exophytic and endophytic tumors 1.0 to 3.2 cm in diameter *(21)*. In this series, the kidney was exposed using both a transperitoneal and retroperitoneal technique. The perirenal fat overlying the tumor was removed and sent for evaluation. An RF probe was positioned into the lesion under laparoscopic visualization to include the lesion and a margin of normal tissue within the spherical treatment zone (Fig. 3). A double RF treatment cycle was applied for coagulation. The probe was then withdrawn and the tumor along with a 0.5- to 1.0-cm margin of normal parenchyma was excised using sharp or ultrasonic dissection. The cut surface was coagulated as necessary using fibrin glue, the argon beam coagulator, or oxidized cellulose. Median operative time was 170 min and median blood loss was 125 mL. No perioperative complications occurred.

One advantage of radiofrequency ablation (RFA) is that although it is an ablative modality it does not alter the histological architecture of the specimen *(32)*. As a result, as opposed to *in situ* ablation, LPN using RF coagulation yields tissue for pathological analysis and determination of resection margins. Although RF-assisted LPN also offers the ability to treat partially endophytic and midpole tumors, it does not provide adequate hemostasis for resecting central tumors or those tumors crossing the corticomedullary junction.

### *Exiting the Abdomen and Closure*

Fibrin glue, oxidized cellulose, electrocautery, and argon beam coagulation can clearly be used as an adjunct to hemostasis based on the preference of the surgeon. Once adequate hemostasis is achieved, the pneumoperitoneum or pneumoretroperitoneum is reduced to 5 mm Hg and any remaining bleeding at the operative site is controlled. Whenever possible, the perinephric fat should be replaced around the kidney, and Gerota's fascia re-approximated. The laparoscopic ports are removed under direct vision and the port sites inspected for hemostasis.

## MORBIDITY

The impetus for developing LPN stems from the potential reduction in morbidity offered by laparoscopic techniques. Laparoscopic surgical approaches can lead to decreased postoperative pain, shorter hospital stays, and shorter convalescence when compared to similar open surgery. Reduced morbidity has clearly been demonstrated for laparoscopic radical nephrectomy compared to open radical nephrectomy *(33,34)*.

LPN is currently in the early stages of technical evolution, and although reduced morbidity is anticipated, it has not yet been definitively demonstrated. The open technique sets the standard by which LPN must be judged with respect to surgical complications and patient recovery. Duque et al. reported complications encountered over a 10-yr experience with open partial nephrectomy, which included 66 partial nephrectomies in 64 patients *(35)*. A peak in creatinine level was the most commonly reported complication (15.1%), followed by urine leak (9.1%) and postoperative hemorrhage (4.5%). Mean hospital stay fell from 8 d during the initial 7 yr of the study, to 4 d during the final 3 yr. Shekarriz et al. also reported complications in a series of 60 open partial nephrectomies over a 7-yr period *(36)*. EBL was 415 mL and 18% of patients required a blood transfusion. Urine leak occurred in 8.3% of patients and one patient suffered a fatal pulmonary embolus. No postoperative hemorrhage was reported. Mean hospital stay was 6 d. Comparatively, in their series of 50 LPNs duplicating the open technique, Gill et al. reported an EBL of 270.4 cc, one intraoperative hemorrhage (2%), and one (2%) postoperative hemorrhage *(11)*. Urine leak was reported in one patient (2%). Mean hospital stay was 2.1 d. These results and those of other LPN series (Table 1) compare favorably with those reported for the open technique.

Convalescence has been reported in only two studies. Janetschek et al. reported "return to normal activity" occurred in 7–21 d *(24)*. Yoshimura et al. reported "full convalescence" ranged from 7 to 25 d,

Table 1
**Operative Results for LPN Series**

| *Author (reference)* | *Total pts* | *Mean size (cm)* | *OR time (min)* | *Mean blood loss (mL)* | *Mean warm ischemia time (min)* | *Mean hosp stay (d)* |
|---|---|---|---|---|---|---|
| Gill et al. *(11)* | 50 | 3 | 180 | 270 | 23 | 2.2 |
| Stifelman et al. *(15)* | 11 | <4 | 274 | 319 | None (local compression) | 3.3 |
| Janetschek et al. *(16)* | 7 | <2.0 | 150–300 | 190–280 | None | 3.6 |
| Hoznek et al. *(17)* | 13 | | 113 | 72 | <10 | 6.1 |
| Cadeddu and Corwin *(20)* | 1 | 3 | 210 | <100 | 12 × 2 (local, distal to tie) | |
| Gill et al. *(21)* | 1 | | | | Local, distal to loop | |
| Harmon et al. *(23)* | 15 | 2.3 | 170 | 368 | None | 2.6 |
| Yoshimura et al. *(28)* | 6 | <2.5 | 186 | <50 | None | Criteria met in 2 d |
| Gettman et al. *(30)* | 10 | 2.1 | 170 | 125 | None | |
| Corwin and Cadeddu *(29)* | 1 | 1.5 | | None | None | 1 |
| Rassweiler et al. *(36)* | 53 | 2.4 | 191 | 725 | | 5.4 |

Reference *36* contains data from refs. *16* and *17*.

OR = operating room.

with a median of 9 d *(19)*. Together, these data suggest that LPN reduces morbidity when compared to open partial nephrectomy. However, a randomized, prospective study is needed to clearly establish improved morbidity in a contemporary series.

## ONCOLOGIC RESULTS

The long term-efficacy for LPN remains to be defined. Results for open partial nephrectomy have demonstrated long-term local control and cure of small renal tumors. With a median followup of 10 yr (range 1–19), Herr reported 98.5% of patients had no local recurrence and 97% were free of metastasis *(7)*. Similarly, Lee et al. showed no significant difference in disease-specific, disease-free, and overall survival between partial nephrectomy and radical nephrectomy for small (<4 cm) renal tumors *(10)*. These results set the standard by which all of the laparoscopic techniques must be judged.

To date, only short-term oncologic results are available, but these have been encouraging (Table 2). Gill et al. reported a negative surgical margin in all 34 of the patients with renal cell carcinoma in their series. During mean followup of 7.2 mo, no recurrence or metastatic disease was seen *(11)*. With short-term followup of 8 mo, Stifelman et al. also reported no recurrences in 9 cancer patients *(13)*. Harmon et al. also reported no recurrences in 12 patients with a mean followup period of 8 mo *(17)*. Most importantly, Rassweiler et al. reviewed the results from five European centers performing LPN, and reported no recurrences with a median followup of 24 mo, and an actuarial disease-free survival of 100% *(37)*. Although the average followup is short, none of the reports evaluating LPN has demonstrated tumor recurrence or metastasis. These early results are promising, but longer followup is necessary.

## CONTROVERSIAL ISSUES

Although the experience to date demonstrates LPN as feasible, the utility of LPN in the general treatment of patients is unclear. In reviewing NSS for renal tumors, Uzzo and Novick expressed concern regarding LPN as a reproducible cancer operation *(38)*. They cited the difficulty in reproducing the essential elements of open partial nephrectomy, namely early and complete vascular control, surface hypothermia, complete tumor excision, meticulous hemostasis, and precise reconstruction of the urinary collecting system and renal remnant. They also considered the prolonged operative time disadvantageous and the complication rate unacceptable. They concluded that it is too early to consider LPN to be a reproducible cancer operation, and it should be

**Table 2**
**Oncologic Results for LPN Series with Stated Followup**

| *Author (reference)* | *Total patients* | *Patients with cancer* | *Mean followup* | *Recurrence* |
|---|---|---|---|---|
| Gill et al. *(11)* | 50 | 34 | 7.2 mo | None |
| Stifelman et al. *(15)* | 11 | 4 | 8 mo | None |
| Janetschek et al. *(16)* | 7 | 5 | 7–35 mo | None |
| Hoznek et al. *(17)* | 13 | 3 | 22 mo | None |
| Harmon et al. *(23)* | 15 | 12 | 8 mo | None |
| Yoshimura et al. *(28)* | 6 | 5 | 3–4 mo | None |
| Rassweiler et al. *(36)* | 53 | 37 | 24 mo | None |

Reference *36* contains data from refs. *16* and *17*.

performed only at specialized tertiary care institutions. We currently agree that LPN should be limited to tertiary care centers as an evolving oncologic treatment option.

The technical challenges of LPN also limit its widespread application. Although laparoscopic urology is currently practiced at many academic centers and is making its way into the common urologic surgical armamentarium, laparoscopy remains a technique that requires a unique skill set and procedure-specific training. LPN is a particularly complex and technically challenging procedure. This challenge currently precludes the procedure from widespread application. Improvements in instrumentation and technology may facilitate the transition of LPN from an experimental treatment available only at specialized academic centers to a commonly practiced NSS approach to renal tumors.

Other minimally invasive NSS approaches are also currently under development. Clinical series employing renal cryotherapy *(39–41)* and RFA *(42,43)* using minimally invasive techniques are in progress. With little or no tissue resection, these alternative procedures are being developed in an effort to minimize the morbidity inherent in resection of renal parenchyma. However, these procedures carry the primary disadvantage of leaving the ablated tumor in situ with no direct evaluation of ablation margins. However, should long-term data show acceptable efficacy with reduced morbidity in treating renal malignancies, these approaches may render LPN obsolete.

## SUMMARY

LPN is an evolving procedure for treating small renal tumors with NSS. Currently, no consensus exists as to the best approach to the procedure. Hemostasis and closure of the collecting system remain the primary challenges to safety and feasibility of LPN. The procedure must maintain oncologic adequacy and offer distinct advantages, namely reduced morbidity, over conventional therapy in order to be accepted as an alternative treatment. These advantages are anticipated, but have yet to be clearly demonstrated. Only longer followup and increased application will demonstrate the efficacy and utility of LPN in modern urologic surgery.

## REFERENCES

1. Clayman RV, Kavoussi LR, Soper NJ, et al. Laparoscopic nephrectomy: initial case report. J Urol 1991; 146: 278–282.
2. Dunn MD, McDougall EM, Clayman RV. Laparoscopic radical nephrectomy. J Endourol 2000; 14: 849–855; discussion 855–857.
3. Hsu TH, Sung GT, Gill IS. Retroperitoneoscopic approach to nephrectomy. J Endourol 1999; 13: 713–718; discussion 718–720.

4. Fadden PT, Nakada SY. Hand-assisted laparoscopic renal surgery. Urol Clin North Am 2001; 28: 167–176, xi.
5. Licht MR, Novick AC. Nephron sparing surgery for renal cell carcinoma. J Urol 1993; 149: 1–7.
6. Morgan WR, Zincke H. Progression and survival after renal-conserving surgery for renal cell carcinoma: experience in 104 patients and extended followup. J Urol 1990; 144: 852–857; discussion 857–858.
7. Herr HW. Partial nephrectomy for unilateral renal carcinoma and a normal contralateral kidney: 10-year followup. J Urol 1999; 161: 33–34; discussion 34–35.
8. Novick AC, Streem SB. Surgery of the Kidney. In *Campbell's Urology, 7th ed.* (Walsh PC, Retik AB, Vaughan ED, Wein AJ, eds.), W. B. Saunders, Philadelphia, 1998, pp. 2973–3061.
9. Butler BP, Novick AC, Miller DP, et al. Management of small unilateral renal cell carcinomas: radical versus nephron-sparing surgery. Urology 1995; 45: 34–40; discussion 40–41.
10. Lee CT, Katz J, Shi W, et al. Surgical management of renal tumors 4 cm. or less in a contemporary cohort. J Urol 2000; 163: 730–736.
11. Gill IS, Desai MM, Kaouk JH, et al. Laparoscopic partial nephrectomy for renal tumor: duplicating open surgical techniques. J Urol 2002; 167: 469–467; discussion 475–476.
12. Cadeddu JA. Laparoscopic Partial Nephrectomy. In *Atlas of Laparoscopic Retroperitoneal Surgery.* (Bishoff JT, Kavoussi LR, eds.), W. B. Saunders, Philadelphia, 2000, pp. 83–104.
13. Stifelman MD, Sosa RE, Nakada SY, et al. Hand-assisted laparoscopic partial nephrectomy. J Endourol 2001; 15: 161–164.
14. Cadeddu JA, Corwin TS. Cable tie compression to facilitate laparoscopic partial nephrectomy. J Urol 2001; 165: 177–178.
15. Gill IS, Munch LC, Clayman RV, et al. A new renal tourniquet for open and laparoscopic partial nephrectomy. J Urol 1995; 154: 1113–1116.
16. Collyer W, Landman J, Olweny E, et al. Use of a novel electrosurgical snare to perform laparoscopic partial nephrectomy in a porcine model. J Urol 2001; 165(5S): 20.
17. Harmon WJ, Kavoussi LR, Bishoff JT. Laparoscopic nephron-sparing surgery for solid renal masses using the ultrasonic shears. Urology 2000; 56: 754–759.
18. Shekarriz H, Shekarriz B, Upadhyay J, et al. Hydro-jet assisted laparoscopic partial nephrectomy: initial experience in a porcine model. J Urol 2000; 163: 1005–1008.
19. Yoshimura K, Okubo K, Ichioka K, et al. Laparoscopic partial nephrectomy with a microwave tissue coagulator for small renal tumor. J Urol 2001; 165: 1893–1896.
20. Corwin TS, Cadeddu JA. Radio frequency coagulation to facilitate laparoscopic partial nephrectomy. J Urol 2001; 165: 175–176.
21. Gettman MT, Bishoff JT, Su LM, et al. Hemostatic laparoscopic partial nephrectomy: initial experience with the radiofrequency coagulation-assisted technique. Urology 2001; 58: 8–11.
22. Wolf JS, Jr. Re: Editorial comment on open donor, laparoscopic donor and hand assisted laparoscopic donor nephrectomy: a comparison of outcomes. J Urol 2002; 168: 199–.
23. Wolf JS, Jr, Moon TD, Nakada SY. Hand assisted laparoscopic nephrectomy: comparison to standard laparoscopic nephrectomy. J Urol 1998; 160: 22–27.

24. Janetschek G, Daffner P, Peschel R, et al. Laparoscopic nephron sparing surgery for small renal cell carcinoma. J Urol 1998; 159: 1152–1155.
25. Hoznek A, Salomon L, Antiphon P, et al. Partial nephrectomy with retroperitoneal laparoscopy. J Urol 1999; 162: 1922–1926.
26. McDougall EM, Clayman RV, Chandhoke PS, et al. Laparoscopic partial nephrectomy in the pig model. J Urol 1993; 149: 1633–1636.
27. Cadeddu JA, Corwin TS, Traxer O, et al. Hemostatic laparoscopic partial nephrectomy: cable-tie compression. Urology 2001; 57: 562–566.
28. Campbell SC, Novick AC, Streem SB, et al. Complications of nephron sparing surgery for renal tumors. J Urol 1994; 151: 1177–1180.
29. Basting RF, Djakovic N, Widmann P. Use of water jet resection in organ-sparing kidney surgery. J Endourol 2000; 14: 501–505.
30. Nakada SY, Johnson DB. Advances in needle invasive and noninvasive tissue ablation. AUA Update Series 2001; 20.
31. Muraki J, Cord J, Addonizio JC, et al. Application of microwave tissue coagulation in partial nephrectomy. Urology 1991; 37: 282–287.
32. Zlotta AR, Wildschutz T, Raviv G, et al. Radiofrequency interstitial tumor ablation (RITA) is a possible new modality for treatment of renal cancer: ex vivo and in vivo experience. J Endourol 1997; 11: 251–258.
33. McDougall E, Clayman RV, Elashry OM. Laparoscopic radical nephrectomy for renal tumor: the Washington University experience. J Urol 1996; 155: 1180–1185.
34. Ono Y, Katoh N, Kinukawa T, et al. Laparoscopic radical nephrectomy: the Nagoya experience. J Urol 1997; 158: 719–723.
35. Duque JL, Loughlin KR, O'Leary MP, et al. Partial nephrectomy: alternative treatment for selected patients with renal cell carcinoma. Urology 1998; 52: 584–590.
36. Shekarriz B, Upadhyay J, Shekarriz H, et al. Comparison of costs and complications of radical and partial nephrectomy for treatment of localized renal cell carcinoma. Urology 2002; 59: 211–215.
37. Rassweiler JJ, Abbou C, Janetschek G, et al. Laparoscopic partial nephrectomy. The European experience. Urol Clin North Am 2000; 27: 721–736.
38. Uzzo RG, Novick AC. Nephron sparing surgery for renal tumors: indications, techniques and outcomes. J Urol 2001; 166: 6–18.
39. Gill IS, Novick AC, Soble JJ, et al. Laparoscopic renal cryoablation: initial clinical series. Urology 1998; 52: 543–551.
40. Sung GT, Meraney AM, Schweizer DK, et al. Laparoscopic Renal Cryoablation in 50 Patients: Intermediate Follow-up. J Urol 2001; 165(S): 158.
41. Shingleton WS, Sewell PE: Percutaneous Renal Cryoablation for Renal Tumors: One-Yar Follow-Up. J Urol 2001; 165(S): 186.
42. McGovern FJ, McDougal WS, Gervais D et al: Percutaneous Radiofrequency Ablation of Human Renal Cell Carcinoma. J Urol 2001; 165(S): 157.
43. Pavlovich CP, Walther MM, Choyke PL et al: Percutaneous radio frequency ablation of small renal tumors: initial results. J Urol 2002; 167: 10–15.

# 7 Laparoscopic and Minimally Invasive Renal Tumor Ablation

## *Cryotherapy and Radiofrequency Techniques*

*Steven M. Baughman,* MD
*and Jay T. Bishoff,* MD, FACS

*CONTENTS*

INTRODUCTION
INDICATIONS AND CONTRAINDICATIONS
MECHANISM OF ACTION: CRYOABLATION AND RFA
OVERVIEW OF TECHNIQUE
ADJUVANT TECHNIQUES
RESULTS
MORBIDITY/COMPLICATIONS
RADIOGRAPHIC CHANGES
HISTOLOGIC CHANGES
CONCLUSION
REFERENCES

## INTRODUCTION

Early radiographic identification of small renal masses has led to a lower stage at the time of initial diagnosis *(1)*. This stage migration, coupled with the advancement of nephron-sparing surgical techniques, has focused attention toward the development of minimally invasive technologies for the treatment of small renal tumors. Open nephron-sparing surgery (NSS) has proven efficacy among patients with tumors less than 4 cm in diameter, despite normal contralateral kidneys *(2,3)*. Additionally, with the low (3.7%) chance of multicentricity of small

From: *Laparoscopic Urologic Oncology*
Edited by: J. A. Cadeddu © Humana Press Inc., Totowa, NJ

renal cell cancers and evidence of increasing rates of renal insufficiency with radical nephrectomy, the argument in favor of NSS is strengthened *(4,5)*. The progressive development of minimally invasive techniques for urologic malignancies has revealed two systems with unique mechanisms and utility—cryotherapy and radiofrequency ablation (RFA). Cryotherapy and RFA produce their respective tissue destruction via cellular freezing or molecular agitation leading to heat production with overall molecular and cellular destruction. Although cellular destruction from freezing has been used for dermatologic lesions for more than 150 years *(6)*, the advent of the cryosurgical apparatus in the 1960s and modern day probe delivery systems have made possible the use of cryosurgical precision for some liver, breast, lung, cervical, and prostatic malignancies *(7–10)*. From the first renal percutaneous cryosurgery by Uchida *(11)* and the well-established uses of RFA in aberrant cardiac pathways, hepatic, and other lesions, energy-based therapy has an accepted utility today. In this chapter, we present the current mechanisms of cryotherapy and RFA, their indications and contraindications, the adjuvant techniques, and results of these new technologies.

## INDICATIONS AND CONTRAINDICATIONS

Although the fundamental mechanism of cryotherapy and RFA are literally opposite, they share similar indications and contraindications (Table 1). Paramount to the use of these alternative surgical therapies is attention to appropriate patient selection. Optimal renal lesions for either cryotherapy or RFA are peripherally based, enhancing, well-circumscribed, distant from the collecting system or other perirenal structures (i.e., bowel, vasculature), and less than or equal to 4 cm in size *(8,12–19)*. Unique populations of patients with a predisposition to renal tumors, such as von Hippel-Lindau disease, tuberous sclerosis, and hereditary papillary renal cell carcinoma (RCC), may be optimal candidates for these less invasive ablative techniques *(6,15,18–20)*. As an alternative to open procedures or observation, patient proclivity for minimally invasive techniques in an effort to obviate, or delay symptoms, has also been recognized *(9,18,19)*. Although animal models have shown that cryotherapy near, and into, the collecting system does not herald a negative outcome, this is one of the few relative contraindications to both forms of treatment *(21,22)*. Incidental "stray" energy from either a cryoprobe, or RFA probe can result in significant injury to pararenal structures, but the protected posterior and lateral renal fat layer may decrease these complications. Relative contraindications reported in the current literature also include uncorrected bleeding diatheses, lesions

Table 1
**Indications and Contraindications to Cryotherapy and RFA**

| *Indications* | *Contraindications* |
|---|---|
| *Lesion Characteristics* | ■ Bleeding diatheses |
| ■ Peripherally based, away from the collecting system and hilar vasculature | ■ Centrally located renal lesions (contiguous with bowel, great vessels, renal sinus, or being near [or into] the collecting system) |
| ■ Well-circumscribed lesion | ■ Lesion size of 5 cm or greater |
| ■ Enhancement on computed tomography, | |
| ■ Less than 4 cm; Robson Stage I, AJCC (1997) Stage T1 | |
| *Patient Characteristics* | |
| ■ Solitary renal unit | |
| ■ Bilateral tumors | |
| ■ Significant renal insufficiency, including compromised contralateral renal function and comorbid disease that could develop into renal insufficiency | |
| ■ Native kidney lesion in a dialysis patient | |
| ■ Previous renal surgery | |
| ■ Obesity | |
| ■ Elderly | |
| ■ Marked comorbid disease | |
| ■ Patient's request | |

AJCC = American Joint Commission on Cancer

contiguous with bowel, great vessels, or renal sinus, and tumor size of at least 5 cm (although larger tumors may be treated with the use of multiply placed cryo- or RFA probes) *(13,15,17–19)*.

## MECHANISM OF ACTION: CRYOABLATION AND RFA

Cryotherapeutic mechanisms of tissue destruction are seen when cryoprobe (typically liquid argon or nitrogen [$LN_2$]-based) deployment causes extraction of the latent heat of boiling from its immediate environment, with 209 Joules of heat energy extracted from each one gram of LN2 that is converted to gas at the probe tips *(13)*. Within 2 to 3 min, the cryoprobe can reach a temperature of –195°C, well below the reported temperature necessary for tissue destruction of –20 to –50°C *(11,13,23,24)*. The effect of this rapid freezing is cellular dehydration, intra- and extracellular ice crystallization, cytosolic organelle destruction, uncoupling of oxidative phosphorylation, protein denaturation, rupturing of cytoplasmic membranes, and endothelial destruction with microvascular thrombosis resulting in local tissue ischemia *(13,23–25)*. Furthermore, cryo-immunologic activity has been proposed as a possible mediator toward inhibition of tumor (re)growth after cryodestruction of tissue through the exposure of possible tumor antigenic moieties to the immune system and subsequent tumor-antibody formation *(11,24,26)*.

Monopolar low-frequency RF energy, generated from alternating current generators, can produce up to 200 watts (current of 1500–1800 mA) of heat energy and raise tissue temperatures to 50–100°C *(15,17,27)*. The sustained temperatures produced by the RF energy result in cellular damage through the induction of ionic agitation and molecular frictional heat causing denaturation of proteins, melting of lipid membranes, and resultant coagulative necrosis *(17,19,25)*.

## OVERVIEW OF TECHNIQUE

The minimally invasive surgeon can readily gain the basic understanding regarding the operation of both cryotherapy and RFA. Open, laparoscopic, and percutaneous deployment of these energies have been successfully reported *(14,16,23,27,28)*. Despite a high degree of variability with regard to the techniques used, a number of underlying tenants must be kept in mind when learning and using cryotherapy and RFA (Table 2). Appropriate patient selection includes complete radiographic and metastatic evaluation. The location of the lesion is of great importance due to the need to avoid surrounding structures, primarily the bowel, collecting system, and vasculature. Posterolateral lesion can easily be approached via a posterior percutaneous or retroperitoneoscopic approach,

**Table 2**
**Critical Steps Toward Successful Cryotherapy and RFA and Their Adjunctive Diagnostics/Techniques**

| *Cryotherapy* | *Radiofrequency ablation* |
|---|---|
| ■ Open or laparoscopic approach recommended | ■ Percutaneous, laparoscopic, retroperitoneoscopic, or open approach acceptable |
| ■ Adequate anesthesia | ■ Adequate anesthesia |
| ■ Mobilization of kidney within Gerota's fascia | ■ Preoperative CT with confirmation of RFA needle placement or intraoperative ultrasound confirmation of the same |
| ■ Excision of overlying perirenal fat | ■ RF deployment with temperature and impedance monitoring |
| ■ Placement and evaluation with *in situ* ultrasonograpy | ■ Postoperative CT imaging |
| ■ Visual and ultrasound-guided needle biopsy | ■ Use of RFA probe for hemostasis assurance |
| ■ Puncture placement/placement of cryoprobe and thermosensors | |
| ■ Assuring avoidance of contiguous structures | |
| ■ Real-time observation of cryolesion development | |
| ■ Hemostasis confirmation | |
| *Adjuvant techniques* | |
| ■ Radiographic: CT, MRI, intraoperative ultrasound | |
| ■ Thermocouple monitoring | |
| ■ Impedance monitoring | |
| ■ Bipolar RF for larger lesions, or two eccentrically placed probes for the same | |
| ■ Infrared imaging with RFA | |

CT = computed tomography; RFA = radiofrequency ablation; MRI = magnetic resonance imaging; RF = radiofrequency.

whereas anterolateral-based lesions may be approached via a tranperitoneal technique *(6,14,23)*. In fact, little to no perihilar dissection is necessary in the majority of these lesions using either approach *(3,21)*.

Both cryotherapy and RFA can be delivered with technical simplicity. Accepted techniques of adequate tissue destruction with cryotherapy include two to three, 2- to 5-min rapid freeze–slow thaw–rapid freeze cycles *(3,21,23,25)* with RFA having a similar ablate–quiescence–ablate cycle *(29)*. Although the freeze–thaw–freeze method is the most frequently reported technique, single freeze techniques (for up to 15 min) have shown equal efficacy *(6,23)*.

Cryotherapy lends itself to use through an open or laparoscopic approach so as to ensure no collateral complications. Steps to cryotherapeutic success include (1) appropriate anatomic approach, (2) mobilization of kidney within Gerota's fascia, (3) excision of overlying perirenal fat, (4) use of *in situ* ultrasonograpy, (5) visual and ultrasound (US)-guided needle biopsy, (6) puncture placement of cryoprobe under ultrasonographic and visual guidance, (7) real-time observation of cryoprobe deployment with US and thermocouple monitoring, and (8) hemostasis *(3,14,23,24,30)*.

Cryotherapy in the kidney is both anatomically and technically easily delivered when compared to other urologic uses such prostate *(14)*. Each basic step of renal cryosurgery has specific highlights. Prior to actual cryoablation, ideal renal mobilization for direct and US visualization of the lesion is needed, as is evaluating the lesion size, exposing the possibility of satellite lesions, and the proximity to vessels and collecting system *(3)*. Minimal hilar dissection is necessary, and typically there is no practical advantage to occluding hilar vessels *(13)*. Needle and wire placement for the cryoprobe can be performed either intraoperatively under US guidance, or as a preoperative percutaneous procedure under similar visualization *(30)*. Once the cryoablation cycle starts, the target tissue temperature must be well below the accepted temperature (–20 to –40°C) needed for cellular destruction *(11,13,23)*. Gill et al. noted various temperature gradients seen at the advancing edge of an ablative therapy via the use of thermosensors placed within and at a lesion's edge *(3)*. A temperature of 0°C at the advancing edge was observed, with the inner 4–6 mm of the cryolesion being the needed –20 to –40°C. It is now generally accepted that an advancing edge of a cryolesion needs to be visualized ultrasonographically and extend at least 1 cm beyond the edge of the tumor *(3,14)*.

There appears to be a lack of consensus regarding the timing of the slow-thaw phase of cryoablation, but the current thought is to await the disappearance of the cryolesion on ultrasound, then refreeze for another

2–3 min *(3,23)*. During the second freeze cycle, the advancing ice ball may not be seen via US until its advancing edge is seen outside what was the first cryolesion's perimeter *(3)*. This stresses the significance of direct visualization as one may see significant subcapsular hemorrhage as a purplish-blue lesion with cryolesion advancement *(3,20)* either during the primary freeze, or during the second freeze that can lead to perirenal tissue damage.

Two final considerations with cryotherapy include the removal of the cryoprobe and resolution of any possible hemorrhage. Patience on the part of the surgeon is required to allow the probe to disengage itself from surrounding renal tissue during thawing. Forcing an attached or adherent frozen probe from its ablation site can fracture the kidney. The final thaw of the cryolesion will allow the tissue to release the cryoprobe, and due to pressure of gas used during laparoscopy there may not be any significant bleeding *(3,8)*. While the probe insertion site is still frozen, hemostatic agents such as Surgicell ™ or Gel Foam ™ can be packed into the resulting hole to assist with hemostasis once the region returns to body temperature *(3,8)*.

RF ablative therapies have been successfully deployed using open, laparoscopic, and percutaneous approaches *(16,19,27,28)*. Electrodes of varying configuration are used to produce an ablated area of tissue, with a deployable umbrella configuration being the most commonly used method secondary to its ability to produce a spherical lesion with little intralesional movement. Current RFA technology has proven the ability to successfully ablate a renal volume of up to 5 cm with a single probe with even greater ablative volumes with the use of concomitant, concentrically placed multi-electrode arrays *(4,7,15,19)*. Monopolar probes are used typically for the smaller, superficial lesions, whereas the bipolar technology can be used for larger lesions with a larger ovoid, or pillow-shaped ablation zones between the two electrodes *(27)*. Caution should be used as tumors are ablated in close proximity to the renal collecting system or adjacent structures *(16)*.

Once the probe is correctly placed, the electrosurgical generator will assist with recording the total energies delivered, the impedance generated, target probe temperatures, and the total times of the procedure *(19,29)*. Because tissue destruction occurs when temperatures exceed 50°C, using probes that reach and maintain temperatures of approx 70°C are recommended. Reports in the literature use ablation–quiescence–ablation cycles up to 10–12 min (ablation); 5–10 min (quiescence); 10–12 min (ablation), with deep medullary tumors undergoing a third ablation *(19)*. Crowley et al. showed that equivalent tissue desiccation was seen with a more limited 3 min–5 min–3 min cycle using

2-cm probes *(29)*. After ablation, few hemorrhagic problems arise secondary to the local tissue and vascular destruction resulting in acute thrombosis. Gettman et al. showed that local intrarenal hemostasis was assured during a post-RFA partial nephrectomy (with a 0.5–1 cm diameter margin) with the assumption being that the RFA adequately coagulated the local tissue, resulting in local hemostasis *(31)*. However, this does not assure probe tract hemostasis and as a result some investigators use decreased wattage (15 W) with the RFA probe during its withdrawal to fulgerate the probe tract *(16,19)*.

## ADJUVANT TECHNIQUES

Adjuvant technologies assist with access to renal lesions, assure safe and adequate tissue desiccation, and maintain hemostasis (Table 2). Cryotherapy and RFA have immediate physical limitations with regard to the volume of local tissue destruction based on the type and size of probe deployed and the ability of imagining techniques to accurately monitor the size of the lesion created *(29)*. Intraoperative US lesion measurements have shown a 13% smaller size compared to computed tomography (CT) images of the same lesion *(14)*. Therefore, adequate tissue destruction must be regulated in other ways including the use of temperature sensors, real-time intraoperative imaging (seen primarily with cryoablation) or and impedance monitors *(15,25)*.

Percutaneous access has been reported using both CT and magnetic resonance imaging (MRI) guidance *(9,32)*. Although CT or MRI are the primary modalities for preoperative radiographic evaluation, intraoperative US is the principal modality for adequate immediate pre-, intra- and immediate postoperative monitoring for both open and laparoscopic cryotherapy *(13,14,20,23,30)*. Ultrasonography allows for real-time observation of the biopsy needle, probe placement, margin of frozen tissue, relationship to surrounding structures, monitoring of the actual ablation, and possible identification of lesions that were not seen with other preoperative images *(13,14,20,23,33)*. Steerable, laparoscopic, color-flow Doppler US, within an end-fire probe, allows one to see the actual margins of the cryolesion as identified by a hyperechoic advancing crescentic lesion with posterior acoustic shadowing and loss of intralesion color-flow, characteristic for vascular and cellular destruction *(13,14,20,23,34)*.

Compared to cyrotherapy, the use of real-time US for RFA is less helpful. Tissue destruction during an RFA cycle can been seen on US as an intense echogenicity spreading from the electrode tip, with little margin identification, leaving an unclear heterogenous echotecture, thought to be microbubbles produced from the ablation *(15,27,28,34)*. The use of US may be of some utility in the evaluation of the postoperative color-flow Doppler characteristics. With local tissue destruction and disruption of the vascular supply, there is loss of blood flow within a radiolesion. Although the use of intraoperative US holds little promise from monitoring RFA lesions, the use of laparoscopic infrared imaging system, correlating with surface temperatures and thermocouple measurements, provides a possible real-time assessment of adequate tumor desiccation *(35)*.

Thermocouple technology has been used in both cryotherapy and RFA in an attempt to predict adequate tumor destruction. Temperatures associated with tissue cell death can be measured with thermocouples immediately within, at the margin, and just outside the margin of a lesion *(8,9,24,25)*. The kidney's blood supply protects the parenchyma from cooling and heating. Observations during RFA show that temperatures recorded at the edge of the ablation zone can be 20–30°C cooler than temperatures recorded at the RFA probe, making sufficient tissue desiccation uncertain with RFA. For this reason, some authors favor an impedance-based system. The higher the electrical impedance the more the tissue acts as a thermal insulator, blocking the flow of RF energy and subsequent tissue destruction. Therefore, the intra- and perilesional placement of RF impedance monitors will assist in assuring adequate marginal destruction. Impedance (to approx 200 Ω) suggests that the tissue is desiccated and that continued lesion growth is unlikely *(27,36)*. "Dry" renal tissue shows a higher impedance vs tissue that is exposed to hypertonic saline at the RFA probe tip and the use of this local saline has proven to be of assistance in increasing the size of lesion created *(25)*. Furthermore, there is a known phenomenon of micro-bubble formation at the site of a radiolesion, which has also been shown to increase local tissue impedance, which only 30 to 60 s of RF quiescence seems to alleviate. This is the basis of the RF free time between ablative maneuvers. Rendon et al. showed in a porcine model that there may be a "thermal blanketing" phenomenon produced by injected saline (hydrodissection) or $CO_2$ (gas dissection) within the perirenal space, resulting in higher temperatures, and possible greater ease of destruction within various peripheral lesions *(37)*.

## RESULTS

Uchida and Zlotta were the pioneers for the clinical application of cryoablation and RFA, respectively *(11,27)*. Both investigators attempted to define the safety, technical , and early followup characteristics of their respective energy system. Uchida's work aided in the understanding of the needed –20°C needed for in vivo tissue desiccation with cryoablation, but their patient selection (two patients with advanced RCC) was of little benefit in determining long-term clinical outcomes *(11)*. Similarly, Zlotta showed that extensive tumor and parenchymal necrosis results from the in vivo RFA experience, under both open and percutaneous applications, with the later performed under local anesthesia *(27)*.

There is a lack of published prospective trials comparing cryoablation or RFA to stage-matched open or laparoscopic renal tumor extirpation. Outcomes studies of these technologies are limited to only prospective trials using radiographic followup and limited histologic evaluation. Although outcome data are limited, the information currently available is optimistic. Operatively, both techniques have proven compatibility with laparoscopic equipment, minimal risk of operative, or delayed blood loss *(12,19,32,37)*. Percutaneous delivery is possible under intravenous sedation and local anesthesia, with patients having less than 24 h of hospital stay *(15,19,27,37)*. No studies report any conversion to an open procedure with either cryoablation or RFA.

Although long-term cancer-free and overall survival data is lacking with both cryoablation and RFA, the current short-term data are encouraging (Table 3–5) *(38–41)*. Gill et al. have the largest series of cryoablation with 32 patients and 23 followup CT-guided biopsies at 3–6 mo, with no radiographic local or port-site recurrence in a mean followup time of 16.2 mo *(14)*. Levin et al. reported the results of their experience in 39 patients, showing 1 patient who underwent renal biopsy 9 mo after treatment when a suspicious nodule was discovered on protocol MRI. The biopsy revealed RCC; the patient underwent laparoscopic radical nephrectomy (LRN) for a 1.3-cm clear cell RCC *(42)*. In our own experience in eight patients with small (mean 2 cm diameter) renal tumors, one patient, at his 9-mo CT followup, was found to have an enhancing lesion in the area of cryoablation and underwent a successful LRN.

Studies using RFA have shown similar results. Walther et al. explored 14 tumors of less than 5cm in diameter in four patients with multiple renal lesions and performed RF immediately prior to surgical excision. Complete, immediate treatment effect was noted in 10 of 11 patients; in the final case, only 35% of the tumor was ablated *(43)*. Rendon et al. recently showed an underestimation of the RFA ablative volume with

Table 3
Outcomes of Renal Cryoablation and RFA

| *Year* | *Author (reference)* | *Contribution* |
|---|---|---|
| *Cryoablation* | | |
| 1995 | Uchida et al. *(11)* | Percutaneous renal cryoablation |
| 1996 | Delworth et al. *(20)* | First human cryoablation |
| 1998 | Gill et al. *(13)* | Initial cryoabaltion series |
| 2000 | Rodriguez et al. *(41)* | Open and laparoscopic cryoablation |
| 1998 | Zegel et al. *(33)* | Utility of ultrasound with cryoablation |
| 2000 | Gill et al. *(14)* | Laparoscopic cryoablation, largest series to date |
| 2000 | Remer et al. *(37a)* | Utility of MRI with cryoablation |
| 2001 | Rukstalis et al. *(38)* | Open cryoablation experience |
| 2001 | Shingleton et al. *(32)* | Pertcutaneous cryoablation with MRI |
| 1999 | Bishoff et al. *(23)* | Laparoscopic renal cryoablation series |
| 2002 | Kim et al. *(39)* | Laparoscopic renal cryoablation series |
| *RFA* | | |
| 1998 | Zlotta et al. *(27)* | Early percutaneous and intraoperative renal RFA |
| 2000 | Gervais et al. *(15)* | Early renal RFA experience |
| 2000 | Walther et al. *(43)* | RFA pathologic correlation |
| 2001 | Crowley et al. *(29)* | Successful laparoscopic deployment in porcine model |
| 2002 | Pavlovitch et al. *(19)* | Percutaneous RFA |
| 2002 | Rendon et al. *(34)* | RFA pathologic correlation |
| 2002 | Su et al. *(40)* | Percutaneous RFA series |

MRI = magnetic resonance imaging; RFA = radiofrequency ablation

7 of 11 (64%) lesions having more than 5% tumor residual on gross inspection *(34)*.

Recently, there has been histopathologic evidence of incomplete ablation following RFA in certain patient populations. Gervais et al. presented data predicting the size and location of tumors most likely to recur, or have incomplete initial treatment. In their series, central, large (>5 cm diameter) tumors recurred with more frequency than the smaller (<3 cm diameter) exophytic peripheral lesions, but statistical significance was not met. This observation is supported by the improved cellular destruction with exophytic, peripherally based tumors secondary to the "oven effect" of the surrounding perirenal fat. Conversely, intraparyenchemal tumors may have less destruction secondary to the possible heat dissipation, or "heat sink," developed by the surrounding dense vasculature. Those patients, who had enhancement on followup CT, were assumed to have been inadequately treated and were electively retreated, and followed again with serial imaging *(15)*.

Table 4
Features of Current Cryoablation Outcomes

| *Author (reference)* | *Uchida et al. (11)* | *Delworth et al.(20)* | *Gill et al. (13)* | *Zegel et al. (33)* | *Bishoff et al. (23)* | *Rodriguez et al. (41)* | *Gill et al. (14)* | *Remer et al. (37a)* | *Rukstalis et al. (38)* | *Shingleton et al. (32)* | *Kim et al. (39)* |
|---|---|---|---|---|---|---|---|---|---|---|---|
| No. pts. | 2 | 2 | 10 | 6 | 8 | 7 | 32 | 21 | 29 | 20 | 12 |
| No. lesions/ ablations | 2 (both with advanced RCC) | 3 | 11 | 14 | 8 | 7 | 34 | 23 | 29 | 22 | 12 |
| Mean tumor diameter (cm) | NR | 4.3 | 1.9 | NR | 2.05 | 2.2+/–0.2 | 2.3 (preop) 2.0 (intraop | <4 | 2.2 | 3 | 2.21 |
| Mean operative time | NR | 4 h | 2.4 h | NR | 210 min | 234 min | 2.9 h | NR | NR | 97 min | NR |
| Cryoablative time | Single 22.5 | NR | Double freeze-thaw at 12.9 min | NR (7–15 min) | One, 15-cycle or two, 5-min cycles | 14.9 +/- 1.5 min single or double freezing | 15.1 min | NR | Two cryoablative cycles, but mean NR | Three cryoablative cycles, but mean NR | Double freeze–thaw |
| Mean blood loss (mL) | NR | 450 | 75 | NR | 140 | 111 | 66.8 | NR/NA | 150 | NR/NA | 60.4 |
| Mean probe temp | –20°C | –180°C | –186°C | –180°C | –180°C | –180°C | –185°C | –185 to –195°C | –140 to 180°C central temperature with –40°C at periphery of mass | NR | NR |
| Hospital stay | NR | 5 d | 9/10 <23 h | NR | 3.5 d | .4.4 +/– 0.6 d | 1.8 d (<23 hrs in 24/32 pts) | NR | 3 | < 24 h | 3.25 d |
| Followup (mo) | CT at 1 and 8 mo | MRI or CT at 1 and 3 mo | Serial CT or MRI at postop d 1 and 1,2 and 3 mo | Serial CT o r MRI at 3 and 22 mo post-operatively | 7.7 mo clinical & 5 mo radiographic | 142 +/- 4.6 mo in 6/7 pts | Sequential MRI CT-guided biopsy negative in 23/23 pts | Sequential MRI at 1, 3, 6 and 12 mo | Sequential CT or MRI to a mean of 16 mo | Sequential MRI Mean = 9.1 mo | Radiographic Mean = 305.2 d |
| Recurrence | Both died secondary to metastatic | 10% enlargement of angiomyolipoma at mo on CT | None with 3 of 3 negative followup CT-guided biopsies | None, 3 and 22 mo after cryoablation | None | No interval growth or recurrence | None at 162 mo, including port sites | 18/23 imaged with no recurrence at 6 mo | One biopsy proven recurrence | 1 patient | 2/3 pts biopsied revealed tumor |

NR = not reported; NA = not applicable; RCC = renal cell carcinoma.

Table 5
Features of Current Radiofrequency Ablation Techniques

| *Author (reference)* | *Zlotta et al. (27)* *In vivo* | *Gervais et al. (15)* | *Walther et al. (43)* | *Pavlovitch) et al. (19)* | *Rendon et al. (34)* | *Su et al. (40)* |
|---|---|---|---|---|---|---|
| No. pts.<br>No. lesions/ ablations | 3<br>3 | 8<br>9 | 4<br>14 | 21<br>24 | 10<br>11 | 17<br>22 |
| Tumor size (cm) | 3, 2.5, and 5 tumors | 3.3 | NR | 2.4 | 2.4 radiologic<br>2.2 grossly | 1.9 ± 0.6 |
| Mean operative time | NR | | NR | NR | NR | NR |
| RFA time | 12 min | 12 min | Single 5-min or two 5-min trials until 60°C in tissue was met | 2, 10–12 min ablation cycles | 17 min, 15 s | NR |
| Mean blood loss (mL) | NR | NR | NR | NR | NR | NR |
| Mean probe temp | NR | NR | 60°C | 70°C | NR | NR |
| Hospital stay | NR | NR | NR | <24 h | 4 h for percutaneous group | NR |
| Followup | 1-wk CT | Serial CTor MRI<br>Mean = 10.3 mo | CT scanning<br>(mean NR) | 2 mo with<br>mean size<br>20 cm | Pathologic | Radiographic f/ug mo.<br>*M* = 3.2 |
| Recurrence | NR | 5 lesions with persistent enchancement after single RFA | No metastatic disease with lesion <3cm | NR | 5% residual tumor in 7 of 11 (64%) tumors s/p RFA | 1/21 had repeat RFA secondary to enchancement at 3 mo |

NR = not reported; NA = not applicable; RFA = radiofrequency ablation; CT = computed tomography; MRI = magnetic resonance imaging; F/U = followup.

Table 6
Reported Complications Specific for Cryoablation and RFA

| *Cryoablation* | *RFA* |
|---|---|
| ■ Intra- and postoperative hemorrhage | ■ Intra- and postoperative hemorrhage |
| ■ Complete small bowel obstruction | ■ Damage to any surrounding structure and RF-induced ischemic injury |
| ■ Urine leak and potential fistulazation | |
| ■ Obstructive stricture of the ureteropelvic junction | ■ Microscopic or gross hematuria |
| ■ Port-site infection | |

RFA, radiofrequency ablation

## MORBIDITY/COMPLICATIONS

Low complication rates have been reported with cryoablation or RFA in the kidney (Table 6). Both systems have the risk of direct contact and subsequent energy transfer to surrounding structures *(44)*. Complications specific to cryoablative technique including mild intraoperative bleeding from a cracked cryolesion (easily controlled with Gelfoam™ and hemostatic sutures *[6]*), poorly understood rising abdominal pressures during the thaw cycle *(8)*, laparoscopic port-site infection *(32)*, intra- or postoperative hematoma *(3,25)*, and inability to adequately see a primary tumor or the cryolesion on US *(19)*.

The slightest contact to any surrounding tissue by the cryoprobe can have catastrophic effects. For example, cryoprobe contact with the surrounding bowel or collecting system can result in respective obstruction or urine leak and fistulization *(14,25)*. Savage et al. and Sung et al. showed that intentional freezing of the collecting system demonstrated urothelial sloughing to the lamina propria, with complete regrowth, and no leak or extravasation on retrograde pyelography *(21,22)*. Additionally, Bishoff et al. also noted in a porcine model that dense adhesions without bowel injury or fistula were seen between cryoablated kidney and overlying bowel in nonretroperitonealized kidneys. However, there were no complications reported with retroperitonealized kidneys *(23)*. Campbell et al. and Gill et al. describe the complication of obstructive stricture of the ureteropelvic junction *(13,14,45)*.

Cryoablation has a reported theoretic, but not proven, risk of tumor seeding secondary to probe manipulation during ablation *(25)*. However, a stronger theoretical risk of tumor seeding has been cited with RFA. Through the heat generated with the RF probe, local vasodilatation just outside the ablative zone may become more receptive to possible tumor spillage, resulting in hematogenous metastases *(16,27)*. Concurrently, both modalities carry the risk of local needle tract, or port-site tumor implantation—again, cited as a potential complication, but not proven *(27)*.

Compared to the 10% conversion rate from laparoscopic to open nephrectomy reported in older literature *(8)*, laparoscopic deployment of cryoprobes or RFA have not been associated with reported conversion to open surgery.

## RADIOGRAPHIC CHANGES

US, fluoroscopy, CT, and MRI have all been used for preoperative assessment, patient positioning, intraoperative assessment, and serial followup for cryoablation and RFA. Each energy therapy has quite different intra- and postoperative radiographic characteristics. Notwithstanding, preoperative assessment is required either through adequate enhanced cross-sectional CT scanning, or MRI with patients having compromised renal function.

Adequate cryoablation requires intraoperative monitoring of the "ice ball." To date, CT and MRI have not proven to be reliable modalities for detecting progression of this cryolesion. Using US, however, the cryoablated region appears with a hyperechoic crescentic rim (cryolesion edge), hypoechogenicity within the center of the lesion, and demonstration of a loss of normal color-flow characteristics—all characteristics demarcating the size and location of the ice ball *(13,20,23,45)*. Open cryoablation permits the use of standard US probes and equipment, whereas laparoscopy requires the intraoperative laparoscopic ultrasound (IOLUS), which can be used to monitor the progression of the cryolesion, to ensure a complete rim of normal renal parenchyma, to avoid injury of the collecting system, and to evaluate the kidney for other concomitant lesions not apparent on preoperative imaging. Large lesions may require multiple passes with multiple probes to achieve adequate ablation.

Serial radiographic evaluation following cryoablation is warranted to assure no persistent enhancement (a possible sign of persistent tumor) or enlargement. Serially enhanced CT scanning or MRI are adequate in this followup. Postoperative CT evaluation of cryolesions at 1 and 3 mo reveals persistent hypointense defects in the area of the ice ball, and eventual cortical defects consistent with tissue loss (Fig. 1) *(23)*. On serial followup, MRI reveals some ambiguity with regard to the signal characteristics of some cryolesions *(3,14,24,32,45)*. However, it is otherwise accepted that the "hallmark" is an initial and prolonged "punched-out," avascular lesion with loss of signal with gadolinium-enhanced MRI, characteristic of lesion eradication *(3,14,24,32)*. Decreasing size of the ablation area should be noted. Gill et al. reported mean percent

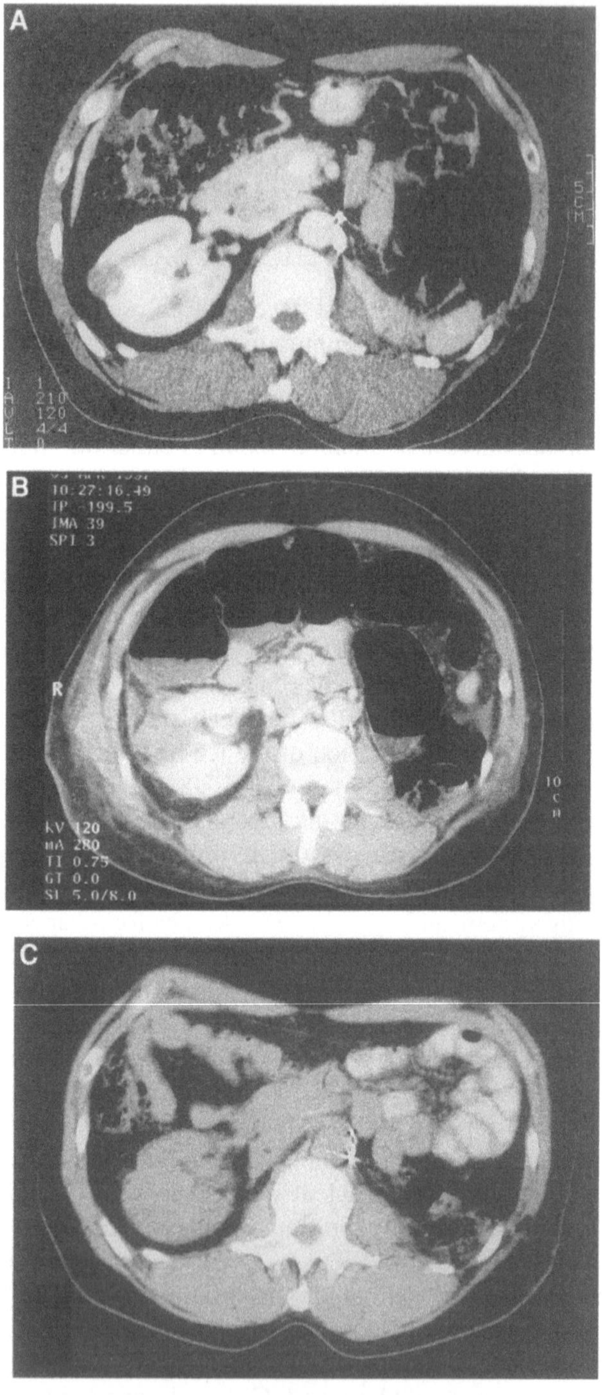


**Fig. 1**

decreases in size of 20.5%, 33–63.3% *(32)*, and 41% at postoperative d-1, 1-mo, and 3-mo CT or MRI evaluations, respectively *(3)*. Eventual loss of lesion identification and enhancement with either CT or MRI at 6–10 mo suggests complete eradication *(32)*. Persistent enhancement, perseverance (without diminishing size), or enlargement of the renal lesion on either CT or MRI followup should prompt one to obtain a percutaneous or laparoscopic needle biopsy to rule out recurrence.

Although US, fluoroscopy, CT, and MRI have all been used for patient positioning and percutaneous placement of RF probes, none of these modalities has proven reliable for the intraoperative monitoring of the RF lesion. On US imaging, there is no immediate change in the echotexture in the area of RF ablation, and color and power Doppler are of no added benefit secondary to the variable and inconsistent findings *(29)*. Moreover, RF treatment can sometimes disturb US imaging, creating a marked scatter of the echoes, secondary to micro-bubble formation as noted previously in this chapter *(15,27,28,34,37)*. Crowley et al. found CT scanning to be an excellent modality for positioning of the patient and probe and for immediate posttreatment imaging, but it was not utilized for intraoperative monitoring (Fig. 2) *(29)*. Lewin et al. and Merkle et al. used MRI to monitor real-time tissue destruction with RF. These groups demonstrated a zone of decreased signal surrounded by a rim of hyperintensity on T2-weighted and turbo short inversion-time inversion recovery images *(36,46)*. However, confirmatory images obtained after conclusion of the ablation session revealed a propensity for these T2-weighted images to underestimate the size of the RF lesion *(36)*. Thus, insofar as intraoperative monitoring for RF is concerned, there is no imaging modality that can, in real time, ensure a sufficient extent of tissue ablation while avoiding injury to normal, adjacent parenchyma and structures.

The solution may lie in the perfection of what Zlotta calls "forecast ablation" *(27)*. This is the correlation between the size of the lesion predicted by the diameter of the prongs on the RF electrode and the actual observation of the RF lesion. Both the low frequency of RF energy and its vulnerability to the dissipating effects of blood flow permit the creation of very localized lesions. It is therefore possible to sculpt a lesion with numerous applications of the RF probe. Zlotta et al. performed RFA in both ex vivo and in vivo human kidneys, comparing probe size to lesion volume. In the in vivo model, the size of the lesion correlated closely with

---

**Fig. 1.** *(from opposite page)* **(A)** Prior to renal cryoablation the computed tomography (CT) image shows a mass in the right kidney. **(B)** CT image obtained in the immediate postoperative period reveals a wedge-shaped defect in the area of the ablated mass, with surrounding edema and perirenal inflammatory reaction. **(C)** One year following cryoablation the CT shows only a subtle residueal renal defect.

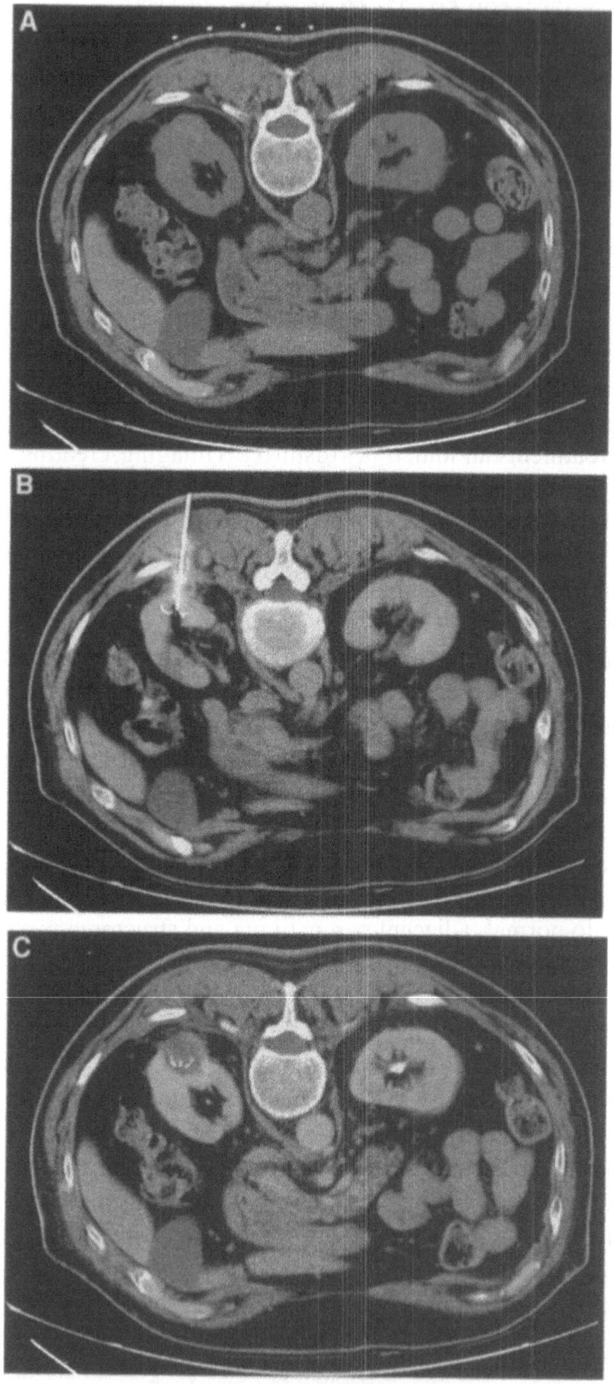


**Fig. 2**

the diameter of the prongs deployed on the electrode probe: treatment with a 2-cm prong resulting in a lesion measuring 2 × 1.8 cm *(27)*.

## HISTOLOGIC CHANGES

Immediate and delayed histopathologic changes have been studied following cryoablation and RFA. At 1 h, a cryolesion contains a well-demarcated interstitial hemorrhage *(12,13,23)* with vascular congestion and early coagulative necrosis, primarily in the tubular epithelial cells *(13,47)*. Electron microscopic studies of these lesions revealed irreversible signs of cellular destruction with partial fragmentation and vacuolization of cytoplasmic membranes, chromatin condensation, nuclear membrane dissipation, and thrombi in glomerular capillaries *(13)*. At 24 h, complete coagulative necrosis is seen with a peripheral zone of partial necrosis, deemed the "zone of sublethal destruction or demarcation," a topic of concern as this may contain viable, nondesiccated carcinoma *(13,14,47)*.

The zone of sublethal destruction may correlate with one of the four layers Bishoff et al. described where, at 7 d, the histology shows a central necrosis, an inflammatory infiltrative process, residual hemorrhage, and fibrosis with tubular regeneration—the latter of which may correlate with an incomplete zone of tissue desiccation (Fig. 3) *(12,23)*. Varying degrees of chronic inflammation, hemosiderosis, fibrosis, necrosis, and regeneration are seen from 3 wk to 3 mo after initial cryoablation *(13,23)* with ultimate spontaneous resorption of the cryolesion to a water-tight lesion at approx 3 mo *(3)*. Histologic specimen 3 to 6 mo after laparoscopic cryoablation reveal degrees of hemosiderin deposition, fibrosis, inflammation, necrosis, or even recurrence—with the latter being seen after an enhancing renal mass was identified on MRI followup *(42)*.

RFA-treated lesions are quite different in that they are typically wedge-shaped secondary to their endothelial destruction, and subsequent segmental vascular thrombosis and ischemia. Ischemia likely augments the primary histopathologic destruction from the RF heat

**Fig. 2.** *(from opposite page)* **(A)** Preoperative CT images show mass in the posterior aspect of the right kidney. The patient is placed in the supine position and skin markers have been positioned to assist with placement of the radiofrequency probe. **(B)** The radiofrequency probe has been positioned inside the mass and the tines deployed. **(C)** Immediately after completion of the ablation cycle, a CT image with intravenous contrast shows decreased enhancement in the area of ablation and normal enhancement of surrounding renal parenchyma.

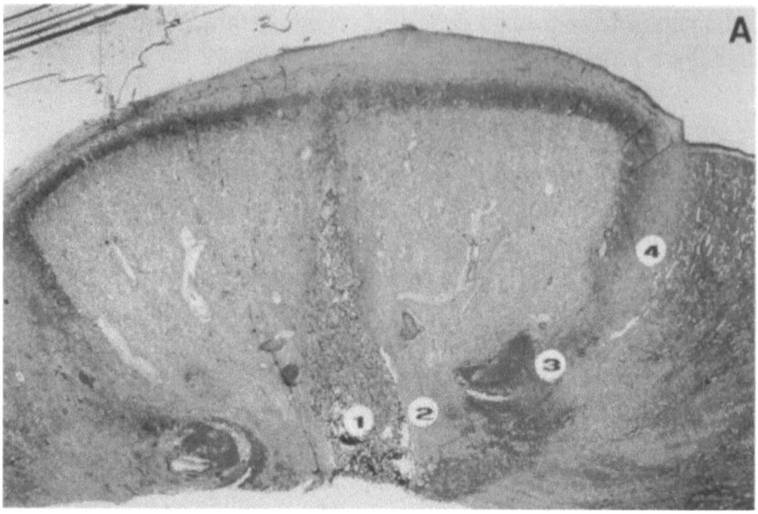


**Fig. 3.** (**A**) One week after cryoablation, pig kidney contains wedge-shaped defect with four distinct zones of histopathologic change: complete necrosis (1), inflammatory infiltrate (2), hemorrhage (3), and fibrosis and regeneration (4). (**B**) Thirteen weeks after cryoablation, pig kidney shows resorption of necrotic tissue with thickened renal capsule and marked interstitial fibrosis with scattered shrunken glomeruli. Outside well-demarcated cryoablation lesion, renal parenchyma is unchanged.

energy itself, which results in characteristic hypereosinophilia (unknown mechanism), pynknosis, stromal edema, loss of nuclear and nucleoli architecture, and coagulative necrosis *(19,27)*.

## CONCLUSION

New minimally invasive therapies represent exciting advances for patients with small renal lesions, or significant comorbidities, that would otherwise force one to recommend observation. One of the main controversies with these treatments lies in the lack of long-term cancer-free and overall survival data. With further refinements of both energy delivery systems and deployment strategies, one can hopefully witness a new era of progressive minimally invasive surgery. In the future it may be possible to use "tailored" probes that can be conformed to a specific pathologic type, size, and located renal lesion. Additionally, alternative ablative energy sources such as microwave thermoablation, high-intensity focused ultrasound, and interstitial photon radiation ablation are being studied as future competitors in the arena of minimally invasive

NSS. Overall, cautious optimism is recommended when considering the incorporation of either cryoablation or RFA into one's surgical armamentarium. Excluding any technical and radiographic inconsistencies in any of the short-term results of cryoablation or RFA, early treatment failure needs to be put into the context of long-term, prospective clinical trials. Any new techniques for the treatment of small renal tumors must show clinical and pathologic success compared to open NSS.

## ACKNOWLEDGMENT

The views expressed in this chapter are those of the authors and do not reflect the official policy of the Department of Defense or other departments of the U.S. government.

## REFERENCES

1. Lee CT, Katz J, Shi W, Thaler HT, Reuter VE, Russo P. Surgical management of renal tumors 4 cm or less in a contemporary cohort. J Urol 2000; 163: 730–736.
2. Clayman RV, Kavoussi LR, Soper NJ, et al. Laparoscopic nephrectomy: Initial case report. J Urol 1991; 146: 278–282.
3. Gill IS, Novick AC. Renal cryosurgery. Urology 1999; 54: 215–219.
4. Nissenkorn I, Burnheim J. Multricentricity in renal cell carcinoma. J Urol 1995; 153: 620–622.
5. McKiernan J, Simmons R, Katz J, Russo P. Natural history of chronic renal insufficiency after partial and radical nephrectomy. Urology 2002; 59(6): 816–820.
6. Cozzi PJ, Lynch WJ, Collins S, Vonthethoff L, Morris DL. Renal cryotherapy in a sheep model; a feasibility study. J Urol 1997; 157: 710–712.
7. Dupuy DE. Radiofrequency ablation: An outpatient percutaneous treatment. Med and Health/Rhode Island 1999; 82(6): 213–216.
8. Johnson DB, Nakada SY. Laparoscopic cryoablation for renal-cell cancer. J Endourol 2000; 14(10): 873–878.
9. Finter L. Cancer cryosurgery potentially 'hot' for patients, new markets. J National Cancer Institute 2000; 92(18): 1464–1466.
10. Uhlschmid G, Kolb E, Largiader F. Cryosurgery of pulmonary metastases. Cryobiology 1979; 16(2): 171–178.
11. Uchida M, Imaide Y, Sugimoto K, Uehara H, Watanabe H. Percutaneous cryosurgery for renal tumors. Br J Urol 1995; 75: 132–136.
12. Stephenson RA, King DK, Rohr LR. Renal Cryoablation in a Canine Model. Urology 1996; 41: 772–776.
13. Gill IS, Novick AC, Soble JJ, et al. Laparoscopic renal cryoablation: initial clinical series. Urology 1998; 52: 543–541.
14. Gill IS, Novick AC, Meraney AM, et al. Laparoscopic renal cryoablation in 32 patients. Urology 2000; 56: 748–753.
15. Gervais DA, McGovern FJ, Wood BJ, Goldberg SN, McDougal WS, Mueller, PR. Radio-frequency ablation of renal cell carcinoma: early clinical experience. Radiology 2000; 217: 665–672.
16. Yohannes P, Pinto P, Rotariu P, Smith AD, Lee BR. Retroperitoneoscopic radiofrequency ablation of a solid renal mass. J Endourol 2001; 15(8): 845–849.

17. Zagoria RJ, Chen MY, Kavanagh PV, Torti FM. Radio frequency ablation of lung metastases from renal cell carcinoma. J Urol 2001; 166: 1827–1828.
18. Shingleton WB, Sewell PE. Percutaneous renal cryoablation of renal tumors in patients with von Hippel-Lindau Disease. J Urol 2002; 167: 1268–1270.
19. Pavlovich CP, Walther MM, Choyke PL, et al. Percutaneous radio frequency ablation of small renal tumors: initial results. J Urol 2002; 167: 10–15.
20. Delworth MG, Pisters LL, Fornage BD, von Eschenbach AC. Cryotherapy for renal cell carcinoma and angiomyolipoma. J Urol 1996; 155: 252–254.
21. Savage SJ, Gill IS. Renal tumor ablation: energy-based technologies. World J Urol 2000; 18: 283–288.
22. Sung GT, Gill IS. Effect of intentional cryoinjury to the renal collecting system. (abstract) J Endourol 1999; 13(S1): A14.
23. Bishoff JT, Chen RB, Lee BR, et al. Laparoscopic renal cryoablation: Acute and long-term clinical, radiographic, and pathologic effects in an animal and application in a clinical trial. J Endourol 1999; 13(4): 233–239.
24. Chen RN, Novick AC, Gill IS. Laparoscopic cryoablation of renal masses. Urol Clin N Amer 2000; 27(4): 813–820.
25. Murphy DP, Gill IS. Energy-based renal tumor ablation: A review. Sem in Urol Onc 2001; 19(2): 133–140.
26. Alder AB. Cryosurgery in Urology. Brit J Urol 1970; 42(6): 744.
27. Zlotta AR, Wildschutz T, Raviv G, et al. Radiofrequency interstitial tumor ablation (RITA) is a possible new modality for treatment of renal cancer: ex vivo and in vivo experience. J of Endourol 1998; 11(4): 251–258.
28. Pautler SE, Pavlovich CP, Mikityansky I, et al. Retroperitoneoscopic-guided radiofrequency ablation of renal tumors. Canad J Urol 2001; 8(4): 1330–1333.
29. Crowley JD, Shelton J, Iverson AJ, Burton MP, Dalrymple NC, Bishoff JT. Laparoscopic and computed tomography-guided percutaneous radio-frequency ablation of renal tissue: acute and chronic effects in an animal model. Urology 2001; 57: 976–980.
30. Feld RI, McGinnis DE, Needleman L, Segal SR, Strup SE, Nazarian LN. A novel application for the end-fire sonographic probe: Guidance during cryoablation of renal masses. Am J Roentgen 173: 652–654.
31. Gettman MT, Bishoff JT, Su LM, et al. Hemostatic laparoscopic partial nephrectomy: Initial experience with the radiofrequency coagulation-assisted technique. Urology 2001; 58: 8–11.
32. Shingleton WB, Sewell PE. Percutaneous renal tumor cryoablation with magnetic resonance imaging guidance. J Urol 2001; 165: 773–776.
33. Zegel HG, Holland GA, Jennings SB, Chong WK, Cohen JK. Intraoperative ultrasonography guided cryoablation of renal masses: Initial experience. J Ultrasound Med 1998; 17: 571–576.
34. Rendon RA, Kachura JR, Sweet JM, et al. The uncertainty of radio frequency treatment of renal cell carcinoma: findings at immediate and delayed nephrectomy. J Urol 2002; 167; 1587–1592.
35. Roberts WW, Fugita OE, Ryan BP, Kavoussi LR, Cadeddu JA. Infrared imaging of laparoscopic renal radiofrequency ablation in a porcine model. (abstract) J Urol 2002; 167(4): 18.
36. Lewin JS, Connell CF, Duerk JL, et al. Interactive MRI-guided radiofrequency interstitial thermal ablation of abdominal tumors: Clinical trial for evaluation of safety and feasibility. J of Mag Res Imag 1998; 8:40–47.

37. Rendon RA, Gertner MR, Sherar MD, et al. Development of a radiofrequency based thermal therapy technique in an in vivo porcine model for the treatment of small renal masses. J Urol 2001; 166: 292–298.
37a. Remer EM, Weinberg EJ, Oto A, O'Malley CM, Gill IS. MR imaging of the kidneys after laparoscopic cryoblation. Am J Roentgen 2000; 174(3): 635–640.
38. Rukstalis DB, Khorsandi M, Garcia FU, Hoenig DM, Cohen JK. Clinical experience with open renal cryoablation. Urology 2001; 57: 34–39.
39. Kim SC, Rubenstein J, Yap RL, et al. Laparoscopic renal cryosurgery: The Northwestern Experience. (abstract) J Urol 2002; 167(4): 1.
40. Su LM, Jarrett TW, Kavoussi LR, Solomon SB. Percutaneous CT-guided radiofrequency ablatin of small renal masses in poor surgical risk patients: preliminary results. (abstract) J Urol 2002; 167(4): 1.
41. Rodriguez R, Chan DY, Bishoff JT, et al. Renal ablative cryosurgery in select patients with peripheral renal masses. Urology 2000; 55(1): 25–30.
42. Levin HS, Meraney AM, Novick AC, Gill IS. Needle biopsy histology for renal tumors 3–6 months after laparoscopic renal cryoablation. J Urol 2000; 163(S682): 153.
43. Walther MM, Shawker TH, Libutti SK, et al. A phase 2 study of radio frequency interstitial tissue ablation of localized renal tumors. J Urol 2000; 163:1424–1427.
44. Yohannes P, Rotariu P, Pinto P, Liatsikos EN, Smith A, Lee B. Transperitoneal laparoscopic radiofrequency ablation of a solid renal mass: free of complications? J Urol 2002; 167(4): 16.
45. Campbell SC, Krishnamurthi V, Chow G, Hale J, Novick AC. Renal cryosurgery: Experimental evaluation of treatment parameters. Urology 1998; 52: 29–33.
46. Merkle EM, Shonk JR, Duerk JL, Jacobs GH, Lewin JS. MR-guided RF thermal ablation of the kidney in a porcine model. Amer J Radiology 1999; 173: 645–651.
47. Edmunds TB, Schulsinger DA, Durand DB, Waltzer WC. Acute histologic changes in human renal tumors after cryoablation. J Endourol 2000; 14(2): 139–143.

# 8 Percutaneous Radiofrequency Tumor Ablation

*Francis J. McGovern, MD,*
*Debra A. Gervais, MD, and Peter R. Mueller, MD*

*CONTENTS*

INTRODUCTION
HISTORICAL BACKGROUND
MECHANISM OF ACTION AND TECHNICAL INNOVATIONS TO INCREASE VOLUME OF COAGULATION NECROSIS
RENAL TUMORS IDEALLY SUITED FOR RFA
EARLY INDICATIONS AND CLINICAL EXPERIENCE WITH RFA IN TREATMENT OF RCC
IMAGING AND RFA
OTHER USES OF RFA IN THE TREATMENT OF RCC
PATIENT TOLERANCE AND COMPLICATIONS
CONTROVERSIES, CURRENT LIMITATIONS, AND FUTURE DIRECTIONS
CONCLUSIONS
REFERENCES

## INTRODUCTION

During the last decade, promising alternatives to the historical standard of open nephrectomy for the treatment of renal cell carcinoma (RCC) have been developed and evaluated *(1–6)*. These new techniques have been developed with the aims of diminishing morbidity, shorten-

From: *Laparoscopic Urologic Oncology*
Edited by: J. A. Cadeddu © Humana Press Inc., Totowa, NJ

ing the postoperative recovery period, and performing nephron-sparing procedures in patients with either limited renal function or predisposition to multiple tumors as occurs in von Hippel-Lindau (VHL) disease or hereditary RCC. The most recent of these therapeutic interventions to undergo clinical evaluation are the ablative therapies, cryoablation and radiofrequency ablation (RFA), which use cold and heat, respectively, to kill tumor cells. This chapter reviews the application of RF thermal ablation and its current status in the treatment of RCC.

## HISTORICAL BACKGROUND

The use of RFA in medicine is not new. The technology is familiar to all surgeons in a common operating room tool—the electrical coagulator used for local hemostasis. The term radiofrequency ablation is derived from the use of electrical energy in the RF range, usually 460 kHz alternating current. Throughout the 1980s and early 1990s, RFA was refined for application via catheters to ablate aberrant cardiac conduction pathways, and via needle electrodes to treat trigeminal neuralgia and osteoid osteomas *(7–9)*. The latter are benign painful osseous lesions, usually small, previously treated by surgical resection.

These applications—surgical hemostasis by coagulation of small vessels, ablation of the trigeminal ganglion, cardiac ablation, and ablation of osteoid osteomas—are all similar with respect to the small volume of tissue coagulation required for therapeutic effectiveness. Interest in the application of RFA to treat soft tissue tumors appeared in the early 1990s *(10)*. These tumors are larger than the foci ablated in prior clinical applications. The next several years saw the development of multiple technical innovations to increase the volume of necrosis achieved with application of RF electrical energy *(11–20)*.

## MECHANISM OF ACTION AND TECHNICAL INNOVATIONS TO INCREASE VOLUME OF COAGULATION NECROSIS

RFA of soft tissue tumors is applied clinically using a monopolar needle electrode in the tissue of interest with the circuit completed by grounding pads placed on the skin, usually on the thighs. Electrical current density is highest near the needle electrode where local hyperthermia is induced by ion agitation in tissues surrounding the electrode. Ideal temperatures for tissue death are between 60°C and 100°C. In this range, there is practically instantaneous protein coagulation and irreversible damage to key intracellular enzymes and nucleic-acid complexes *(21)*.

The pathological changes induced by RFA are known as coagulation necrosis, a combination of coagulative necrosis and other irreversible changes inducing cell death *(21)*. Although cell death will occur between 46°C and 60°C, the time needed to induce cytotoxicity is markedly reduced above 60°C. Temperatures above 100°C to 105°C result in tissue vaporization and carbonization (charring). Formation of gas bubbles and charred tissue diminish energy transmission and deposition by increasing the impedance of the tissues to the flow of electrical current. Gas bubbles also form a thermal insulator limiting the spread of thermal energy. Therefore, avoidance of these extreme temperatures is desirable.

Coagulation necrosis caused by a single 17 G needle electrode heated to 90°C for 6 min is cylindrical in shape and measures a maximum of 1.6 cm in diameter *(11)*.

However, for practical purposes, ablation of soft tissue tumors requires necrosis of regions larger than 1 to 2 cm in diameter. Investigators seeking to increase the volume of coagulation necrosis turned to the bioheat equation delineated by Pennes in 1948 *(22)*. The equation takes into account all the factors that influence tissue heating. For practical purposes, the equation can be simplified to:

Coagulation necrosis = energy deposited × local tissue interactions – heat lost *(23)*

Theoretical and practical means to improve the equation in favor of increasing coagulation necrosis are described here *(23)*:

### *Energy Deposition*

Energy deposition can be increased by the following mechanisms:

- Multiple applications of a single electrode
- An array of electrodes
- A single electrode that deploys into an array (umbrella electrode)
- An electrode with multiple needles mounted on a single handle (cluster electrode)
- Internally cooled electrodes
- Pulsed current

Multiple applications of an electrode are commonly performed in current clinical applications of RFA to assure complete three-dimensional coagulation necrosis of an entire tumor. However, for tumors larger than 2 to 3 cm, this approach is time-consuming. An array of individual electrodes could shorten the time to achieve complete necrosis *(16)*. However, precise placement of equidistant electrodes is difficult, and so this strategy is not used in current practice. Instead, modifications of

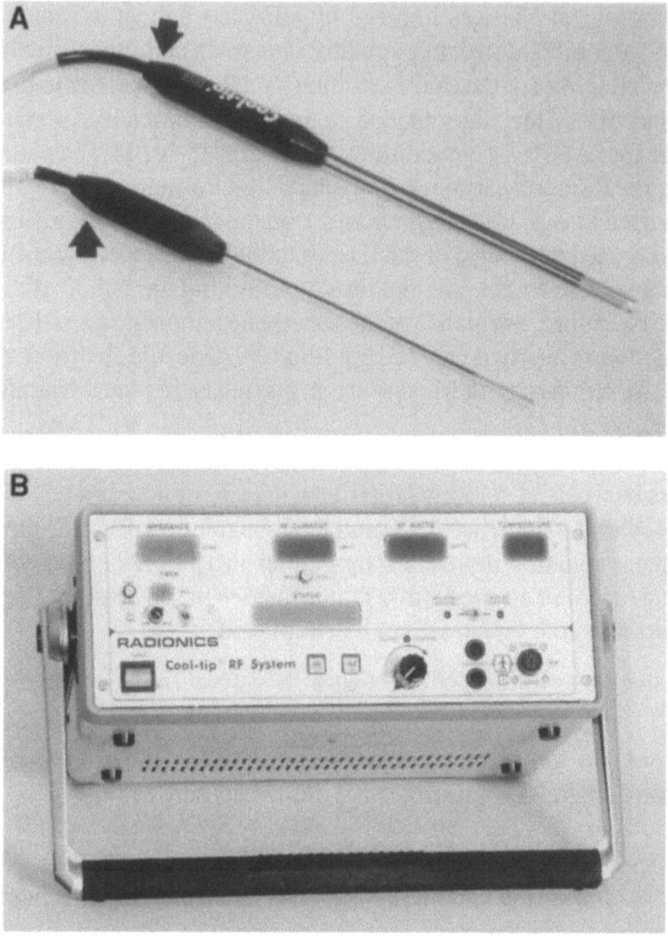


**Fig. 1. (A)** Single and cluster internally cooled electrodes. The handle (arrows) of the needle electrode connects to electrical wiring and two ports for inflow and outflow of cooled fluid. **(B)** Radiofrequency generator (Radionics, Burlington, MA). The current is controlled by the operator with the display of temperature, impedance, and current on the generator face. Optional switches allow setting of a timer and automated pulsing of current.

single electrodes have been developed to allow multifocal ablation with a single percutaneous application. One modification is to mount three needle electrodes together for simultaneous application of RFA. This arrangement is referred to as a cluster electrode (Radionics, Burlington, MA) (Fig. 1). Another modification is to place a coaxial introducer through which a hooked, or umbrella, array of multiple electrodes is deployed (Fig. 2). As with single electrodes, cluster or umbrella array

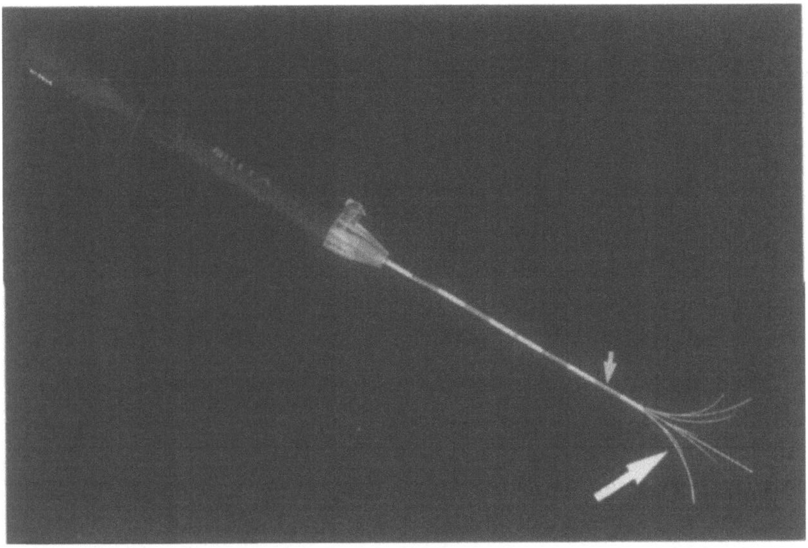

**Fig. 2.** A needle electrode with a coaxial introducer needle (short arrow) allowing deployment of an "umbrella" array (long arrow) inside the target tumor.

electrodes can be applied in more than one location during an ablation session to achieve complete coagulation necrosis of an entire tumor.

Other strategies to increase energy deposition are internal cooling of electrodes and pulsing of current *(14,18,20)*. Internal cooling, seemingly a paradox, is based on the distribution of heat in the tissues adjacent to the electrode. The highest temperatures are in the immediate vicinity of the electrode and diminish as radial distance from the electrode increases. Thus, the easiest portion of a tumor to kill is in the center of the necrosis region, and the hardest is at the periphery. Similarly, the region at highest risk for vaporization and carbonization, which increase impedance to electrical current, is tissue in the immediate vicinity of the electrode. Internal cooling of the electrode maximizes energy deposition at the periphery of the tumor by limiting vaporization and carbonization in the center. In practice, this is achieved by perfusion of chilled saline or water via two internal lumens within the needle electrode, which allow inflow and outflow of the fluid. Pulsing of electrical current has also been shown to increase the zone of necrosis *(20)*. When a rapid rise in tissue impedance is detected, the current is diminished to minimize vaporization and carbonation and to allow time for dissipation of gas bubbles. The current is then increased and maximal energy deposition resumes. The use of internally cooled electrodes and the pulsing of current together results in a synergistic effect in increasing the volume of coagulation necrosis

*(20)*. Internally cooled electrodes are commercially available with a 200 Watt generator that provides automated pulsing of current via a computer chip (Radionics, Burlington, MA) (Fig.1).

### *Local Tissue Interactions*

Local tissue interactions can be optimized by the following mechanisms *(23)*:

- Increase electrical and heat conduction in the treated tissue
- Decrease tissue heat conduction in the surrounding tissue
- Decrease tissue heat tolerance to facilitate cell death

The simplest and most extensively studied means of improving tissue conduction is injection of saline into the tissues *(13)*. The injected saline conducts heat farther and faster than soft tissue, and likely increases current flow as well by increasing ion density. In liver tumors, Livraghi et al. showed increased ablation size with the use of injected saline, but the lesions created were more irregular and less predictable in shape than those created without saline injection *(13)*.

Although conduction of heat to the periphery of the treated tumor is good, conduction of heat away from the tumor is undesirable. Thus, the ideal tumor conducts heat and current, but is surrounded by insulating tissues. In practice, this theory has been validated by Livraghi et al. who described the "oven effect" in the RFA of hepatocellular carcinoma in cirrhotic liver *(24)*. Cirrhotic tissue insulates the tumor and allows higher temperatures to be maintained. Similarly, Dupuy et al. showed that cortical bone can serve as an insulator allowing ablation of vertebral body tumors without damaging the spinal cord *(25)*. With respect to the kidney, the presence of perinephric fat around a tumor should likewise facilitate thermally induced cytotoxicity.

Mechanisms to decrease heat tolerance of tissues to optimize results of RFA are experimental at this time *(23)*.

### *Heat Loss*

Experimental RFA of ex vivo liver produces regions of coagulation necrosis that are reproducible in size and shape. Results in in vivo liver, however, show smaller regions of necrosis and greater variability in size *(17)*. Perfusion-mediated tissue cooling from blood flow is thought to be responsible for the discrepancy *(17)*. Flowing blood serves as a heat sink removing heated blood from the region and constantly supplying cool (body temperature) blood. In practice, perfusion-mediated tissue cooling results in diminished necrosis in vascular regions of a tumor, at the tumor interface with a vascular organ, or in regions of tumor adjacent to large vessels.

## RENAL TUMORS IDEALLY SUITED FOR RFA

Based on the experimental and clinical work just summarized, both tumor size and tumor location are considered when determining the ideal RCC for treatment with RFA. Small tumors, 3 cm or less, are ideal in that they fall into the size range of coaguluation necrosis that can be achieved with current RFA systems. Furthermore, effectiveness of RFA is enhanced when the target tissue is surrounded by insulating tissues—the so-called oven effect—and so exophytic tumors surrounded by perirenal fat would be expected to respond favorably because of the insulating properties of fat *(24)*. The intraparenchymal component of the tumor would fare less well given vascularity of adjacent renal parenchyma, but complete ablation of 3 cm tumors would be expected based on in vivo experience with RF of liver tumors *(24)*. Finally, the hardest lesion to treat would be a tumor in the renal sinus adjacent to large blood vessels that serve as heat sinks *(17)*. Therefore, the ideal lesion is an exophytic tumor 3 cm or less (Fig. 3). Based on these considerations, we have previously proposed a categorization scheme by location. Exophytic tumors have a component extending beyond parenchyma, whereas central tumors have a component within the renal sinus. Mixed tumors have both central and exophtytic components, and parenchymal tumors are limited to the renal parenchyma without extension into the perinephric fat or renal sinus (Figs. 3 and 4). When assessing reports of the success of RFA in achieving coagulation necrosis of RCC left *in situ*, both size and location must be considered.

### *Currently Available Systems and Applications*

Currently, three RFA systems are commercially available for clinical applications in the United States. These are the Radionics 200 Watt generator with internally cooled electrodes available as single needles or in a cluster array (Radionics, Burlington, MA) (Fig.1). The length of the uninsulated electrically active tip ranges from 2 to 3 cm. The generator provides the option of automated pulsing of current. The other two systems provide umbrella-type electrodes placed via an introducer needle (RITA Medical Systems, Inc., Mountain View, CA; and Radiotherapeutics, Mountain View, CA) (Fig. 2). These latter two systems do not allow for internal cooling or pulsing of electrical current.

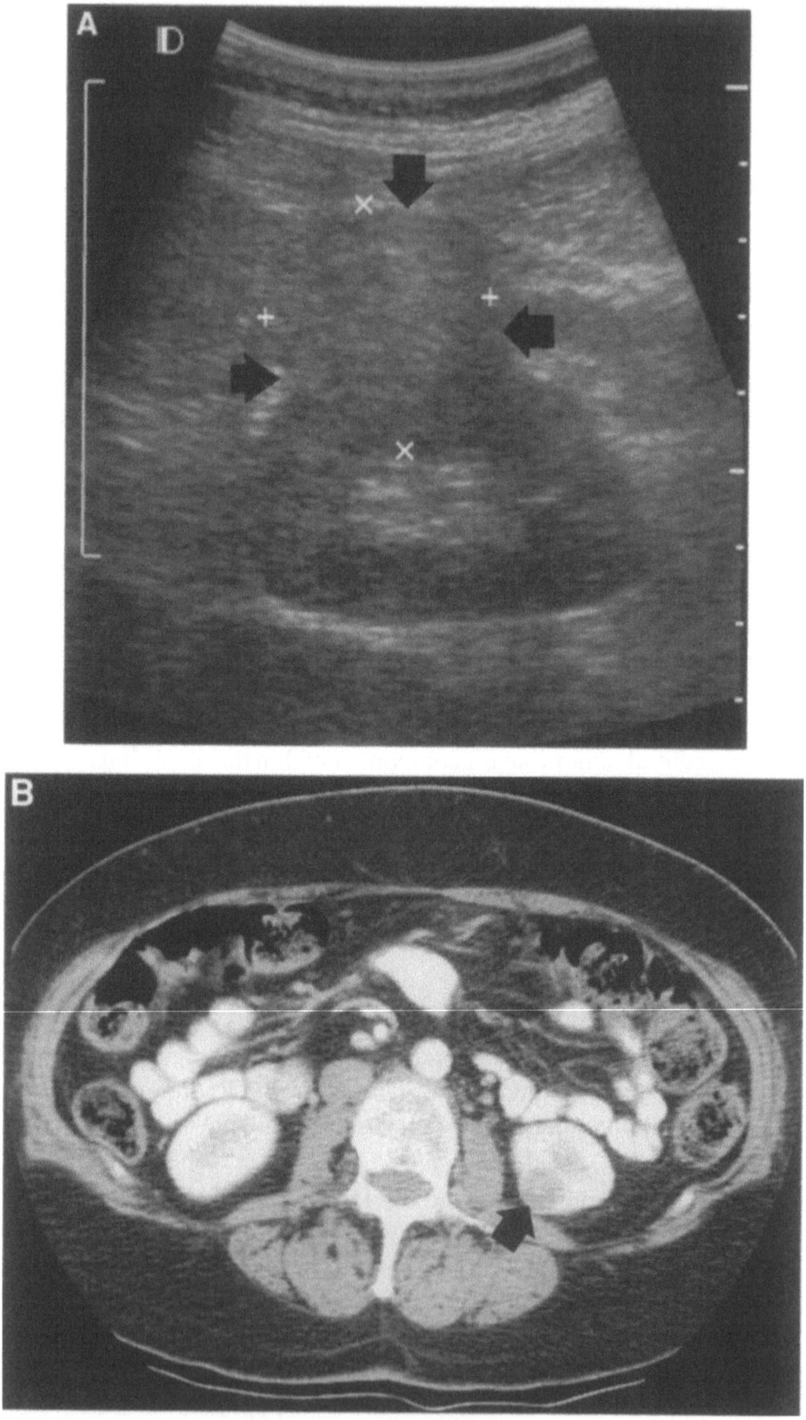
A
D
B

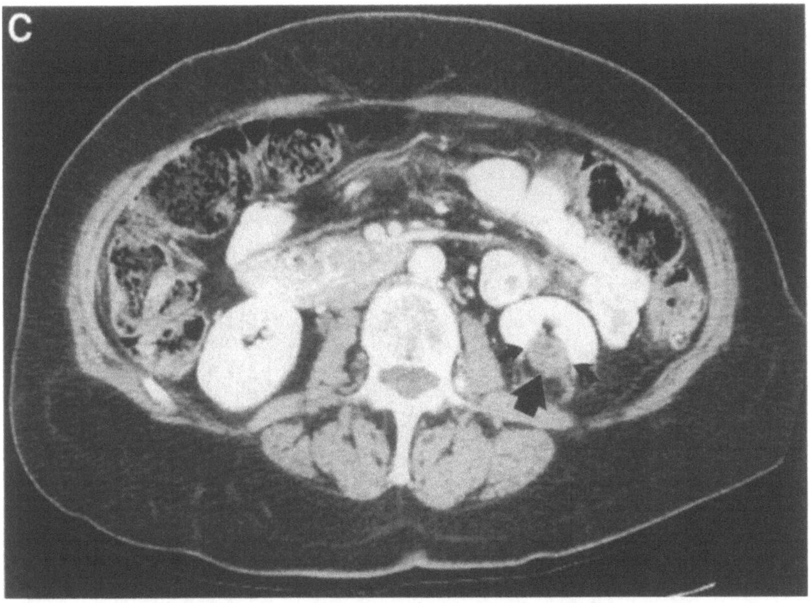


**Fig. 3.** **(A)** Ultrasound of a 3.5 × 2.9 cm exophytic biopsy proven renal cell carcinoma (arrows). The tumor is surrounded by perirenal fat with only a small component of its surface adjacent to renal parenchyma. This is an ideal tumor location for treatment with radiofrequency ablation (RFA). RFA successfully eliminated tumor enhancement on CT (not shown). **(B)** CT scan in another patient with a small lower pole exophytic renal cell carcinoma (arrow). This tumor is in part surrounded by fat but also by renal parenchyma over much of its surface. Still, it is not adjacent to large blood vessels in the renal sinus. It too, is a good candidate for RFA. **(C)** CT scan in the same patient 1 yr following RFA shows no enhancement in the tumor (arrow). There is also some fat at the tumor–kidney interface (curved arrows).

All three electrodes can be accurately deployed with ultrasound (US) or computed tomography (CT) imaging guidance. Imaging guidance is crucial for successful ablation no matter which system is employed. Meticulous attention to the placement of the electrode for treatment is necessary to ensure coagulation necrosis of the entire tumor. Additionally, the operator must assess the overall tumor volume and geometry and ensure that, if needed, multiple overlapping ablations are performed. Finally, the operator must ensure that electrode placement minimizes risk of thermal injury to adjacent structures such as bowel or ureter. In cases with bowel or ureter immediately adjacent to tumor, a laparoscopic approach may be useful to allow mobilization and separation of the tumor from other structures.

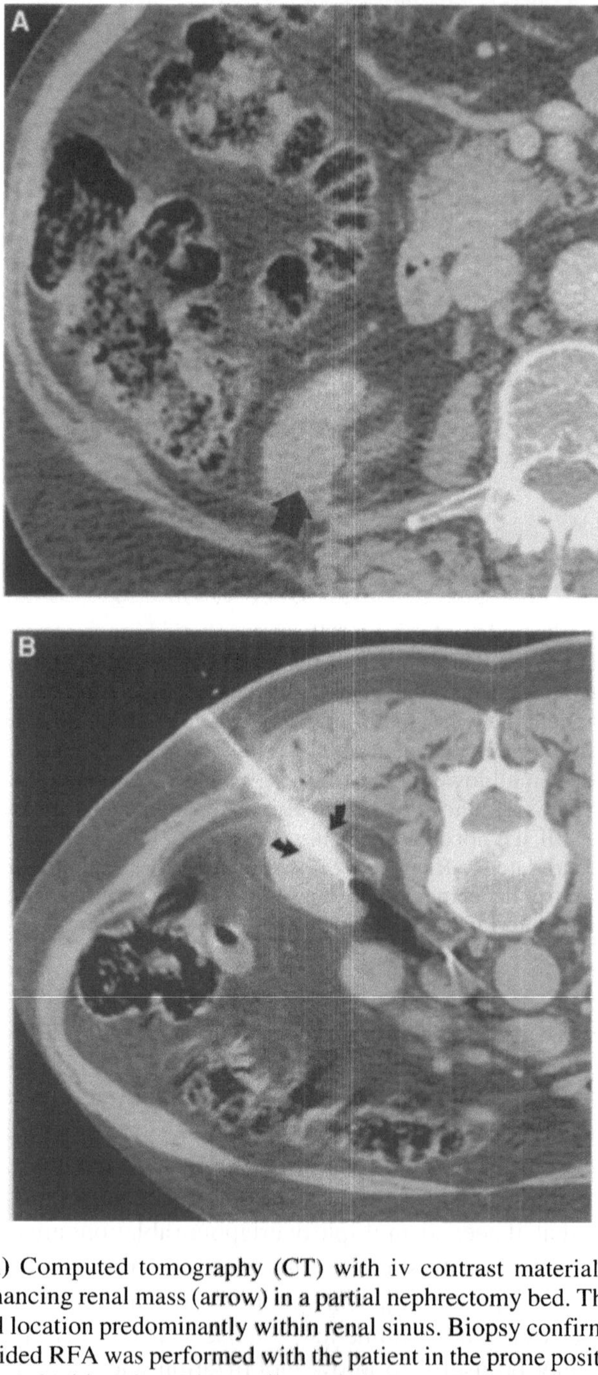

**Fig. 4. (A)** Computed tomography (CT) with iv contrast material shows a 3.4 cm enhancing renal mass (arrow) in a partial nephrectomy bed. The mass is in a central location predominantly within renal sinus. Biopsy confirmed RCC. **(B)** CT-guided RFA was performed with the patient in the prone position. RFA was performed with a cluster internally cooled electrode (arrows). Subsequent CT scans (not shown) showed no enhancement and no growth over 2 yr.

# EARLY INDICATIONS AND CLINICAL EXPERIENCE WITH RFA IN TREATMENT OF RCC

## *Early Applications*

The application of RFA to treat human RCC was first reported by Zlotta et al. who reported three patients who underwent RFA of small RCC's prior to nephrectomy *(26)*. One patient underwent percutaneous US-guided ablation 1 wk prior to nephrectomy. The other two patients underwent intraoperative ablation just prior to nephrectomy. Percutaneous ablation was well tolerated with local analgesia, and necrosis was confirmed at pathology. Subsequently, McGovern et al. reported a case of RCC treated with RFA and left *in situ (27)*. The initial postablation scan showed no enhancement in the tumor. Further followup was not available at the time of that report. Hall et al. later reported combined catheter arterial embolization and RFA of a large RCC in a nonoperative candidate with imaging evidence of coagulation necrosis *(28)*.

## *Expanded Series and Indications*

In 2000, Gervais et al. reported nine tumors in eight patients treated with image-guided percutaneous RFA and followed by imaging over a mean period of 10.3 mo with a range of 3 to 21 mo and with 6-mo followup in seven of the eight patients *(29)*.

In this initial series, RFA thus far has been limited to patients who are poor candidates for surgery because of comorbidities and/or patients who have a life expectancy of greater than 1 yr but less than 10 yr. This series of patients has been expanded to 42 tumors in 36 patients with all exophytic and parenchymal tumors up to 5 cm showing complete necrosis by imaging criteria *(30)*. Six-month followup was available in 20 patients without evidence of recurrent disease following complete coagulation necrosis. Additionally, another population was included—patients with VHL disease who are predisposed to multiple RCCs. In the past, tumors 3 cm or larger in patients with VHL were removed. However, surgery becomes progressively more difficult because of scarring induced by prior surgeries, and ultimately nephrectomies are often needed. As a result, patients become dialysis-dependent. Percutaneous RFA is a very attractive option in these patients to defer dialysis as long as possible.

In the initial Gervais series, RFA was performed with internally cooled electrodes with pulsed current. The choice of single or cluster electrodes was based on tumor size. In this series, three of the nine tumors fit the ideal characteristics of the small (<3 cm) exophytic tumor and all three were completely ablated with a single session. As tumor size increased or as the lesions became central, the tumors became more difficult to ablate completely. Nevertheless, all five exophytic tumors (up to 3.5 cm) were completely ablated. The larger exophytic tumors required more ablations, and one of the large exophytic tumors required a staged approach. All three central tumors in the Gervais series were also larger than 3 cm, and only one of these (3.4 cm) was free of enhancement following ablation. A single tumor with both central and exophytic components was also completely ablated. In our ongoing series, complications include two perinephric hematomas, one ureteral clot obstruction, one inreteral stricture, and one grounding pad burn.

With particular attention to the VHL population, Pavlovich et al. reported results of RFA in 24 tumors all less than 3 cm in diameter *(31)*. Twenty-two tumors were in patients with VHL disease, and two were in patients with hereditary papillary renal carcinoma. In these patients, RFA provides a promising minimally invasive nephron-sparing procedure that can be reapplied to new tumors as needed. In the Pavlovich series, all ablations were performed under intravenous (iv) sedation with a RITA 50 Watt Model 500 generator, and all patients had a minimum of 2 mo of followup by CT scan *(31)*. Of the 24 tumors, 19 (79%) were free of CT enhancement suggesting complete coagulation necrosis, whereas the remaining 5 tumors demonstrated focal areas of persistent enhancement. The lower rate of complete coagulation necrosis for these small tumors compared to the series of Gervais et al. may be related to the less powerful generator used in the Pavlovich series *(29,31)*. Alternatively, a more central tumor location may have limited coagulation necrosis in the five failures in the Pavlovich series because four of these five tumors were not exophytic *(31)*.

Comparison of the Gervais and Pavlovich series illustrates some of the limitations inherent in comparing the early reports of RFA. Different generators and different electrode design may produce different results. Additionally, the 50 Watt RITA generator used in the Pavlovich series has been replaced by a new 150 Watt generator that itself is likely to be upgraded in the future. Thus, constantly evolving technology limits generalizations based on past reports of RFA in the treatment of RCC.

## IMAGING AND RFA

The importance of image guidance during RFA has been emphasized. Equally important is imaging followup of RCC treated by RFA as imaging is the only noninvasive way to assess for residual active tumor. Because a tumor mass remains *in situ* with little decrease in size, active enhancement is the marker for live residual tumor *(29)*. This practice is based on extrapolation from radiological–patholigical correlation work in liver tumors *(21)*. Findings indicative of coagulation necrosis are absence of enhancement in previously enhancing tumor. CT is performed without and with iv contrast material. In patients with renal insufficiency, magnetic resonance imaging (MRI) without and with gadolineum-chelate enhancement can be performed.

## OTHER USES OF RFA IN THE TREATMENT OF RCC

Since the introduction of RFA for treatment of human RCC by Zlotta in 1997, other investigators have assessed the application of RFA for purposes other than primary tumor eradication. Two of these new applications take advantage of the cauterizing effects of RFA. In 2001, Wood et al. reported the use of RFA to treat a case of gross hematuria complicating a 7 cm RCC that invaded the urinary collecting system in a patient with a solitary kidney *(32)*. Selective arterial trans-catheter embolizaton had failed to control hematuria, and the patient underwent RFA with resolution of gross hematuria in 24 h. At our own institution, we have successfully treated a similar patient following multiple hospitalizations for gross hematuria. RFA, therefore, can be considered in cases of intractable hematuria in which surgical or other percutaneous alternatives would likely result in dialysis.

In a second application utilizing the coagulative effects of RFA, Gettmen et al., in 2001, reported their experience in the use of RF coagulation to produce hemostasis in the setting of laparoscopic partial nephrectomy (LPN) *(33)*. Ten patients with mean tumor size of 2.1 cm (range 1 to 3.2) underwent RFA of the tumor periphery with one of two RF generators (RITA Medical System, Mountain View, CA or RadioTherapeutics, Mountain View, CA) prior to laparoscopic removal of the tumor. RFA in this setting minimized blood loss and improved visualization of the operative region, thus facilitating the tumor removal. All but one patient had 300 mL or less of intraoperative blood loss. In this report, Gettman et al. anticipate the use of RFA in this setting may increase the scope of patients eligible for LPN, a procedure in which hemorrhagic problems are not uncommon *(5,33)*.

Reports of application of RFA to treat isolated foci of metastatic RCC appeared in 2001. Zagoria et al. reported a case of a RFA to treat two focal RCC metastasis to the lung *(34)*. Over 16 mo of followup there was no local recurrence or new metastases on CT. Gervais et al. presented two cases of isolated retrocrural lymph nodes with metastatic RCC treated with RFA with induction of complete coagulation necrosis at imaging and no local recurrence over 7 to 12 mo *(35)*. Clinical experience and followup in this application of RFA remains limited, and further studies will be needed to determine the ultimate role of RFA in the treatment of metastatic RCC. The use of RFA will likely be limited to a small subset of patients with isolated foci of disease because multifocal disease becomes impractical to treat with a local therapy. Although rigid limits are difficult to define, in practice, percutaneous application of RFA to more than three to five separate tumors is usually not performed as several ablation sessions are often needed depending on the size of the individual tumors.

## PATIENT TOLERANCE AND COMPLICATIONS

In both the Gervais and Pavlovich series, percutaneous image-guided RFA of RCC was generally well tolerated by patients *(29,31)*. Gervais et al. performed RFA as an outpatient procedure with hospital admissions reserved for patients with severe coagulation abnormalities, patients in the hospital for other indications who also have incidentally discovered RCC, and patients who experience complications following ablation *(29)*. Pavlovich et al. admitted their patients for a minimum of one night with most recovering uneventfully by the next morning *(31)*.

Pavlovich et al. reported no major complications in their series of 24 tumors *(31)*. Gervais et al. reported one major hemorrhage both into the perirenal space and into the collecting system of a solitary kidney following RFA of a large central tumor *(29)*. The patient required placement of a ureteral stent as the hemorrhage resulted in obstruction. These preliminary reports suggest that hemorrhagic complications may be more likely in large central tumors *(29,31)*.

## CONTROVERSIES, CURRENT LIMITATIONS, AND FUTURE DIRECTIONS

Early reports of RFA to treat small RCC are encouraging. Given the increase in incidentally discovered RCC in the aging population, minimally invasive techniques such as RFA are likely to continue to generate interest. However, the major hurdle for RFA remains to achieve longer followup periods. A minimum of 5-yr followup is needed to allow comparison of RFA to the results of the standards of nephrectomy and partial nephrectomy *(5)*. Given concerns about any therapeutic modality that leaves tumor *in situ*, more experience is needed to identify possible predictors of success or failure in achieving complete coagulation necrosis. Knowledge of these predictors in turn would facilitate triaging of patients to the most appropriate treatment modality. Finally, new technical developments in electrode design and in more powerful RF generators may overcome some limitations described in early reports.

Other technical developments involve the use of MRI-compatible ablation systems for percutaneous MRI-guided ablation. Preliminary reports of this technology have proved it safe *(36)*. Early results suggest that intraprocedural MRI imaging may allow mapping of residual non-necrotic tumor, thus guiding subsequent electrode placement and minimizing the likelihood of residual disease remaining *in situ* following ablation. Findings at the time of ablation under US or CT guidance have not been shown to predict residual disease reliably, and so a followup contrast-enhanced CT is used to assess the initial result *(29)*. MRI guidance may provide reliable assessment of residual tumor and allow electrode positioning as needed to coagulate larger tumors in a single ablation session, eliminating the need for a staged approach in larger tumors. At this time, MRI-compatible ablation systems are not commercially available in the United States, and most practitioners who perform percutaneous RFA use US or CT for imaging guidance. Finally, cryoablation of RCC is a competitive ablative therapy with recent technical developments that include development of percutaneous needles. Historically, cryoablation required an open approach. However, even with percutaneous application, cryoablation systems are more expensive and cumbersome than RFA systems.

## CONCLUSIONS

Early applications of RFA in the treatment of RCC have produced encouraging results, especially in the treatment of small, exophytic tumors. Five-year followup of RFA in the treatment of primary RCC is awaited. New developments that may reliably produce complete coagulation necrosis of larger and/or central tumors include more powerful RF generators, technical improvements in electrode design, and possibly intraprocedural MRI guidance. Additional applications of RFA in selected cases of RCC show promise. These other roles for RFA include control of gross hematuria from invasion of the collecting system, improved hemostasis during laparoscopic nephrectomy, and local control of isolated foci of metastatic disease.

## REFERENCES

1. Duque JL, Loughlin KR, O'Leary MP, Kumar S, Richie JP. Partial nephrectomy: alternative treatment of selected patients with renal cell carcinoma. Urology 1998; 52: 584–590.

2. Novick AC. Nephron-sparing surgery for renal cell carcinoma. Br J Urol 1998; 82: 321–324.
3. Gill IS. Retroperitoneal laparoscopic nephrectomy. Urol Clin North Am 1998; 25: 343–360.
4. Nakada SY, McDougall EM, Clayman RV. Laparoscopic extirpation of renal cell cancer: feasibility, questions, and concerns. Semin Surg Oncol 1996; 12: 100–112.
5. Uzzo RG, Novick AC. Nephron sparing surgery for renal tumors: Indications, techniques and outcomes. J Urol 2001; 166: 6–18.
6. Reddan DN, Raj GV, Polascik TJ. Management of small renal tumors: an overview. Am J Med 2001; 110: 58–562.
7. Moulton L, Grant J, Miller B, Moulton K. Radiofrequency catheter ablation for supraventricular tachycardia. Heart Lung 1993; 22: 3–14.
8. Moraci A, Buonaituo C, Punzo A, Parlato C, Amalfi R. Trigeminal neuralgia treated by percutaneous thermocoagulation. Comparative analysis of percutaneous thermocoagulation and other surgical procedures. Neurochirurgia 1992; 35: 48–53.
9. Rosenthal DI, Alexander A, Rosenberg AE, Springfield D. Ablation of osteoid osteomas with a percutaneously placed electrode: a new procedure. Radiology 1992; 183: 29–33.
10. McGahan JP, Browning PD, Brock JM, Tesluk H. Hepatic ablation using radiofrequency electrocautery. Invest Radiol 1990; 25: 267–270.
11. Goldberg SN, Gazelle GS, Halpern EF, Rittman WJ, Mueller PR, Rosenthal DI. Radiofrequency tissue ablation: importance of local temperature along the electrode tip exposure in determining lesion shape and size. Acad Radiol 1996; 3: 212–218.
12. Goldberg SN, Gazelle GS, Solbiati L, Rittman WJ, Mueller PR. Radiofrequency tissue ablation: increased lesion diameter with a perfusion electrode. Acad Radiol 1996; 3: 636–644.
13. Livraghi T, Goldberg SN, Monti F, et al. Saline-enhanced radiofrequency tissue ablation in the treatment of liver metastases. Radiology 1997; 202: 205–210.
14. Solbiati L, Goldberg SN, Ierace T, et al. Hepatic metastases: percutaneous radiofrequency ablation with cooled-tip electrodes. Radiology 1997; 205: 367–373.
15. Goldberg SN, Gazelle GS, Dawson SL, Rittman WJ, Mueller PR, Rosenthal DI. Tissue ablation with radiofrequency: effect of probe size, gauge, duration, and temperature on lesion volume. Acad Radiol 1995; 2: 399–404.
16. Goldberg SN, Gazelle GS, Dawson SL, Rittman WJ, Mueller PR, Rosenthal DI. Tissue ablation with radiofrequency using multiprobe arrays. Acad Radiol 1995; 2: 670–674.
17. Goldberg SN, Hahn PF, Tanabe KK, et al. Percutaneous radiofrequency tissue ablation: does perfusion mediated tisuse cooling limit coagulation necrosis? J Vasc Interv Radiol 1998; 9: 101–111.
18. Goldberg SN, Solbiati L, Hahn PF, et al. Large-volume tissue ablation with radio frequency by using a clustered internally cooled electrode technique: laboratory and clinical experience in liver metastases. Radiology 1998; 209: 371–379.
19. Goldberg SN, Hahn PF, Halpern EF, Fogle RM, Gazelle GS. Radio-frequency tissue ablation: effect of pharmacologic modulation of blood flow on coagulation diameter. Radiology 1998; 209: 761–767.
20. Goldberg SN, Stein MC, Gazelle GS, Sheiman RG, Kruskal JB, Clouse ME. Percutaneous radiofrequency tissue ablation: optimization of pulsed radiofrequency technique to increase coagulation necrosis. J Vasc Interv Radiol 1999; 10: 907–916.

21. Goldberg SN, Gazelle GS, Compton CC, Mueller PR, Tanabe KK. Treatment of intrahepeatic malignancy with radiofrequency ablation: radiologic-pathologic correlation. Cancer 2000; 88: 2452–2463.
22. Pennes HH. Analysis of tissue and arterial blood temperatures in the resting human forearm. J Appl Physiol 1948; 84: 1245–1248.
23. Goldberg SN, Gazelle GS, Mueller PR. Thermal ablation therapy for focal malignancy: a unifed approach to underlying principles, techniques, and diagnostic imaging guidance. AJR Am J Roentgenol 2000; 174: 323–331.
24. Livraghi T, Goldberg SN, Lazzaroni S, Meloni F, Solbiati L, Gazelle GS. Small hepatocellular carcinoma: treatment with radiofrequency ablation versus ethanol injection. Radiology 1999; 210: 655–661.
25. Dupuy DE, Hong R, Oliver B, Goldberg SN. Radiofrequency ablation of spinal tumors: temperature distribution in the spinal canal. AJR Am J Roentgenol 2000; 175: 1262–1266.
26. Zlotta AR, Wildschutz T, Raviv G, et al. Radiofrequency interstitial tumor ablation (RITA) is a possible new modality for treat.ment of renal cancer: ex vivo and in vivo experience. J Endourol 1997; 11: 251–258.
27. McGovern FJ, Wood BJ, Goldberg SN, Mueller PR. Radio frequency ablation of renal cell carcinoma via image guided needle electrodes. J Urol 1999; 161: 599–600.
28. Hall WH, McGahan JP, Link DP, deVere White RW. Combinded embolization and percutaneous radiofrequency ablation of a solid renal tumor. AJR Am J Roentgenol 2000; 174: 1592–1594.
29. Gervais DA, McGovern FJ, Wood BJ, Goldberg SN, McDougal WS, Mueller PR. Radio-frequency ablation of renal cell carcinoma: early clinical experience. Radiology 2000; 217: 665–672.
30. Gervais DA, Arellano R, McGovern FJ, McDougal WS, Mueller PR. Radio-frequency (RF) ablation of renal tumors: Logistics of initiating a program, triaging/radiologic management, and clinical follow-up—lessons learned over 4 years and 90 ablations. Radiology 2001; 221(P): 261.
31. Pavlovich CP, Walther MM, Choyke PL, et al. Percutaneous radio frequency ablation of small renal tumors: initial results. J Urol 2002; 167: 10–15.
32. Wood BJ, Grippo J, Pavlovich CP. Percutaneous radio frequency ablation for hematuria. J Urol 2001; 166: 2303–2304.
33. Gettman MT, Bishoff JT, Su LM, et al. Hemostatic laparoscopic partial nephrectomy: initial experience with the radiofrequency coagulation-assisted technique . Urology 2001; 58: 8–11.
34. Zagoria RJ, Chen MY, Kavanagh PV, Torti FM. Radio frequency ablation of lung metastases from renal cell carcinoma. J Urol 2001; 166: 1827–1828.
35. Gervais DA, Arellano R, McDougal WS, McGovern FJ, Mueller PR. Radiofrequency (RF) ablation of metastatic soft tissue tumors of the genitourinary system: indications, results, and the role of RFA after failed conventional therapies. Radiology 2001; 221(P): 261.
36. Lewin JS, Connell CF, Duerk JL, et al. Interactive MRI-guided radiofrequency interstitial thermal ablation of abdominal tumors: clinical trial for evaluation of safety and feasibility. J Magn Reson Imaging 1998; 8: 40–47.

# II

# Transitional Cell Carcinoma of the Ureter and Renal Pelvis

# 9 Laparoscopic Nephroureterectomy

*Herkanwal S. Khaira,* MD
*and J. Stuart Wolf, Jr.,* MD

*CONTENTS*

INTRODUCTION
INDICATIONS
TECHNIQUE
PREOPERATIVE PREPARATION
TRANSPERITONEAL LNU
HALNU
RETROPERITONEOSCOPIC NEPHROURETERECTOMY
MANAGEMENT OF THE DISTAL URETER
RESULTS
SUMMARY
REFERENCES

## INTRODUCTION

Upper urinary tract urothelial carcinoma is an uncommon entity composing 4.5–9% of all renal malignancies and 5–6% of all urothelial tumors *(1–5)*. The current treatment standard is *en bloc* removal of the kidney, ureter, ipsilateral ureteral orifice, and a surrounding 1-cm bladder cuff *(6)*. Surgical treatment has traditionally been performed through an open approach; this involves either a large flank incision extending toward the pubis, or two incisions, one involving the flank and the other

From: *Laparoscopic Urologic Oncology*
Edited by: J. A. Cadeddu © Humana Press Inc., Totowa, NJ

the lower abdomen. In 1991, Clayman and colleagues described the first laparoscopic nephroureterectomy (LNU) *(7)*. Today, LNU is an effective alternative to open surgery with advantages that include shorter convalescence and decreased postoperative discomfort.

## INDICATIONS

The indications for LNU are similar to those for the open surgery. The most common indication is organ-confined urothelial carcinoma involving the renal pelvis and/or ureter. Nephroureterectomy is also appropriate for end-stage upper tract disease secondary to tuberculosis and vesicoureteral reflux. The procedure has been successfully performed in both adult and pediatric populations *(8–10)*. This chapter focuses on the oncologic indications, techniques, and outcomes of LNU. The oncologic principles of LNU are detailed with attention on distal ureteral management techniques.

Appropriate planning necessitates that the surgeon considers treatment alternatives to nephroureterectomy. For low-grade solitary tumors both antegrade and retrograde endoscopic treatment have been used effectively *(11)*. Patients with solitary kidneys, renal insufficiency, bilateral tumors or high anesthetic risks should be considered for endoscopic therapy *(12–15)*.

The contraindications to LNU are similar to those of open nephroureterectomy. As with the open procedure, the urothelial carcinoma should be organ confined. Once urothelial carcinoma is diagnosed, preoperative evaluation includes abdominal computed tomography (CT), chest radiography, a complete blood count, and complete serum chemistry. A bone scan is performed if there is bone pain, the alkaline phosphatase is elevated, or if bony abnormalities are seen on other imaging studies. A careful discussion of risks, benefits, and consequences of surgery should be held with the patient prior to the laparoscopic procedure. Notably, patients should be forewarned of the potential for worsening renal function, especially among those with preoperative renal insufficiency. The risks of any major surgical procedure (cardiovascular complications, infection, organ injury, need for re-operation, etc.) should be discussed, as well as the complications unique to laparoscopic intervention (gas embolus, hypercapnia, and potential for conversion to open surgery). Distal ureteral tumors should be approached very cautiously with LNU; the technique is better suited for more proximal lesions. Particularly, the choice of bladder cuff management technique should minimize potential leak of urine containing malignant cells.

Morcellation in an entrapment is not advised following nephroureterectomy for urothelial carcinoma. Unlike renal cell carcinoma

(RCC), the pathological stage of urothelial carcinoma might suggest need for adjuvant chemotherapy. Additionally, urothelial carcinoma more so than RCC has the potential for implantation into wounds. These considerations argue for intact specimen removal. The specimen may be extracted via an incision at the end of a pure LNU or through the hand incision site for hand-assisted laparoscopic nephroureterectomy (HALNU).

## TECHNIQUE

Nephroureterectomy may be accomplished laparoscopically via a standard transperitoneal approach, with hand assistance, or with retroperitoneoscopy. Each method has merits and varying degrees of difficulty. Retroperitoneoscopic nephroureterectomy avoids entering the peritoneum and offers rapid access to the renal hilum, but is rendered difficult by the limited working space and unfamiliar anatomic approach. Standard transperitoneal laparoscopy offers clearer landmarks, a larger working space, and better access to the distal ureter. HALNU (transperitoneal) offers the same advantages as the standard transperitoneal approach, but with technical simplification that reduces operative time for most surgeons. It does, however, require a larger incision than might otherwise be required only for specimen extraction.

## PREOPERATIVE PREPARATION

For transperitoneal approaches, the patient is instructed to start a clear liquid diet 24 h prior to surgery. The patient takes an oral laxative such as Fleet's Phosphasoda or magnesium citrate the day before surgery. For retroperitoneoscopic nephroureterectomy, a bowel preparation is not necessary. Because the bladder will be addressed in some manner, intravenous (iv) antibiotics are recommended. Positioning depends on the approach to the nephrectomy portion of the procedure, and whether the ureter is addressed before or after the nephrectomy.

## TRANSPERITONEAL LNU

For the nephrectomy portion, the patient is placed in the flank or semi-flank position. Some authors recommend flexing the table and raising the kidney rest, but we have found that this does not improve exposure, and moreover increases the risk of neuromuscular injury *(16)*. A Foley catheter and orogastric tube are inserted and secured. Standard transperitoneal LNU may be performed with three to five trocar ports. A five-port configuration is typical; four 12-mm ports are used: (1)

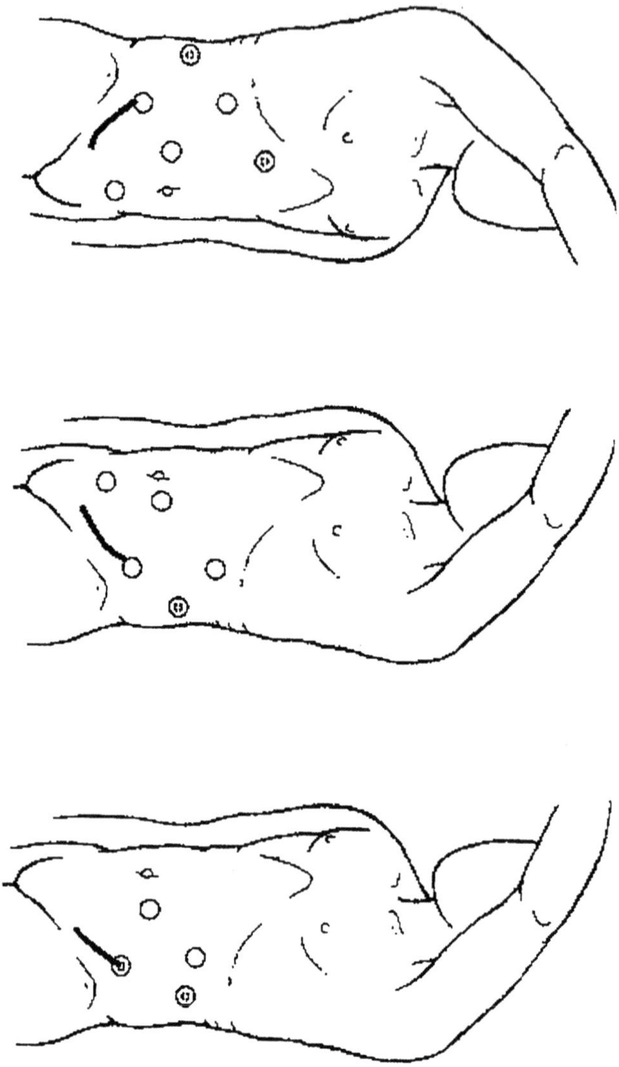

**Fig. 1.** Transperitoneal nephroureterectomy port location sites (open circle = 12 mm, dotted circle = 5 mm). Reproduced from ref. *17*.

supraumbilical midclavicular line, (2) subcostal anterior axillary line, (3) anterior axillary line above the iliac crest, (4) lower midline, with a 5-mm fifth port in the posterior axillary line *(17)* (Fig. 1). The nephrectomy portion of all the procedures follows the basic principles for standard laparoscopic nephrectomy.

The peritoneum is incised at the line of Toldt and the colon is reflected infero-medially. The gonadal vein is transected and the ureter is freed from the retroperitoneal tissue. Generally, the ureter can be dissected below the iliac vessels, proximal to the ureterovesical junction (UVJ). Care is taken to maintain generous periureteral tissue, which helps prevent violations of the ureteral lumen and ensure negative margins. The lower and upper poles of the kidney are then freed of attachments. Dissection is performed to maintain the integrity of Gerota's fascia if there is any concern for invasive disease *(18)*. If the upper pole is uninvolved the adrenal can be spared. Nodal dissection aids pathologic staging, but is not necessary if metastatic disease is not suspected *(19,20)*. The renal artery is ligated with endoscopic clips and incised. The renal vein is taken with the endoscopic vascular stapler. The kidney is then freed of all lateral and superior attachments. A clip is placed on the proximal ureter for patients with renal pelvic tumors to reduce the risk of malignant urine extravasation during distal ureteral dissection. Following management of the distal ureter (discussed later), the specimen is removed intact via a Pfannenstiel, Gibson, or midline incision.

## HALNU

Hand assistance allows the surgeon to maintain better tactile connection with the operative field, improves laparoscopic proprioception, facilitates the surgeon's ability to manipulate the intra-abdominal contents, and perhaps most importantly provides the surgeon with better control, especially early in the surgeon's laparoscopic experience. Even accomplished laparoscopists, however, feel the hand-assisted approach is optimal for a procedure that requires intact specimen removal, such as nephroureterectomy for malignancy. This is the preferred laparoscopic approach for nephroureterectomy at the authors' institution. The inevitable incision is utilized throughout the procedure via placement of a hand-assistance device, rather than making it at the conclusion of an otherwise standard laparoscopic procedure. Additionally, the hand-assistance port may be used for distal ureteral management, which is discussed later.

For HALNU, various positions and port configurations have been reported, some of which involve intraoperative repositioning. We place the patient in a modified flank position at 45° with the ipsilateral arm supported on an arm board anterior to the patient. Preparation is otherwise identical to the transperitoneal procedure.

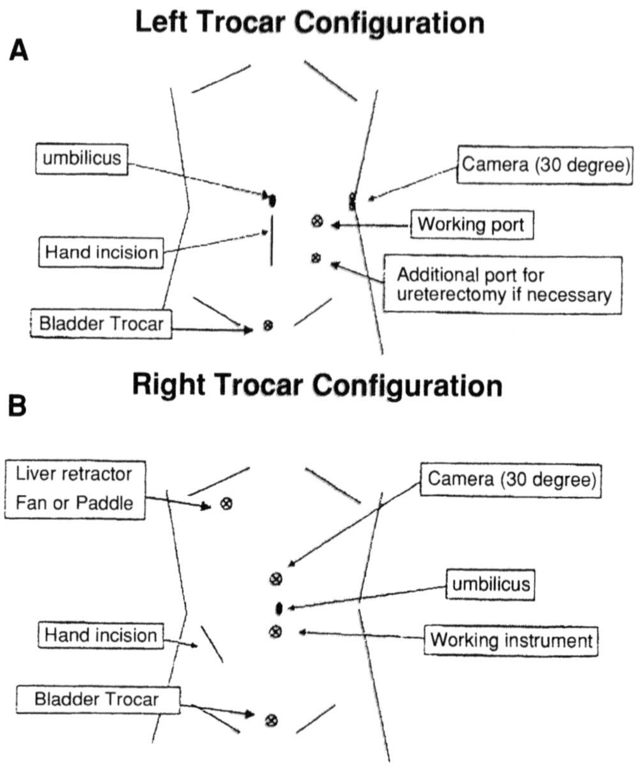


**Fig. 2. (A)** Left and **(B)** right. Trocar and incision placement location for hand-assisted nephroureterectomy. Reprinted form ref. *47*.

Typically, the HALNU incision is 7–9 cm in length, made midline around the umbilicus. A commercially available hand-assistance device is inserted, to maintain pneumoperitoneum. When open bladder cuff management is anticipated, a lower midline or Gibson (oblique, lower abdominal) incision may be used *(21)*. The laparoscopic trocars are placed in the following locations: a 12-mm anterior axillary line port at the level of the umbilicus, which will serve as the camera site, an upper midclavicular line 12-mm port, and a lower midclavicular line 5 mm port (Fig. 2). The nephrectomy and proximal ureteral dissection then proceed in standard fashion, and the ureteral cuff is managed with one of the techniques discussed later. Specimen extraction is performed through the incision for the hand-assistance device.

## RETROPERITONEOSCOPIC NEPHROURETERECTOMY

After placing the patient in the flank position with the table flexed (which, as opposed to positioning during the transperitoneal approach, is necessary for optimal exposure and port placement), the retroperitoneum is opened either with a balloon dilator or with blunt finger dissection through an incision below the tip of the 12th rib *(22,23)*. With the balloon dilator, Gerota's fascia is initially mobilized anteriorly. Subsequently, the balloon is placed more caudally and reinflated. The second dilation allows for identification and mobilization of the ureter *(24)*. Once the peritoneum is mobilized anteriorly, a 12-mm port is placed at the initial incision site, a 5-mm port is placed 3 cm above the iliac crest anterior to the midaxillary line, and a 12-mm port at the inferior border of the 12th rib at the erector spinae lateral border *(25)*. A 5- or 10-mm port at the tip of the 11th rib may be needed for retraction (Fig. 3). The ureter is ligated early to prevent accidental spillage of urine. The renal hilum is controlled and the kidney is mobilized external to Gerota's. The ureter is then retracted superiorly and dissected free of the retroperitoneum distally. The bladder cuff is managed in one of the manners indicated later. The entire specimen can then be removed intact through a previous open incision *(26)* or a new Gibson incision.

## MANAGEMENT OF THE DISTAL URETER

There are a variety of management options for securing the distal ureter during LNU. Distal ureterectomy with bladder cuff may precede or follow nephrectomy, depending on the technique used. If a technique that occludes the ureter early in the case is chosen, challenges could arise during a prolonged nephrectomy or if the nephrectomy has to be aborted for some reason. Other considerations include the need for an additional bladder incision, options for repositioning, the specific laparoscopic approach to the nephrectomy portion of the procedure, and surgeon preference. Some of the techniques are better suited for hand-assisted or retroperitoneoscopic approaches, but with modification any of them can be used with any type of LNU. The most important factor in the choice of technique may be the potential for tumor cell spillage. The authors prefer to perform the nephroureterectomy primarily, followed by securement of the distal ureter with a technique that reduces the potential for local tumor spillage *(27)*. Unfortunately, the total popu-

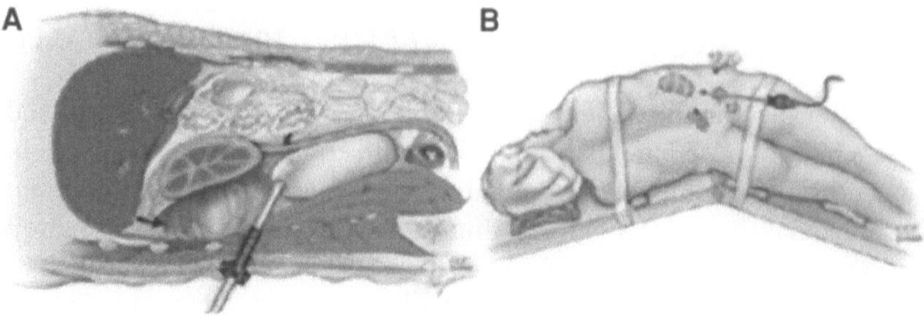


**Fig. 3.** **(A)** Retroperitoneoscopic nephroureterectomy using the dilation technique. Initial balloon dilation is cephalad towards kidney, creating working space (straight arrow). Second balloon dilation is caudally along anterior psoas displacing ureter anteriorly (curved arrow). **(B)** Port placement locations. (Reproduced from ref. *46*.)

lation size and followup period for LNU is limited and therefore long-term comparative analysis of the different techniques is not yet possible.

## *Ureteral Dissection Before Nephrectomy*

### Ureteral Unroofing with Laparoscopic Bladder Cuff Stapling *(28)*

At the onset, the patient is placed in the dorsal lithotomy position and the ipsilateral ureteral orifice is intubated with a guidewire under cystoscopic guidance. A 7 French ureteral balloon dilator (5-mm diameter) is placed over the wire. Under fluoroscopic guidance, dilute contrast material is used to inflate the balloon in the distal ureter to low pressure (1 atmosphere). A 24 French resectoscope with an Orandi electrosurgical knife is used to unroof the ureteral orifice. The intramural ureter is then fulgurated with a rollerball. A balloon occlusion catheter is placed in the renal pelvis and the catheter is secured to a bladder Foley catheter. After the nephrectomy portion, the distal ureter is freed from the peri-ureteral tissue to the level of the bladder. The superior vesicle artery is ligated, as are the medial umbilical ligament and the vas deferens or round ligament. The bladder around the ureteral vesical junction is cleared and the ureter is retracted supero-laterally. The ureteral balloon is deflated and removed and an endoscopic stapler is used to transect the bladder cuff. Integrity of the urinary tract is maintained throughout the procedure if the initial ureteral unroofing incision is not extended too far. Irrigation of the Foley catheter confirms watertight closure and bladder leaks may be suture repaired. The theoretic risk of calculus formation along the staple line has not been demonstrated in more than 2 yr of followup. The group that originated this technique recently noted that

8% of patients developed retroperitoneal metastatic disease postoperatively contrasted by 0% of patients treated with open surgery. A large concern has been whether distal ureteral management was responsible for the recurrence rate disparity *(29)*. Typically, unroofing and stapling should not permit urinary spillage, particularly from the affected ureter. Nevertheless, the group affected measures to further reduce the risk of urinary spillage by proceeding with ureteral unroofing after bladder cuff stapling. Long-term studies will likely delineate the hazards of early vs late ureteral unroofing. Presently, for such small followup, no conclusive determination of increased risk can yet be made.

### Pluck Technique

With initial positioning in lithotomy, the bladder is entered with the resectoscope. The ureteral orifice and intramural ureter are either incised circumferentially with an Orandi knife, or resected with a loop electrode, to the level of the perivesical fat. The patient is then repositioned and the nephrectomy portion proceeds as usual. The ureter is dissected laparoscopically as far caudally as possible. The ureter is then retracted cephalad and the most distal dissection proceeds. Ultimately, the ureter detaches at the site of the previous endoscopic resection. The small cystotomy where the ureter was removed is not closed. The catheter remains for 1 wk, and a cystogram is performed prior to removal to confirm closure. There have been case reports of retrovesical recurrence of the urothelial carcinoma following the pluck procedure, possibly due to extravasation of tumor-laden urine *(30,31)*. Therefore, it is advisable to limit urine leak by prompt occlusion of the detached ureter prior to extraction. A modification of the pluck technique that may reduce urine extravasation involves placement of a balloon occlusion catheter up the ureter into renal pelvis (or below a proximal ureteral tumor if present) which is then snugged down at the ureteropelvic junction. Mitomycin can be instilled into the renal pelvis through this catheter as well *(32)*. This was the method used by the authors in our early experience, but we have now adopted the transvesical bladder cuff technique (discussed later) to further minimize the risk of tumor seeding.

### Transvesical Bladder Cuff Technique—Two Ports

Gill and colleagues have described a technique for bladder cuff management that modifies the pluck technique to prevent urine spillage. The patient is placed in lithotomy, the bladder is endoscopically entered, and the affected ureteral orifice is identified. Two needlescopic 2-mm ports are inserted into the bladder and placed to wall suction *(24)*. A 2-mm endoloop is then placed near the ureteral orifice. Through a cystoscope, a ureteral catheter is passed through the endoloop to intubate the ureteral orifice. The ureteral orifice is retracted anterior-medially with a grasper through a suprapubic port. A Collin's knife is then used endoscopically to circumferentially detach the ureter from the detrusor. The dissection is continued until 3 to 4 cm of the intramural ureter is freed into the bladder; this is accomplished by maintaining continued anterior-medial traction of the ureteral orifice. At this point, the 2-mm endoloop tie is closed occluding the distal ureter. The suprapubic ports are removed, a Foley catheter is placed to drainage, and the nephrectomy proceeds normally after repositioning the patient. When the distal ureter is encountered laparoscopically, it can be removed via the previously described pluck technique. A Foley catheter is left for 1 wk and may be removed after a negative cystogram. The 90° angle between the suprapubic retractors and transurethral endoscope may be challenging and add to the learning curve of this technique *(33)*. Initially, the technique was complicated by irrigant extravasation that necessitated drainage; however, placing the suprapubic ports to suction has eliminated this problem. The technique lengthens operative time by 60–90 min *(34)*, but compared with the standard "pluck" method, this technique better maintains the oncologic principles of the nephroureterectomy by preventing urine spillage.

### Ureteral Intussusception Technique

With initial placement of the patient in lithotomy, a stone basket is inserted in the proximal ureter/renal pelvis cystoscopically. After repositioning and completion of the nephrectomy, the proximal ureter is occluded with laparoscopic clips to prevent urine spillage, and then divided distal to the clips. The proximal end of the ureteral stump is incised longitudinally. The stone basket is advanced, opened, and then used to firmly grasp the two ureteral leaflet edges. Just distal to the basket, the adventia of the ureter is firmly held with the laparoscopic grasper and then the basket is retracted. This intussuscepts the ureter, which may then be completely extracted into the bladder. With the ureter under tension, a resectoscope with an Orandi knife is inserted transurethrally (after repositioning the patient into lithotomy) and used to detach the ureter. Alternatively, prior to placement of the ureteral basket, the bladder around the ureter can be incised with an endoscopic cautery knife. Following the procedure, a Foley catheter should be left in place for 7 d with a negative cystogram performed prior to catheter removal. The intussusception technique should be reserved for patients with renal pelvic tumors. Invasive ureteral tumors may not be completely removed by this technique. If the ureter is fibrosed from prior injury or infection, the intussusception technique may be more challenging or impossible *(35,36)*.

## *Ureteral Dissection After Nephrectomy*

### Open Ureteral Resection *(26)*

Open resection can proceed through a lower midline or through a muscle-splitting Gibson incision after the nephrectomy. The bladder cuff can be resected with an intra or extravesical approach. For the extravesical approach, the bladder cuff is grasped with a right angle clamp and bladder closure sutures are placed. The UVJ is circumferentially incised removing a 1-cm bladder cuff. The distal ureter is then occluded, and the bladder is immediately closed. For the intravesical approach, the bladder is opened anteriorly between stay sutures, the ipsilateral ureteral orifice is pulled up with a suture, and the ureter is sharply dissected out from within the bladder. Both the resection site and the anterior cystotomy are closed with sutures. These techniques do not require intraoperative cystoscopy, and benefit from complete bladder closure, which allows for early catheter removal. Depending on the technique used for the nephrectomy, repositioning may be necessary. The open incision is additionally used for intact specimen extraction. Alternatively, the open bladder cuff incision may be similarly performed as the first stage of an HALNU. This technique entails retroperitoneal management of the distal ureter and bladder cuff *(21)*. Subsequently, the peritoneum is opened through the Gibson incision and this site is used for placement of the hand-assistance device for the nephrectomy portion of the procedure. For any HALNU, the incision for the hand-assistance device can be made in the lower abdomen; this allows open resection of the bladder cuff though the same incision. The lower placement of the incision, however, can make dissection of the kidney, particularly the upper pole, more challenging. Open surgical ureteral management maintains integrity of the urinary tract and avoids spillage of urine potentially laden with malignant cells.

### Laparoscopic Extravesical Cuff with Bladder Closure *(37)*

This technique may be used in conjunction with hand-assisted or standard laparoscopy. Typically, an additional 10-mm trocar will be necessary in the lower abdomen. A ureteral catheter should be placed at the start of the procedure and the ureter should be occluded distal to the level of the tumor. Following nephrectomy, the upper ureter is retracted with a locking grasper. The distal ureter is identified and with electocautery a bladder cuff is incised around the UVJ. The ureteral catheter is identified, divided and the specimen is removed intact. Pneumoperitoneum is re-established and the bladder is then suture closed. The bladder suture may be tied with intracorporeal knot tying or a laparoscopic stitch device may be employed. Potential malignant urine spillage with this technique is minimal because the ureter is occluded proximally prior to removal. The bladder closure reduces the risk of spillage of an undetected bladder tumor, while facilitating earlier removal of the Foley catheter.

### Transvesical Bladder Cuff Technique—One Port *(27)*

Upon completion of the nephrectomy and distal ureteral lysis, including placement of clips on the ureter to occlude it, the surgeon's hand is placed through the hand-assistance port to push the bladder (which has been filled through the Foley catheter) anteriorly. A 10-mm trocar is extraperitoneally placed into the bladder through a small suprapubic incision following confirmation of bladder location with a spinal needle. A 24 Fr nephroscope with offset lens (or resectoscope) is then placed through the port and the ureteral orifice and bladder cuff are excised with a Collin's knife. During this portion, the intra-abdominal hand elevates the bladder for exposure and the bladder is drained through the Foley catheter (Fig. 4). When the cuff is completely detached, the nephroureterectomy specimen is then removed intact through the hand port. The bladder is left to Foley drainage, and an extraperitoneal drain may be placed at the surgeon's discretion. This technique, which has become the first choice of the authors, benefits from the surgeon's hand posterior to the bladder, elevating the hemitrigone and ensuring appropriate size cuff excision. The ureter is occluded, which reduces risk of tumor seeding, and repositioning is not necessary. The only disadvantage is placement of a single port into the bladder. This disadvantage can be obviated by performing the excision transurethrally. One option is to use a flexible cystoscope with an electrocautery probe to excise the bladder cuff. Another alternative is to position the patient in a combined lithotomy—semiflank position, which allows simultaneous laparoscopic nephrectomy and transurethral access with a 24 French resectoscope for the excision *(38)*.

## RESULTS

Laparoscopic approaches for treating upper tract urothelial carcinoma have rapidly developed over the past decade. Immediate and short-term outcomes data demonstrate improved postoperative convalescence and patient comfort. Oncologic outcome data is constrained due to limited long-term followup data. To date, patients treated with LNU have had similar recurrence and survival rates compared with patients treated with open surgery. Specific areas of concern for LNU are the oncologic

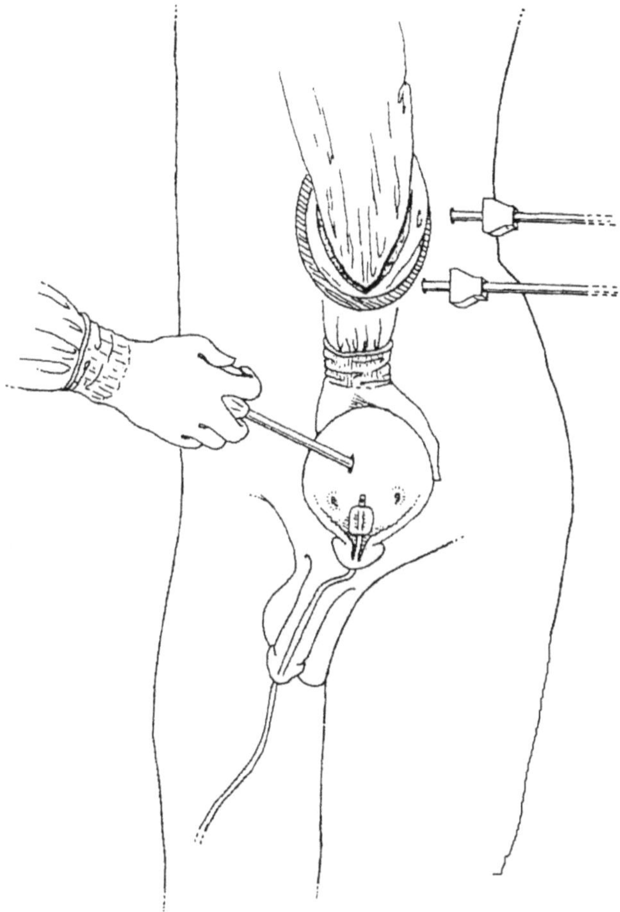

**Fig. 4.** Transvesical bladder cuff technique: 10-mm laparoscopic trocar inserted into distended bladder while surgeon's left hand pushes bladder anteriorly. (Reproduced from ref. *27*.)

efficiency of various distal ureteral management techniques and the hazards of specimen manipulation.

During nephroureterectomy, retroperitoneal and pelvic tumor seeding is a potential adverse consequence. Clearly, higher stage and aggressive grade carcinomas increase the risk for local and distant recurrence *(6)*; both risk factors cannot be fully determined preoperatively. Therefore, management strategy should focus on strict maintenance of oncologic principles. Operative techniques that permit urine to enter the pelvic space have consequently faced great criticism. Sporadic case reports have warned of local recurrence with various distal ureteral

Table 1
Results of Laparoscopic Nephroureterectomy for Urothelial Carcinoma

| *Author (reference)* | *No. pts.* | *Technique* | *Ureteral orifice* | *Age* | *OR time (min)* | *MSO4 (mg)* | *Hosp. (d)* | *Conval. (d)* | *Minor comp (%)* | *Major comp (%)* | *Conv.* | *No. w/ FU* | *FU (mo)* | *Non-vesial recur.* | *Vesical recur.* |
|---|---|---|---|---|---|---|---|---|---|---|---|---|---|---|---|
| McNeill *(45)* | 25 | TP | Pluck, Open | NA | 165 | NA | 9.1 | NA | 16 | 4 | 3 | NA | 32.9 | NA | NA |
| Salomon *(26)* | 4 | RP | Open | 68 | 220 | 10 | 5.7 | NA | 0 | 0 | 0 | 4 | 19 | 1 | 0 |
| Shalhav *(42)* | 25 | TP | Uret unroof | 70 | 462 | 37 | 3.6* | 19.6 | 40 | 8 | 0 | 25 | 39 | 5 | 7 |
| Gill *(46)* | 42 | RP | Endo cuff | 72 | 225 | 26 | 2.3 | 32.9 | 7 | 5 | 2 | 35 | 11.1 | 3 | 8 |
| Stifelman *(47)* | 22 | HALS | Endo cuff | 65 | 272 | 55 | 4.1 | 19 | NA | NA | 0 | 22 | 13 | 2 | 4 |
| Seifman *(32)* | 16 | HALS | Pluck | 71 | 321 | 48 | 3.9 | 18 | 19 | 19 | 1 | 16 | 18 | 0 | 3 |
| McGinnis *(37)* | 32 | HALS | Lap cuff | 67 | 372 | NA | 5.5 | NA | 22 | 9 | 0 | 28 | 13 | 0 | 6 |
| Chen *(21)* | 7 | HALS | Open | 67 | 224 | 38 | 7.3 | 26 | NA | NA | 0 | NA | 7.8 | 0 | 1 |
| Jarrett *(48)* | 25 | TP, HALS | Open, Lap cuff | 63 | 329 | NA | 4 | NA | 24 | 12 | 1 | 25 | 24.2 | 4 | 4 |
| Landman *(41)* | 16 | HALS | Uret unroof. open | 66 | 294 | 33 | 4.5 | 25 | 13 | 19 | 1 | 15 | 27.4 | 3 | 4 |
| Totals | 189 | | | 68 | 288.4 | 35.3 | 5.0 | 23.4 | 17.6 | 9.5 | 0.8 | 21 | 20.5 | 2.0 (11%) | 4.1 (23%) |

*excluding two major complications.

Pt = patients; OR = operating room; Hosp. = hospital; conval. = convalescence; comp. = complications; conv. = conversions; FU = followup; recur = recurrence; TP = transperitoneal; RP = retroperitoneal; HALS = hand-assisted laparoscopic surgery; NA = not available.

management techniques. Tumor recurrence at the site of ureteral detachment has been found with traditional "pluck" ureterectomy during open nephroureterectomy *(30,31)*. Similarly, tumor recurrence at the site of an endoscopic resected ureter has been reported with modified open nephroureterectomy *(39)*. The relationship between urine spillage and ureteral management technique, however, has not been firmly established *(40)*. Although local recurrences have been reported with the pluck technique, they have also been seen with open and ureteral unroofing methods *(26,41,42)* that supposedly avoid urine leakage. Nevertheless, the case reports underscore the genuine potential for seeding of the retroperitoneum and pelvis from urine spillage or inadequate bladder cuff margins. As case series numbers expand, the relationship between local recurrence and distal ureteral management technique will better define the risks of urine spillage. Regardless, careful management of the bladder cuff with limited urine spillage, ureteral occlusion when feasible, and generous margins should be routinely employed during all nephroureterectomies.

Port-site recurrence is another potential complication during LNU. Renal bed and subcutaneous recurrence after an uncomplicated, transperitoneal laparoscopic nephroureterectomy with transurethral resection of the ureteral orifice has been reported *(43)*. Despite intact specimen removal, a metastatic recurrence involved the port site 8 mo postoperatively. Port-site metastasis has also been noted following laparoscopic nephrectomy with unsuspected upper tract carcinoma. In this case, the specimen was removed intact with a torn entrapment sack *(44)*. These reports are infrequent, however, port-site metastasis is a genuine risk for laparoscopic nephroureterectomy. In order to reduce the risk, an entrapment sack should always be employed during specimen removal. Morcellation is inappropriate in laparoscopic nephroureterectomy. Pathologic staging is inadequate with morcellation and port-site seeding associated with potential entrapment sack compromise diminishes possible benefits of the procedure.

The followup studies of laparoscopic nephroureterectomy have shown favorable oncologic control and postoperative recovery outcomes (Table 1). When compared with open controls, individual institutional study groups exhibited improved immediate and short-term outcomes. Subjects followed for 7–33 mo demonstrated improvements across the board for immediate operative results and patient comfort measures.

Among studies comparing retroperitoneal, transperitoneal nephroureterctomy, and HALNU with open surgery, there were significant

Table 2
Comparison of Results of Laparoscopic and Open Nephroureterectomy

| *Author (reference)* | *No. pts* | *Route* | *Or time (min)* | *MSO4 (mg)* | *Hospital stay (d)* | *Convalescence (d)* | *Minor complications* | *Major complications* | *Conversions* | *No. with followup* | *Followup (mo)* | *Nonvesical recur* | *% Nonvesical recur* | *Vesical recur* | *% Vesical recur* |
|---|---|---|---|---|---|---|---|---|---|---|---|---|---|---|---|
| Gill *(46)* | 42 | RP | 225 | 26 | 2.3 | 32.9 | 3 | 2 | 2 | 35 | 11.1 | 3 | 8.6% | 8 | 22.9% |
| | 35 | Open | 280 | 228 | 6.6 | 57 | 9 | 1 | | 30 | 34.4 | 4 | 13.3% | 11 | 36.7% |
| | | % Lap over Open | 80% | 11% | 35% | 58% | 28% | 167% | | | | 64% | | 62% | |
| McNeill *(45)* | 25 | TP | 165 | | 9.1 | | 4 | 1 | 3 | | 32.9 | | | | |
| | 42 | Open | 165 | | 10.7 | | 7 | 2 | | | 42.3 | | | | |
| | | % Lap over Open | 100% | | 85% | | 96% | 84% | | | | | | | |
| Shalhav *(42)* | 25 | TP | 462 | 37 | 3.6 | 19.6 | 10 | 2 | 0 | 25 | 39 | 5 | 20% | 7 | 28% |
| | 17 | Open | 234 | 144 | 9.6 | 70 | 5 | 5 | | 13 | 43 | 3 | 23.1% | 7 | 53.8% |
| | | % Lap over Open | 197% | 26% | 38% | 28% | 136% | 27% | | | | 87% | | 52% | |
| Chen *(21)* | 7 | HALS | 224 | 38 | 7.3 | 26 | | | 0 | | 7.8 | 0 | 0% | 1 | 14.3% |
| | 15 | Open | 216 | 70 | 9.1 | 39 | | | | | 6.5 | 0 | 0% | 3 | 20.0% |
| | | % Lap over Open | 104% | 54% | 80% | 67% | | | | | 120% | | | 72% | |
| Seifman *(32)* | 16 | HALS | 321 | 48 | 3.9 | 18 | 3 | 3 | 1 | 16 | 18 | 0 | 0% | 3 | 18.8% |
| | 11 | Open | 199 | 81 | 5.2 | 38 | 5 | 3 | | 11 | 15 | 4 | 36.4% | 3 | 27.3% |
| | | % Lap over Open | 161% | 59% | 75% | 47% | 41% | 69% | | | | 0% | | 69% | |
| Totals | 235 | % Lap over Open | 129% | 38% | 63% | 50% | 75% | 87% | | | | 50% | | 64% | |

Pts = patients; OR = operating room; recur = recurrence; RP = retroperitoneal; TP = transperitoneal; HALS = hand-assisted laparoscopic surgery.

reductions in postoperative analgesia requirements, convalescence, time to oral intake, and hospital stay (Table 2). There were no significant differences in the complication rates between the individual laparoscopic and open groups. Oncologic outcome measures were similar in the groups. Bladder recurrence rates, distant metastasis rates, and cancer-specific survival were equivalent in the limited followup.

Cross-institutional comparisons of the different laparoscopic approaches to nephroureterectomy lack standardization. Therefore, there is limited valid comparative analysis between transperitoneal, retroperitoneal nephroureterectomy, and HALNU. Recently, however, a single institution performed comparison between standard nephroureterectomy and HALNU *(41)*. Operative time trended toward reduction in the hand-assisted procedure. Analgesic requirements, hospital stay, complication rates, blood loss, and time to recovery were equivalent between the two groups. The bladder and distant recurrence rates among the HALNU group were consistent with the rates among standard laparoscopy patients.

## SUMMARY

LNU appears to be an effective technique for the management of upper tract urothelial carcinoma. Presently, the urologic surgeon may choose from a variety of approaches for performing the operation. HALNU, standard transperitoneal, and retroperitoneoscopic nephroureterectomy all demonstrate similar or improved short-term outcomes (duration and intensity of convalescence, complications, and initial oncologic effectiveness) compared with open nephroureterectomy. Management of the distal ureter is still a controversial issue; the techniques that avoid any urine extravasation likely reduce the risk of local recurrence. However in the studies to date, oncologic efficacy of all the laparoscopic procedures appears to rival that of the open surgery. Determination of the ultimate role of these operations will require assessment of long-term oncologic outcomes.

## REFERENCES


1. Cummings KB. Nephroureterectomy: rationale in the management of transitional cell carcinoma of the upper urinary tract. Urol Clin North Am 1980; 7: 569–578.
2. Gittes RF. Management of transitional cell carcinoma of the upper tract: case for conservative local excision. Urol Clin North Am 1980; 7: 559–568.
3. Nocks BN, Heney NM, Daly JJ, et al. Transitional cell carcinoma of renal pelvis. Urology 1982; 19: 472–477.
4. Wagle DG, Moore RH, and Murphy GP. Primary carcinoma of the renal pelvis. Cancer 1974; 33: 1642–1648.

5. Wallace DM, Wallace DM, Whitfield HN, et al. The late results of conservative surgery for upper tract urothelial carcinomas. Br J Urol 1981; 53: 537–547.
6. Hall MC, Womack S, Sagalowsky AI, et al. Prognostic factors, recurrence, and survival in transitional cell carcinoma of the upper urinary tract: a 30-year experience in 252 patients. Urology 1998; 52: 594–601.
7. Clayman RV, Kavoussi LR, Figenshau RS, et al. Laparoscopic nephroureterectomy: initial clinical case report. J Laparoendosc Surg 1991; 1: 343–349.
8. Doehn C, Fornara P, Fricke L, et al. Comparison of laparoscopic and open nephroureterectomy for benign disease. J Urol 1998;159: 732–734.
9. Figenshau RS, Clayman RV, Kerbl K, et al. Laparoscopic nephroureterectomy in the child: initial case report. J Urol 1994;151: 740–741.
10. Janetschek G, Reissigl A, Peschel R, et al. Laparoscopic nephroureterectomy. Br J Urol 1993; 72: 987–988.
11. Elliott DS, Segura JW, Lightner D, et al. Is nephroureterectomy necessary in all cases of upper tract transitional cell carcinoma? Long-term results of conservative endourologic management of upper tract transitional cell carcinoma in individuals with a normal contralateral kidney. Urology 2001; 58: 174–178.
12. Gerber GS, Lyon ES. Endourological management of upper tract urothelial tumors. J Urol 1993; 150: 2–7.
13. Lee BR, Jabbour ME, Marshall FF, et al. 13-year survival comparison of percutaneous and open nephroureterectomy approaches for management of transitional cell carcinoma of renal collecting system: equivalent outcomes. J Endourol 1999; 13: 289–294.
14. Plancke HR, Strijbos WE, Delaere KP. Percutaneous endoscopic treatment of urothelial tumours of the renal pelvis. Br J Urol 1995; 75: 736–739.
15. Stoller ML, Gentle DL, McDonald MW, et al. Endoscopic management of upper tract urothelial tumors. Tech Urol 1997; 3: 152–157.
16. Wolf JS, Jr, Marcovich R, Gill IS, et al. Survey of neuromuscular injuries to the patient and surgeon during urologic laparoscopic surgery. Urology 2000; 55: 831–836.
17. Shalhav AL, Portis AJ, McDougall EM, et al. Laparoscopic nephroureterectomy. A new standard for the surgical management of upper tract transitional cell cancer. Urol Clin North Am 2000; 27: 761–773.
18. McDougall EM, Clayman RV, Elashry O. Laparoscopic nephroureterectomy for upper tract transitional cell cancer: the Washington University experience. J Urol 1995; 154: 975–979.
19. Charbit L, Gendreau MC, Mee S, et al. Tumors of the upper urinary tract: 10 years of experience. J Urol 1991; 146: 1243–1246.
20. Miyake H, Hara I, Gohji K, et al. The significance of lymphadenectomy in transitional cell carcinoma of the upper urinary tract. Br J Urol 1998; 82: 494–498.
21. Chen J, Chueh SC, Hsu WT, et al. Modified approach of hand-assisted laparoscopic nephroureterectomy for transitional cell carcinoma of the upper urinary tract. Urology 2001; 58: 930–934.
22. Gasman D, Saint F, Barthelemy Y, et al. Retroperitoneoscopy: a laparoscopic approach for adrenal and renal surgery. Urology 1996; 47: 801–806.
23. Gill IS, Munch LC, Lucas BA, et al. Initial experience with retroperitoneoscopic nephroureterectomy: use of a double-balloon technique. Urology 1995; 46: 747–750.
24. Gill IS, Soble JJ, Miller SD, et al. A novel technique for management of the en bloc bladder cuff and distal ureter during laparoscopic nephroureterectomy. J Urol 1999; 161: 430–434.

25. Gill IS. Retroperitoneal laparoscopic nephrectomy. Urol Clin North Am 1998; 25: 343–360.
26. Salomon L, Hoznek A, Cicco A, et al. Retroperitoneoscopic nephroureterectomy for renal pelvic tumors with a single iliac incision. J Urol 1999; 161: 541–544.
27. Gonzalez CM, Batler RA, Schoor RA, et al.: A novel endoscopic approach towards resection of the distal ureter with surrounding bladder cuff during hand assisted laparoscopic nephroureterectomy. J Urol 2001; 165: 483–485.
28. Shalhav AL, Elbahnasy AM, McDougall EM, et al. Laparoscopic nephroureterectomy for upper tract transitional-cell cancer: technical aspects. J Endourol 1998; 12: 345–353.
29. Landman J, McDougall EM, Gill IS, et al. Specific laparoscopic procedures. In: *Adult and pediatric urology, 4th ed.* (Gillenwater JY, Grayhack JT, Howards SS, et al., eds.), Lippincott Williams & Wilkins, Baltimore, MD, 2002, pp. 729–731.
30. Hetherington JW, Ewing R, Philp NH. Modified nephroureterectomy: a risk of tumour implantation. Br J Urol 1986; 58: 368–370.
31. Jones DR, Moisey CU. A cautionary tale of the modified "pluck" nephroureterectomy. Br J Urol 1993; 71: 486.
32. Seifman BD, Montie JE, Wolf JS, Jr. Prospective comparison between hand-assisted laparoscopic and open surgical nephroureterectomy for urothelial cell carcinoma. Urology 2001; 57: 133–137.
33. Gill IS. Needlescopic urology: current status. Urol Clin North Am 2001; 28: 71–83.
34. Kaouk JH, Savage SJ, Gill IS. Retroperitoneal laparoscopic nephroureterectomy and management options for the distal ureter. J Endourol 2001; 15: 385–390.
35. Angulo JC, Hontoria J, Sanchez-Chapado M. One-incision nephroureterectomy endoscopically assisted by transurethral ureteral stripping. Urology 1998; 52: 203–207.
36. Matsushita Y, Owari Y, Nozawa T, et al. Transurethral removal of the ureter by the intussusception method in the treatment of renal pelvic and ureteral tumors. Hinyokika Kiyo - Acta Urologica Japonica 2000; 46: 241–245.
37. McGinnis DE, Trabulsi EJ, Gomella LG, et al. Hand-assisted laparoscopic nephroureterectomy: description of technique. Tech Urol 2001; 7: 7–11.
38. Wong C, Leveillee, RJ. Hand-assisted laparoscopic nephroureterectomy with cystoscopic *en bloc* excision of the distal ureter and bladder cuff. J Endourol 2002; 16: 329–332.
39. Arango O, Bielsa O, Carles J, et al. Massive tumor implantation in the endoscopic resected area in modified nephroureterectomy. J Urol 1997; 157: 1839.
40. Laguna MP, de la Rosette JJ. The endoscopic approach to the distal ureter in nephroureterectomy for upper urinary tract tumor. J Urol 2001; 166: 2017–2022.
41. Landman J, Lev RY, Bhayani S, et al. Comparison of hand assisted and standard laparoscopic radical nephroureterectomy for the management of localized transitional cell carcinoma. J Urol 2002; 167: 2387–2391.
42. Shalhav AL, Dunn MD, Portis AJ, et al. Laparoscopic nephroureterectomy for upper tract transitional cell cancer: the Washington University experience. [Review] [19 refs]. J Urol 2000; 163: 1100–1104.
43. Ahmed I, Shaikh NA, Kapadia CR. Track recurrence of renal pelvic transitional cell carcinoma after laparoscopic nephrectomy. Br J Urol 1998; 81: 319.
44. Otani M, Irie S, Tsuji Y. Port site metastasis after laparoscopic nephrectomy: unsuspected transitional cell carcinoma within a tuberculous atrophic kidney. J Urol 1999; 162: 486–487.

45. McNeill SA, Chrisofos M, Tolley DA. The long-term outcome after laparoscopic nephroureterectomy: a comparison with open nephroureterectomy. BJU Int 2000; 86: 619–623.
46. Gill IS, Sung GT, Hobart MG, et al. Laparoscopic radical nephroureterectomy for upper tract transitional cell carcinoma: the Cleveland Clinic experience. J Urol 2000; 164: 1513–1522.
47. Stifelman MD, Sosa RE, Andrade A, et al. Hand-assisted laparoscopic nephroureterectomy for the treatment of transitional cell carcinoma of the upper urinary tract. Urology 2000; 56: 741–747.
48. Jarrett TW, Chan DY, Cadeddu JA, et al. Laparoscopic nephroureterectomy for the treatment of transitional cell carcinoma of the upper urinary tract. Urology 2001; 57: 448–453.

# III Testicular Cancer

# 10 Laparoscopic Retroperitoneal Lymph Node Dissection for Nonseminomatous Germ Cell Tumors of the Testis

*David S. Wang,* MD
*and Howard N. Winfield,* MD

***CONTENTS***

INTRODUCTION
INDICATIONS FOR LAPAROSCOPIC RPLND
SURGICAL TECHNIQUE
POSTOPERATIVE CARE
COMPLICATIONS
OUTCOMES
CONCLUSION
REFERENCES

## INTRODUCTION

The management of testicular cancer has changed dramatically since the early 1980s because of highly effective chemotherapy and improvements in surgical technique. The long-term survival and cure rate even for advanced stages of all germ cell tumors is excellent. As such, there is now increased emphasis on developing treatment regimens that attain a high cure rate while minimizing patient morbidity.

From: *Laparoscopic Urologic Oncology*
Edited by: J. A. Cadeddu © Humana Press Inc., Totowa, NJ

Patients with clinical stage I nonseminomatous germ cell tumors (NSGCT) of the testis have several acceptable treatment options, including surveillance, primary chemotherapy, and retroperitoneal lymph node dissection (RPLND) *(1)*. Surveillance relies on a rigorous followup plan with a highly motivated and compliant patient. Of patients who undergo surveillance, 30% will develop clinical relapse and ultimately require salvage chemotherapy. Fortunately, the survival rate of this subset of patients still exceeds 95% *(2–6)*.

Primary chemotherapy following orchiectomy has been employed for some patients with high-risk stage I NSGCT, as manifested by pathologic evidence of vascular invasion and/or large percentage embryonal carcinoma *(7)*. However, what constitutes high-risk stage I disease is not well-defined. Furthermore, only 20 to 50% of patients with high-risk disease have metastasis *(8)*, suggesting that the rest are treated unnecessarily. Although the morbidity of chemotherapy has decreased tremendously with time, chemotherapy is not without complication and long-term toxicity exists *(9)*.

Open RPLND has become a standard of care as a staging and therapeutic modality for patients with clinical stage I NSGCT, with long-term cure rates of 98% or greater *(9)*. Perioperative morbidity and sexual dysfunction have been minimized with refinements in surgical technique *(10–12)*. Nevertheless, 70% of patients with stage I NSGCT undergo RPLND with no therapeutic benefit.

Laparoscopic RPLND has emerged as a minimally invasive technique to precisely determine the presence of lymph node metastases in patients with clinical stage I NSGCT *(13)*. Several series have been published in the literature *(14–20)*. In its present state, laparoscopic RPLND is considered a diagnostic procedure, and to date the vast majority of patients with pathologically confirmed metastatic retroperitoneal nodes have received adjuvant chemotherapy. Laparoscopic RPLND is a technically advanced procedure with a significant learning curve. It should be performed by surgeons who have substantial experience in other laparoscopic procedures.

This chapter discusses the indications, technique, complications, and results of laparoscopic RPLND for the treatment of NSGCT of the testis.

## INDICATIONS FOR LAPAROSCOPIC RPLND

The goal of laparoscopic RPLND for management of nonseminomatous testicular tumors is to maintain a survival rate equivalent to or greater than that of open surgery while minimizing patient morbidity. Laparoscopic RPLND should be offered to patients who have clinical stage I NSGCT with negative tumor markers following orchiectomy and negative abdominal and pelvic computed tomography (CT) scans. Radiographic evaluation of the chest should also be negative. Additionally, patients should have no absolute contraindications to laparoscopic surgery.

Patients who have clinical evidence of stage II disease by CT scan are not candidates for laparoscopic RPLND as the primary treatment modality. Although open RPLND has been used as a therapeutic modality for patients with stage II disease, the therapeutic value of laparoscopic RPLND has not been tested. All patients who have had pathologic evidence of metastatic disease following laparoscopic RPLND have received adjuvant chemotherapy. The primary role of laparoscopic RPLND at this time is to reliably determine which patients have metastatic disease. Negative findings after laparoscopic RPLND would spare patients chemotherapy and also decrease the rigorous surveillance protocol otherwise required.

More recently, laparoscopic RPLND has been performed in patients who have had isolated persistent retroperitoneal disease following primary chemotherapy for stage IIB or IIC disease *(17,21)*. However, this procedure is technically demanding secondary to the desmoplastic reaction that exists, and should therefore be performed only in centers with experience in standard laparoscopic RPLND.

A summary of general indications for performing laparoscopic RPLND is shown in Table 1.

## SURGICAL TECHNIQUE

### *Preoperative Patient Preparation*

The patient should be fully informed of all other options including surveillance and open RPLND. He should also be advised of all potential complications of laparoscopic RPLND including hemorrhage, infection, injury to other intra-abdominal structures, retrograde ejaculation, and the possibility of conversion to an open operation. Additionally, the patient should be informed of the surgeon's experience with laparoscopic RPLND. Routine blood testing, including type and crossmatching for two units of blood, should be performed along with anesthesia clearance.

A low-fat diet started 1 wk prior to surgery and continued 2 wk postoperatively has been suggested by Janetschek et al. to decrease the risk of chylous ascites *(16)*. The patient undergoes a mechanical bowel preparation the day before surgery with 1 gallon of GoLytely, and has only clear liquids until midnight. Broad spectrum antibiotics are administered on call to the operating room, and pneumatic compression stockings are applied.

Table 1
Indications for Laparoscopic RPLND

| |
|---|
| Clinical Stage I nonseminomatous germ cell tumor of the testis |
| Negative testis tumor markers |
| Patient otherwise considered for surveillance |
| No absolute contraindications to laparoscopic surgery |
| Residual isolated abdominal or pelvic mass following chemotherapy with negative testis tumor markers |

## *Operative Template*

The operative templates for laparoscopic RPLND are based on those described by Weissbach and Boedefeld *(22)* and include all primary landing sites of lymph node metastases. Template modifications have enabled preservation of antegrade ejaculation in nearly all patients. Templates are either right- or left-sided based on the side of the primary testicular tumor. The right-sided template (Fig. 1) is bordered superiorly by the renal vessels, laterally by the right ureter, medially by the anterior surface of the aorta, and inferiorly by the right common iliac artery to where the ureter crosses the iliac artery. The lymph node tissue to be removed should include the precaval, right paracaval, and interaortocaval tissue.

The left-sided template (Fig. 2) is smaller than that for the right. The left-sided template is bordered superiorly by the renal vessels and laterally by the left ureter. The dissection includes all tissue lateral and ventral to the aorta between the renal vessels and origin of the inferior mesenteric artery. The left-sided template does not include the interaortocaval nodes. Caudally, the dissection stops at the inferior mesenteric artery but continues lateral to the aorta over the lateral aspect of the common iliac artery where the ureter crosses.

Controversy exists regarding the removal of tissue behind the lumbar vessels, aorta, and inferior vena cava (IVC). Although this tissue is routinely removed with the split-and-roll technique during open RPLND, there is no evidence that this tissue is the primary landing site for metastatic disease. It is believed that the primary landing site for testicular tumors is the ventral lymph node tissue, obviating need for dissecting the posterior tissue. Moreover, this further decreases operative time and increases safety.

The only contraindications to laparoscopic RPLND are persistently elevated tumor markers after orchiectomy, active infection, and bleeding diathesis. Additionally, any other contraindication to laparoscopic surgery would also apply to laparoscopic RPLND.

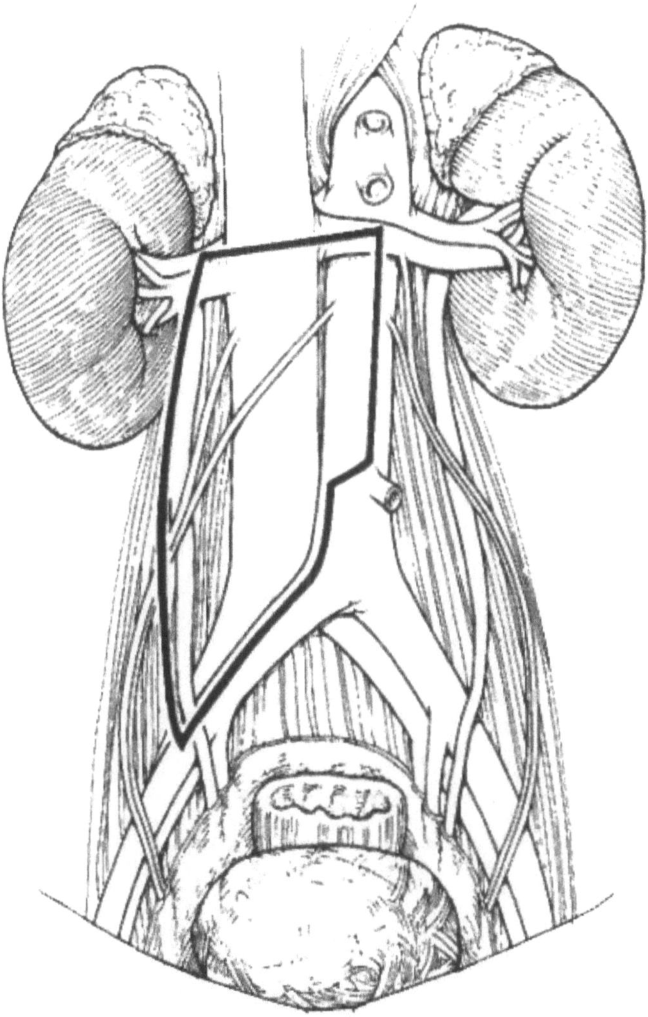

**Fig. 1.** Template for right-sided RPLND.

## *Right-Sided Transperitoneal Laparoscopic RPLND*

After general anesthetic by agents other than nitrous oxide, the patient is positioned with the right side elevated 45° upward and the table slightly flexed at the level of the umbilicus. The patient should be positioned in a beanbag with extensive padding over pressure points. Next, the patient should be secured with tape to allow the table to be tilted side to side to facilitate exposure. A catheter is placed to drain the bladder, and an orogastric tube to decompress the stomach.

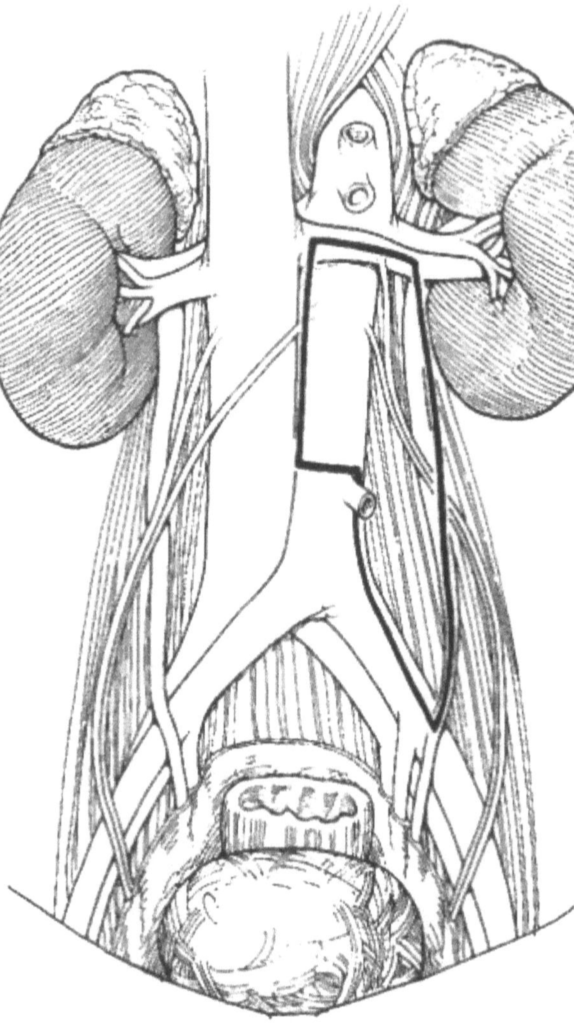

**Fig. 2.** Template for left-sided RPLND.

Four or five 10-mm trocars are required as depicted in Fig. 3. The camera is introduced via the umbilical port. Two additional midline ports are placed, one above and one below the umbilical port. One or two additional ports can be placed to aid in retraction either laterally or in the suprapubic area to assist with retraction as necessary.

The first step after successful pneumoperitoneum involves access to the retroperitoneum by incising the peritoneum along the line of Toldt from the cecum to the hepatic flexure. The incision is extended cephalad

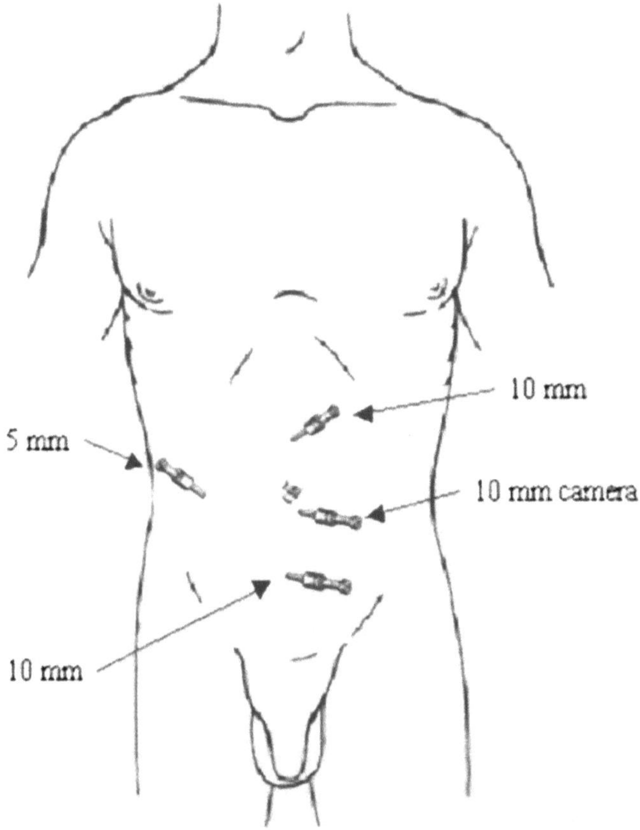


**Fig. 3.** Port placement for right-sided laparoscopic RPLND.

above the level of the transverse colon along the IVC to the hepatoduodenal ligament. Mobilization around the hepatic flexure is extended around the liver out toward the triangular ligaments, so that the liver can be mobilized upward and medially. This allows adequate exposure of the IVC. The peritoneal incision is continued caudally along the spermatic vessels to the internal inguinal ring.

Next, the colon and duodenum are reflected medially to expose the anterior surface of the IVC, aorta, and left renal vein. The spermatic vein is then fully dissected free down to the right internal ring. The stump of the testicular vessels is then dissected free, identifying the nonabsorbable stitch placed at the time of radical orchiectomy. The testicular vessels are then dissected cephalad toward the IVC and aorta. Care must be taken during mobilization of the testicular vessels to prevent inadvertent avulsion at the level of the IVC. The ureter should be carefully identified prior to completing the dissection of the testicular vessels. The remnants of the testicular vessels are then doubly ligated proximally and delivered intact through a laparoscopic port.

Next, the lymphatic tissue is dissected off of the IVC. The lymphatic tissue overlying the IVC is split open, and the anterior and lateral surfaces are dissected free. Identification of the right and left renal veins is critical at this point. The right renal artery is then exposed lateral to the IVC. The lymphatic tissue is freed from the right common iliac artery to the inferior mesenteric artery and continued in a cephalad fashion, taking care to preserve the inferior mesenteric artery. The remaining precaval and lateral caval tissue is dissected free. The dissection is continued cranially to the superior border at the level of the right renal artery. The interaortocaval lymphatic tissue is next excised with great care; lumbar vessels, if necessary, should be divided. Finally, the right lateral border of the nodal package should be freed from the ureter.

Once the nodal package is completely separated, it should be placed in a specimen retrieval bag and removed *en bloc*. Assuming adequate hemostasis, the laparoscopic ports are removed under direct vision and fascia closed with the Carter-Thomason fascial closure device. A drain is usually not necessary. The orogastric tube is removed at the conclusion of the procedure.

### *Left-Sided Transperitoneal Laparoscopic RPLND*

The patient is positioned with the left side elevated 45° upward. Port placement is identical to the right-sided dissection, except an additional port can be placed on the left side of the patient if necessary. Four ports are usually sufficient because the bowel does not need to be retracted as extensively as on the right side. The template is significantly smaller, and includes tissue lateral to the aorta and the preaortic tissue cephalad to the inferior mesenteric artery. The interaortocaval nodes are not removed. The nodal packet is bounded superiorly by the renal vessels, laterally by the left ureter, and inferiorly by the crossing of the ureter with the iliac artery.

Again, the first step following pneumoperitoneum is access to the retroperitoneum. The peritoneum is incised along the line of Toldt from the splenic flexure to the pelvic brim, continuing to the level of the internal inguinal ring. The spermatic vein is dissected free from the left renal vein down to the internal ring. Once the ureter is identified, the nodal package is dissected free in a similar fashion as to the right side using the modified template. Often, division of a large lumbar vessel, which joins the left renal vein, is necessary in order to remove all of the nodal tissue around the left renal vein.

## *Laparoscopic RPLND After Chemotherapy for Stage II or III Disease*

Patients with stage IIB, IIC, or III NSGCT disease generally undergo three or four cycles of combination chemotherapy as initial treatment. If there is residual or new tumor mass present with negative tumor markers, then RPLND is recommended for diagnostic and therapeutic purposes. The pathology of the residual mass dictates the need for further chemotherapy vs continued surveillance.

RPLND can be technically challenging, in an open or laparoscopic fashion, due to the desmoplastic reaction around the great vessels that can occur following chemotherapy. The goal is to remove all residual tumor mass. To be considered for postchemotherapy laparoscopic RPLND, patients with stage II or III disease must have negative tumor markers as well as a reduction in size of retroperitoneal lesions indicating a good response to therapy.

Because of the extensive desmoplastic fibrosis that develops after chemotherapy, it is often not possible to follow the traditional templates. Instead, excising residual tumor mass is the objective. Surgical templates for unilateral RPLND are loosely based on standard laparoscopic RPLND, but again it is often impossible to perform traditional template RPLND following chemotherapy. Intraoperatively, meticulous hemostasis is critical; even minimal bleeding must be controlled instantly to provide a bloodless surgical field. The use of bipolar fine grasping forceps has been useful, and fibrin glue or other hemostatic substances can be used.

## *Laparoscopic RPLND Using Retroperitoneal Approach*

The laparoscopic retroperitoneal approach has become widely used in urology, particularly with renal surgery, since introduction of the balloon dissection technique by Gaur *(23)*. However, to date, experience with retroperitoneal laparoscopic RPLND is very limited, with 17 cases reported by Rassweiler et al. *(19)*, who classified the technique as very difficult. The technique differs from transperitoneal laparoscopic RPLND in several key aspects.

Patients are placed in the flank position. A small incision is made in the lumbar triangle between the 12th rib and the iliac crest. Access to the retroperitoneum is obtained by blunt dissection, and balloon dilation is carried out. Pneumoretroperitoneum is then established and the RPLND performed using the same templates as previously described.

Experience with this technique is very limited, even among surgeons with considerable skill in retroperitoneal laparoscopy. The technique is among the most challenging of all retroperitoneal laparoscopic procedures. Therefore, it should be performed only in limited centers with a large experience in retroperitoneal laparoscopy.

## POSTOPERATIVE CARE

The benefits of laparoscopic RPLND are apparent immediately postoperatively. The orogastric tube is typically removed at the end of the operation. Bowel function returns usually within 24 h, and diet is advanced on the first postoperative day. Discharge is usually in 2 to 4 d, with return to full activity requiring 2 to 3 wk.

## COMPLICATIONS

Intraoperative hemorrhage is the most frequent complication of laparoscopic RPLND. Troublesome bleeding can occur from lumbar or other small branches of the IVC as well as from vasa vasorum of the aorta. In most cases, hemorrhage can be controlled with the judicious use of bipolar electrocautery. Hemostatic substances such as Surgicel or fibrin glue and intracorporeal suturing may be required for persistent bleeding.

Conversion to an open procedure is most frequently the result of uncontrollable intraoperative hemorrhage; however, the conversion rate for stage I disease is less than 7%. Other major complications, such as pulmonary and cardiac, appear to be less common than with open RPLND.

One minor complication that has been noted by Janetschek et al. has been chylous ascites *(16)*. This complication is thought to be more related to early resumption of oral intake and not to surgical technique. In all cases, the chylous ascites resolved with dietary modification, and the authors currently institute a low-fat diet 1 wk preoperatively and 2 wk postoperatively to prevent this complication. Lymphocele formation is also a rare minor complication.

## OUTCOMES

### *Laparoscopic RPLND for Stage I NSGCTs*

Laparoscopic RPLND offers the usual benefits of laparoscopic intervention vs open surgery including decreased narcotic requirement, faster return to bowel function, shorter hospital stay, and overall shorter return to normal activity. The morbidity of the procedure continues to decrease as the learning curve is overcome and overall operative time decreases even further *(24)*.

The worldwide published experience with laparoscopic RPLND for clinical stage I disease is summarized in Table 2. The overall low incidence of testicular carcinoma coupled with the complexity of laparoscopic RPLND explain the small sizes of these series. Nevertheless, as more urologists are gaining expertise with laparoscopic surgery, the number of laparoscopic RPLND procedures performed will undoubtedly increase. All authors comment on the need to overcome the learning curve. The current conversion rate is less than 7%, which is reasonable given the complexity of this procedure.

Unlike other genito-urinary cancers, followup for testicular cancer can be considered long-term after as little as 2 to 4 yr. Thus far, there has only been one report of a local retroperitoneal recurrence of tumor following laparoscopic RPLND. However, in this case the original RPLND specimen contained tumor that was, in retrospect, missed on initial pathological examination, and was thus a false-negative. Recurrences following laparoscopic RPLND have been primarily pulmonary metastases. This has occurred in 4–5% of patients post-RPLND. This rate compares favorably with the result obtained from open RPLND.

Laparoscopic RPLND is considered by most clinicians to be a diagnostic, and not therapeutic, procedure. In open RPLND, a subset of patients with minimal lymph node metastasis following RPLND have undergone surveillance strategies without the use of adjuvant chemotherapy. A significant portion of patients with even stage IIB disease will require no further treatment. However, to date, the vast majority of patients with pathologically confirmed lymph node metastasis following laparoscopic RPLND have received adjuvant chemotherapy. As such, the therapeutic value of laparoscopic RPLND for clinical stage I disease is unknown, and the procedure must be considered a diagnostic staging procedure.

Yet, the value of laparoscopic RPLND may lie in its ability to distinguish patients with retroperitoneal metastases from those who have negative nodes. Currently, CT scan is neither sensitive nor specific enough to accomplish this task. Because only 30% of clinical stage I patients relapse on surveillance, open RPLND would be performed without therapeutic benefit in 70% of patients. Even those patients with high-risk stage I disease experience relapse only 50% of the time; thus, half of stage I patients who receive chemotherapy would be given chemotherapy unnecessarily. Laparoscopic RPLND serves as a minimally invasive approach to accurately identify those patients without retroperitoneal metastasis, thus sparing them potentially harmful and unnecessary chemotherapy.

Table 2
Worldwide Experience with Laparoscopic RPLND for Clinical Stage I Nonseminomatous Germ Cell Testicular Cancer

| *Author (reference)* | *No. pts* | *Mean OR time (min)* | *Conversion rate* | *Complications* | *Postop days* | *Recurrence* | *Followup (mo)* | *Survival* |
|---|---|---|---|---|---|---|---|---|
| Gerber et al. *(14)* | 20 | 480 | 10% because of bleeding | Gonadal bleeding requiring laparotomy (2)<br>Subcapsular myonecrosis (1)<br>IMA injury requiring delayed laparotomy (1)<br>Lymphocele (1)<br>Trocar bleeding (1)<br>Retrogade ejaculation | 3 | 0 local<br>2/20 plumonary | 10 | 20/20 |
| Giusti et al. *(15)* | 6 | 325 | 0% | Subcutaneous emphysema, 18 day hospitalization (1) | 4.8 | 0/6 local<br>0/6 distant | 27.1 | 6/6 |
| Janetschek et al. *(16)* | 73 | 297 | 3% | Minor bleeding (3)<br>Small lymphocele (1)<br>Transient lymphedema (1)<br>Transient genitofemoral nerve irritation (1) | 3.3 | 1/73 local (false negative)<br>0/73 distant | 43 | 64/64 |
| Klotz *(25)* | 4 | 285 | 25% | None reported | 1-2 | 0/4 local<br>1/4 pulmonary | – | – |
| Nelson et al. *(18)* | 29 | 258 | 6.9% | | 2.6 | 0/29 local<br>1/29 pulmonary<br>1/29 elevated markers | 16 | 29/29 |
| Rassweiler et al. *(19)* | 34 | 248 | 12%<br>1/34 coverted because of bleeding<br>3/34 converted because of positive frozen section | Ureteral stenosis requiring ureterolysis (1)<br>Retrograde ejaculation (1)<br>Pulmonary embolus (1)<br>Temporary ureteral stent placement (1) | 5.3 | 0/34 local recurrence<br>2/34 with pulmonary metastasis treated with chemotherapy | 40 | 34/34 |
| Rukstalis et al. *(26)* | 1 | 510 | 0 | Minor postoperative bleed | – | 0 | 2 | 1/1 |
| Stone et al. *(27)* | 1 | 360 | 0 | 0 | 3 | 0 | 24 | 1/1 |
| Zhuo et al. *(20)* | 13 | 292 | 8% | 0 | 6.4 | 0/13 local<br>1/13 pulmonary metastasis | 14.6 | 13/13 |

OR = operating room; IMA = inferior mesenteric artery.

### *Postchemotherapy Laparoscopic RPLND for Stage II or III Disease*

The largest published series of postchemotherapy laparoscopic RPLND is by Janetschek et al. from Austria involving 49 patients with stage II NSGCT *(21)*. All patients underwent primary induction therapy with cisplatin-based combination chemotherapy. Inclusion criteria were the normalization of tumor markers and reduction in retroperitoneal tumor size. Additionally, laparoscopic RPLND was performed even if patients had complete remission.

Forty-nine patients with stage II disease underwent laparoscopic RPLND following chemotherapy. Operative time averaged 219 min. Again, the lower operative time in this series reflects the fact that postchemotherapy RPLND was performed after the learning curve was overcome. Pathologic analysis demonstrated necrosis in 30 patients, mature teratomas in 18 patients, and active tumor in 1 patient who received two additional cycles of chemotherapy. The authors report no disease recurrence after a mean followup of 35 mo. The authors conclude that laparoscopic RPLND after chemotherapy is feasible and seemingly effective for tumor control, specifically in the 18 patients with mature teratomas. Longer followup is required to determine the therapeutic benefit of RPLND in these patients.

## CONCLUSION

Laparoscopic RPLND is an advanced procedure that has been successfully performed by a limited number of surgeons in select academic centers. It has been shown to be feasible for clinical stage I NSGCTs and is considered a diagnostic procedure for these patients. Laparoscopic RPLND allows for precise determination of lymph node status for patients with stage I disease. Postchemotherapy RPLND has been performed in select stage II or III patients with residual disease and negative markers. The role of laparoscopic RPLND in nonseminomatous disease warrants further investigation through continued long-term followup.

## REFERENCES

1. Lashley DB, Lowe BA. A rational approach to managing stage I nonseminomatous germ cell cancer. Urol Clin North Am 1998; 25: 405–423.
2. Sogani PC, Perrotti M, Herr HW, Fair WR, Thaler HT, Bosl G. Clinical stage I testis cancer: long-term outcome of patients on surveillance. J Urol 1998; 159: 855–858.
3. Foster RS, Roth BJ. Clinical stage I nonseminoma: surgery versus surveillance. Semin Oncol 1998; 25: 145–153.
4. Nicolai N, Pizzocaro G. A surveillance study of clinical stage I nonseminomatous germ cell tumors of the testis: 10-year followup. J Urol 1995; 154: 1045–1049.

5. Sturgeon JF, Jewett MA, Alison RE, et al. Surveillance after orchidectomy for patients with clinical stage I nonseminomatous testis tumors. J Clin Oncol 1992; 10: 564–568.
6. Gels ME, Hoekstra HJ, Sleijfer DT, et al. Detection of recurrence in patients with clinical stage I nonseminomatous testicular germ cell tumors and consequences for further follow-up: single-center 10-year experience. J Clin Oncol 1995; 13: 1188–1194.
7. Heidenreich A, Sesterhenn IA, Mostofi FK, Moul JW. Prognostic risk factors that identify patients with clinical stage I nonseminomatous germ cell tumors at low risk and high risk for metastasis. Cancer 1998; 83: 1002–1011.
8. Read G, Stenning SP, Cullen MH, et al. Medical Research Council prospective study of surveillance for stage I testicular teratoma. Medical Research Council Testicular Tumors Working Party. J Clin Oncol 1992; 10: 1762–1768.
9. Foster RS, Donohue JP. Retroperitoneal lymph node dissection for the management of clinical stage I nonseminoma. J Urol 2000; 163: 1788–1792.
10. Baniel J, Foster RS, Rowland RG, Bihrle R, Donohue JP. Complications of primary retroperitoneal lymph node dissection. J Urol 1994; 152: 424–427.
11. Donohue JP, Foster RS. Retroperitoneal lymphadenectomy in staging and treatment. The development of nerve-sparing techniques. Urol Clin North Am 1998; 25: 461–468.
12. Donohue JP, Foster RS, Rowland RG, Bihrle R, Jones J, Geier G. Nerve-sparing retroperitoneal lymphadenectomy with preservation of ejaculation. J Urol 1990; 144: 287–291.
13. Winfield HN. Laparoscopic retroperitoneal lymphadenectomy for cancer of the testis. Urol Clin North Am 1998; 25: 469–478.
14. Gerber GS, Bissada NK, Hulbert JC, et al. Laparoscopic retroperitoneal lymphadenectomy: multi-institutional analysis. J Urol 1994; 152: 1188–1191.
15. Giusti G, Beltrami P, Tallarigo C, Bianchi G, Mobilio G. Unilateral laparoscopic retroperitoneal lymphadenectomy for clinical stage I nonseminomatous testicular cancer. J Endourol 1998; 12: 561–566.
16. Janetschek G, Hobisch A, Peschel R, Hittmair A, Bartsch G. Laparoscopic retroperitoneal lymph node dissection for clinical stage I nonseminomatous testicular carcinoma: long-term outcome. J Urol 2000; 163: 1793–1796.
17. Janetschek G, Peschel R, Hobisch A, Bartsch G. Laparoscopic retroperitoneal lymph node dissection. J Endourol 2001; 15: 449–453.
18. Nelson JB, Chen RN, Bishoff JT, et al. Laparoscopic retroperitoneal lymph node dissection for clinical stage I nonseminomatous germ cell testicular tumors. Urology 1999; 54: 1064–1067.
19. Rassweiler JJ, Frede T, Lenz E, Seemann O, Alken P. Long-term experience with laparoscopic retroperitoneal lymph node dissection in the management of low-stage testis cancer. Eur Urol 2000; 37: 251–260.
20. Zhuo Y, Klaen R, Sauter TW, Miller K. Laparoscopic retroperitoneal lymph node dissection in clinical stage I nonseminomatous germ cell tumor: a minimal invasive alternative. Chin Med J (Engl) 1998; 111: 537–541.
21. Janetschek GJ, Hobisch A, Hittmair A, Holtl L, Peschel R, Bartsch G. Laparoscopic retroperitoneal lymphadenectomy after chemotherapy for stage IIB nonseminomatous testicular carcinoma. J Urol 1999; 161: 477–481.
22. Weissbach L, Boedefeld EA. Localization of solitary and multiple metastases in stage II nonseminomatous testis tumor as basis for a modified staging lymph node dissection in stage I. J Urol 1987; 138: 77–82.

23. Gaur DD. Laparoscopic operative retroperitoneoscopy: use of a new device. J Urol 1992; 148: 1137–1139.
24. Janetschek G, Hobisch A, Holtl L, Bartsch G. Retroperitoneal lymphadenectomy for clinical stage I nonseminomatous testicular tumor: laparoscopy versus open surgery and impact of learning curve. J Urol 1996; 156: 89–93.
25. Klotz L. Laparoscopic retroperitoneal lymphadenectomy for high-risk stage 1 nonseminomatous germ cell tumor: report of four cases. Urology 1994; 43: 752–756.
26. Rukstalis DB, Chodak GW. Laparoscopic retroperitoneal lymph node dissection in a patient with stage 1 testicular carcinoma. J Urol 1992; 148: 1907–1909.
27. Stone NN, Schlussel RN, Waterhouse RL, Unger P. Laparoscopic retroperitoneal lymph node dissection in stage A nonseminomatous testis cancer. Urology 1993; 42: 610–614.

# IV Adrenal Adenoma and Carcinoma

# 11 Laparoscopic Adrenalectomy for Benign Disease

*D. Duane Baldwin*, MD
*and S. Duke Herrell*, MD

*CONTENTS*

INTRODUCTION
INDICATIONS AND CONTRAINDICATIONS TO LAPAROSCOPIC ADRENALECTOMY
OVERVIEW OF LAPAROSCOPIC SURGICAL TECHNIQUE
LATERAL TRANSPERITONEAL TECHNIQUE
EXTRAPERITONEAL LAPAROSCOPIC TECHNIQUE
INCIDENTALOMA
PHEOCHROMOCYTOMA
ALDOSTERONOMA
EXCESS CORTISOL PRODUCTION
ADRENOCORTICAL CARCINOMA
METASTATIC ADRENAL TUMORS
NEEDLESCOPIC ADRENALECTOMY
PEDIATRIC ADRENALECTOMY
LAPAROSCOPIC PARTIAL ADRENALECTOMY
MORBIDITY AND RECOVERY
COST
CONTRAINDICATIONS TO THE LAPAROSCOPIC APPROACH
SUMMARY
REFERENCES

From: *Laparoscopic Urologic Oncology*
Edited by: J. A. Cadeddu © Humana Press Inc., Totowa, NJ

## INTRODUCTION

Surgical adrenalectomy has traditionally played a major role in the management of benign and malignant conditions of the adrenal gland. Adrenalectomy is curative in many functional endocrine disorders including pheochromocytoma, primary aldosteronism, and excess cortisol production, and has maintained an important role in the management of these endocrine diseases *(1)*. Conventional open surgical approaches include the subcostal, flank, or posterior approaches *(2)*. Although effective, these open approaches require large, invasive incisions accompanied by long hospitalizations, and a protracted recovery *(1)*.

Since its original report in 1992, the laparoscopic approach has played a major role in minimizing the morbidity associated with adrenal surgery *(3)*. The advantages of laparoscopic adrenalectomy include decreased postoperative pain, a shortened hospitalization, and a more rapid convalescence *(4–9)*. The surgeon benefits from a direct approach to the gland, optical magnification, the tamponade provided by the pneumoperitoneum, and gravity retraction of surrounding structures *(2)*.

The location deep in the retroperitoneum, the small size of most adrenal tumors, and the rare incidence of malignancy, combined with the dramatic decrease in morbidity of the laparoscopic approach has quickly made this the procedure of choice for most adrenal tumors *(9,10)*.

The surgical diseases of the adrenal gland are varied and complex. This chapter provides an overview of surgical adrenal disease and discusses the role of laparoscopic adrenalectomy and the results utilizing the laparoscopic technique. Emphasis is placed on the particular nuances associated with the laparoscopic approach, along with the potential differences between the laparoscopic and open approaches.

## INDICATIONS AND CONTRAINDICATIONS TO LAPAROSCOPIC ADRENALECTOMY

The indications for laparoscopic adrenalectomy have greatly expanded since the original published report in 1992 *(3)*. Although the use of laparoscopic resection is well accepted for most benign adrenal tumors, large primary adrenocortical carcinomas are probably best managed with open surgery. Absolute contraindications to a laparoscopic approach include cranial hypertension, and uncorrected coagulopathy *(11)*. General contraindications for laparoscopic surgery include unacceptable cardiopulmonary risk, abdominal sepsis, and small bowel obstruction *(12)*. Relative contraindications for laparoscopic adrenalectomy include adrenocortical carcinoma with adrenal vein thrombus or local invasion *(9,12)*. Tumors larger than 10 to 12 cm are technically challenging and have an increased incidence of malignancy favoring an open surgical approach. Morbid obesity, increased patient age, and prior abdominal surgery are not contraindications for laparoscopic adrenal surgery *(12,13)*.

## OVERVIEW OF LAPAROSCOPIC SURGICAL TECHNIQUE

Laparoscopic approaches to the adrenal gland include the transperitoneal and the retroperitoneal approach. Advocates of the transperitoneal approach cite a more consistent identification of surgical landmarks, a superior surgical orientation, and the ability to safely remove larger adrenal tumors *(5,14)*. Criticism of the retroperitoneal approach include a smaller working space, difficulty with orientation, and a steeper learning curve *(1)*. Vascular injuries may also be more difficult to control from a retroperitoneal approach. Proponents of the retroperitoneal approach cite shorter operative times, decreased blood loss, reduced analgesic requirements, and shorter hospital stays *(15–18)*.

Comparisons have failed to reveal significant differences in hypercarbia *(19)*, patient outcome, morbidity, or operative time for the two approaches *(20–22)*. Both procedures may be performed safely and the final choice of approach should be determined by the surgeon's familiarity with laparoscopy and each of the surgical approaches.

The transperitoneal approach may be further divided into the anterior, modified lateral and lateral approaches. The anterior supine position does not allow gravity to provide optimal retraction of the surrounding abdominal viscera; therefore additional ports may be required. The only advantage of the anterior supine approach is that bilateral adrenalectomy can be accomplished without patient repositioning *(23)*.

In a comparison of three approaches for laparoscopic adrenalectomy, Suzuki and colleagues found in a nonrandomized study that the lateral transperitoneal approach resulted in a significantly shorter operative time compared to an anterior transperitoneal approach or a lateral retroperitoneal approach. There was also no significant difference in the recovery parameters *(20)*. Similarly, in a small prospective randomized study comparing the transperitoneal and the retroperitoneal approaches, Fernandez-Cruz demonstrated no significant difference in operative times, pain medication requirements, or recovery time *(17)*. The lateral transperitoneal approach provides for maximal gravity retraction of the peritoneal contents and is the authors' preferred approach in the majority of laparoscopic adrenalectomies.

Laparoscopic adrenalectomy is performed under general endotracheal anesthesia. Decompression of the bladder and stomach minimizes distension and potential for injury. Oxygen saturation and end-tidal carbon dioxide are monitored. Lower extremity intermittent compression devices are used to prevent deep venous thrombosis.

## LATERAL TRANSPERITONEAL TECHNIQUE

The patient is positioned in the lateral flank position with the contralateral anterior superior iliac crest located just below the break in the table. Entry into the abdomen may be accomplished using either the open (Hasson) or closed (Veress) techniques *(24)*. A variety of port placements will allow successful removal of the adrenal gland. The authors prefer an open cannulation through a 1.5-cm incision and placement of a 12-mm port in the midclavicular line 2 cm below the costal margin. An additional 10-mm port is placed in the anterior axillary line also 2 cm below the costal margin. Finally two 5-mm ports are placed in the midaxillary line and the posterior axillary line (Fig. 1).

### *Right-Sided Procedures*

In the initial experience, right-sided cases are easier due to the constancy of reliable landmarks. In right-sided procedures an additional 5-mm port may be placed in the midline 2 cm below the xiphoid and used for placement of a liver retractor (Fig. 1). Transection of the triangular ligament and the posterior peritoneum under the liver allows cephalad retraction of the liver for maximal exposure. The vena cava provides a constant landmark establishing the medial extent of the dissection. The peritoneum overlying the vena cava is incised caudally along the anterior surface of the cava down to the take off of the right renal vein. The peritoneum overlying the renal vein is then incised laterally over the upper pole of the kidney forming a backward C-shaped incision. Often, minimal or no dissection of the large bowel or duodenum are required in right-sided cases. The opening in the peritoneum along the anterior surface of the vena cava is then dissected superiorly and posteriorly, from the take off of the renal vein cephalad to the adrenal vein (Fig. 2). The short adrenal vein is circumferentially dissected, secured, and transected (Figs. 3–5). An accessory adrenal vein may be encountered cephalad to the main renal vein and the dissection should proceed carefully allowing for this possibility. After completely dissecting the caval surface of the adrenal, the liver is dissected from the superior surface of

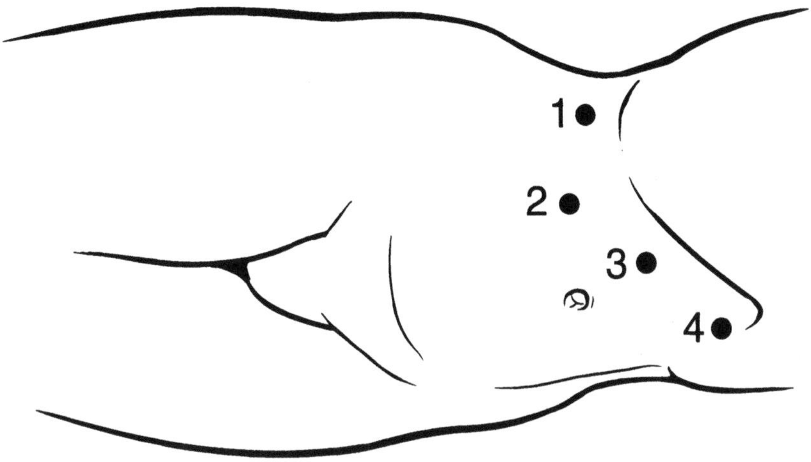


**Fig. 1.** Port site placement for right transperitoneal adrenalectomy.

the gland. The arteries to the adrenal are variable and may be controlled with clips although small arteries may be controlled with electrocautery (Fig. 6). The arteries enter the adrenal gland from three main locations. The medial artery originates from the aorta and enters the medial surface of the gland. The superior artery enters the superior aspect of the gland after branching from the inferior phrenic artery. The inferior arterial branch arises from the renal artery and enters the inferior surface of the gland. After freeing up the cephalad and medial surfaces of the adrenal, the plane between the adrenal gland and the kidney is identified. It is important to preserve the attachment of the adrenal to the kidney until the adrenal gland has been freed from the inferior surface of the liver as traction on the kidney will assist in separating the adrenal gland from the liver. With gentle retraction, the adrenal is rolled laterally and the avascular posterior surface of the adrenal gland is freed with blunt dissection (Fig. 7). The last portion of the adrenal gland to be freed is the avascular lateral surface and attachments to the upper pole of the kidney. The completely mobilized adrenal is then placed in an entrapment sack and removed intact through the 12 mm midclavicular port site. No drains are routinely required.

### *Left-Sided Cases*

Despite a longer vein, left laparoscopic adrenalectomy is complicated by the more variable position of the gland, and the absence of the reliable anatomic landmarks that are present on the right side. The port placement is a mirror image of the right side, except the 5 mm midline

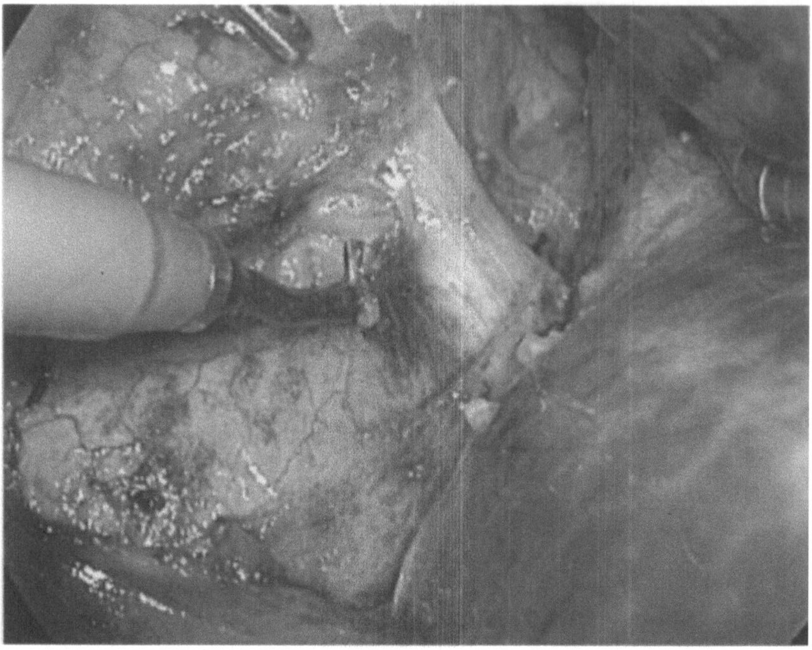

**Fig. 2.** Right adrenalectomy: Dissection along the vena cava exposes the large, short adrenal vein to this 8 cm adrenal mass.

port for liver retraction is omitted (Fig. 8). The most important step in left-sided procedures is complete mobilization of the spleen cephalad and medial until the greater curvature of the stomach is visualized. This mobilization allows the spleen and the tail of the pancreas to rotate cephalad and medially, providing access to the adrenal gland (Figs. 9 and 10). Care must be taken during this dissection to avoid traumatizing the delicate spleen. The dissection to expose the left adrenal gland is sometimes extremely time consuming particularly in obese patients *(25)*. Toldt's fusion fascia is incised from the splenic flexure down several centimeters to expose the upper pole of the left kidney. Dissection of the plane just deep to the pancreas and splenic vein will allow exposure of the left renal vein. The left adrenal vein is identified, secured, and transected (Fig. 11). Cephalad dissection from the left adrenal vein allows identification of the vein joining the inferior phrenic vein. Once these two veins have been transected the medial artery off of the aorta is identified, secured, and transected. Lateral retraction away from the aorta will allow identification of the superior adrenal artery originating from the inferior phrenic artery. The adrenal gland is left attached to the upper pole of the kidney to allow retraction inferiorly while dissecting

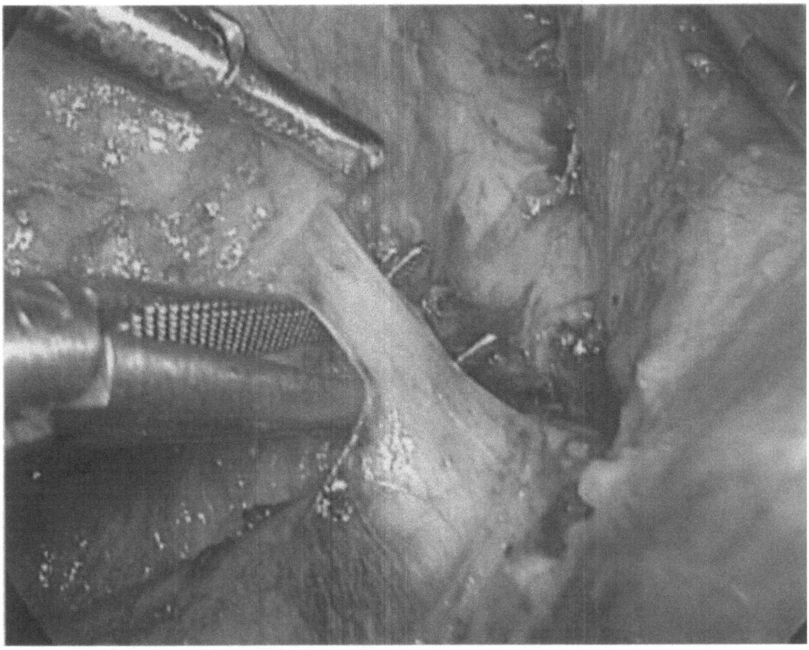

**Fig. 3.** Right adrenalectomy: The adrenal vein is freed circumferentially. Note the importance of the liver retraction in maintaining exposure in right-sided laparoscopic adrenalectomy.

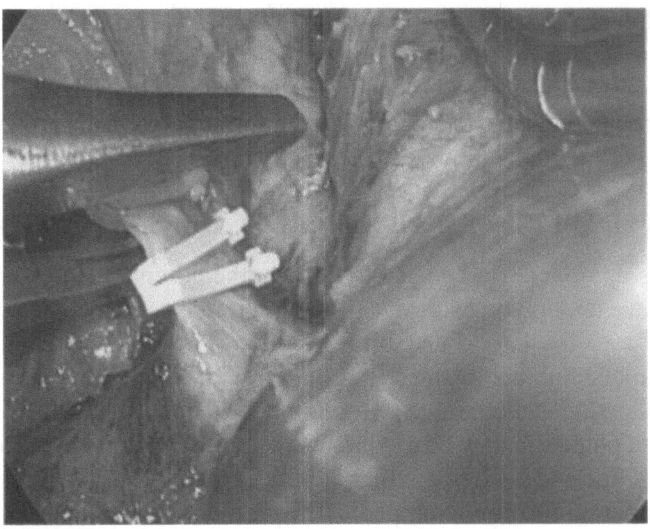

**Fig. 4.** Right adrenalectomy: Hemolock™ clips are applied to the adrenal vein. Alternatively, a stapler may be used for control and ligation.

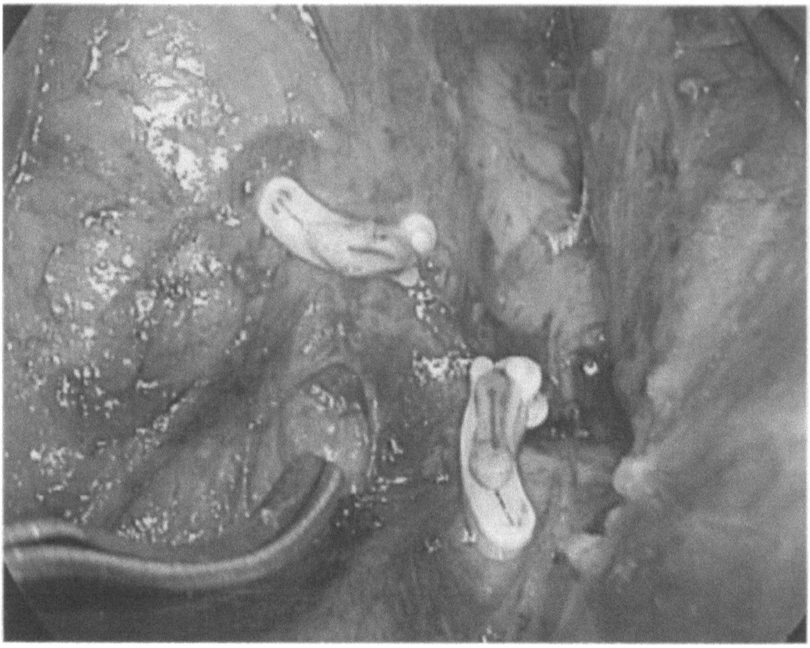

**Fig. 5.** Right adrenalectomy: The adrenal vein is divided. Attachments between the adrenal and kidney are left intact to aid in inferior retraction during superior dissection.

the adrenal off of the diaphragm (Figs. 12–14). Finally, the adrenal gland is separated from the kidney and the lateral and posterior attachments (Figs. 15 and 16). Occasionally, in obese patients, localization of the adrenal gland may be more difficult. Intraoperative ultrasound (US) can assist in localization of the adrenal gland *(26)*.

## EXTRAPERITONEAL LAPAROSCOPIC TECHNIQUE

This approach can be used to remove the adrenal gland in patients who have undergone extensive prior abdominal surgery. The patient is placed into the lateral decubitus position. A 1.5-cm incision in the midaxillary line below the costal margin is incised down through the lumbodorsal fascia into the retroperitoneal space. Blunt finger dissection and palpation may be used to insert additional ports in the anterior axillary line and posterior axillary lines. Gerota's fascia is incised from the diaphragm to the renal pedical from the posterior approach. The renal pedical may be identified by the pulsations of the renal artery. Prior to mobilization of the adrenal gland the adrenal vein is identified,

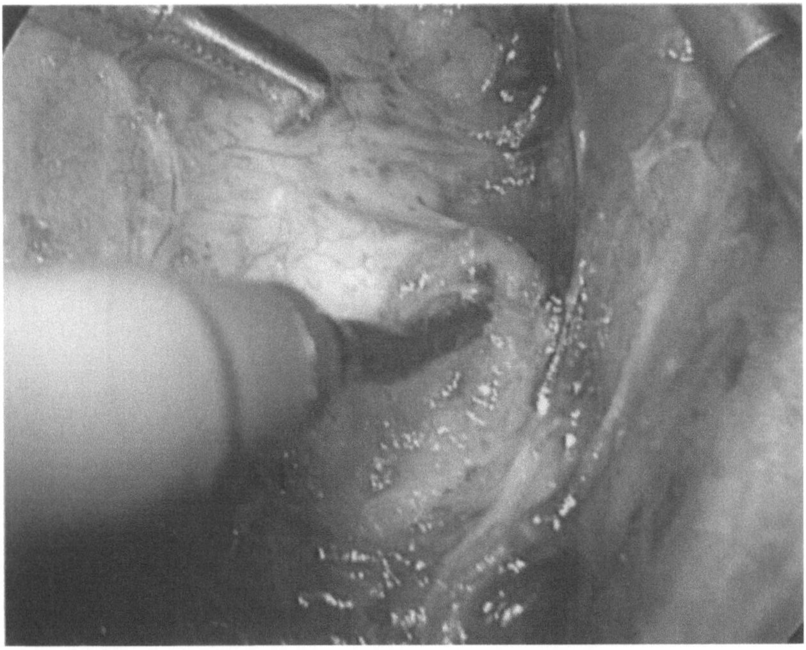

**Fig. 6.** Right adrenalectomy: Dissection along the superior aspect of the adrenal gland exposes the short arterial branches supplying the gland. Electrocautery or small clips may be utilized for hemostasis.

controlled, and transected. In right-sided dissections, the vena cava is identified and followed toward the renal hilum allowing the identification of the adrenal vein. On the left side, dissection of the renal vein will allow identification of the adrenal vein and allow its control and transection. Following transection of the main adrenal vein, the kidney and adrenal are pushed caudally and the adrenal attachments to the diaphragm are taken down. Then the peritoneal attachments and the renal attachments are taken down. Specimen removal is similar to transperitoneal approaches. Due to the retroperitoneal location of the port sites no muscular closure may be necessary although the larger 15-mm incision may require two figure-of-8 fascial sutures as dehiscence has been reported *(27)*.

## INCIDENTALOMA

Incidental adrenal masses are detected at an increased frequency due to the increased utilization of abdominal imaging including US, computed tomography (CT), and magnetic resonance imaging (MRI) in the

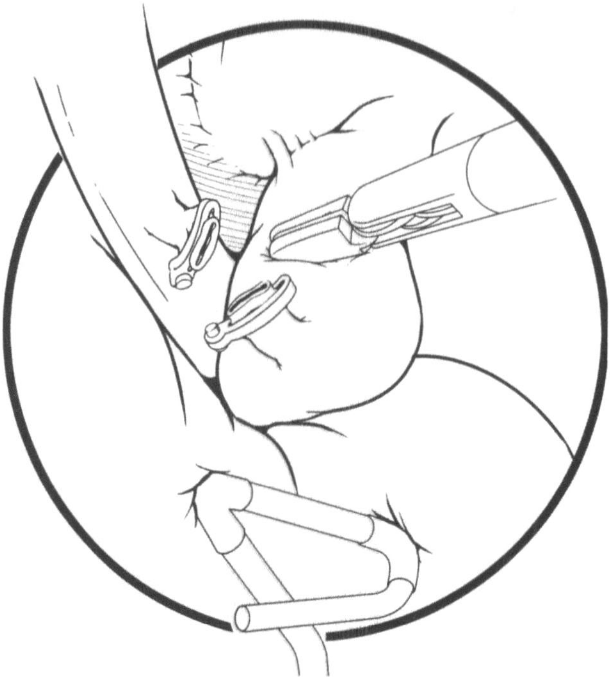

**Fig. 7.** Schematic diagram shows liver retracted and right adrenal view divided between Hemlock™ clips.

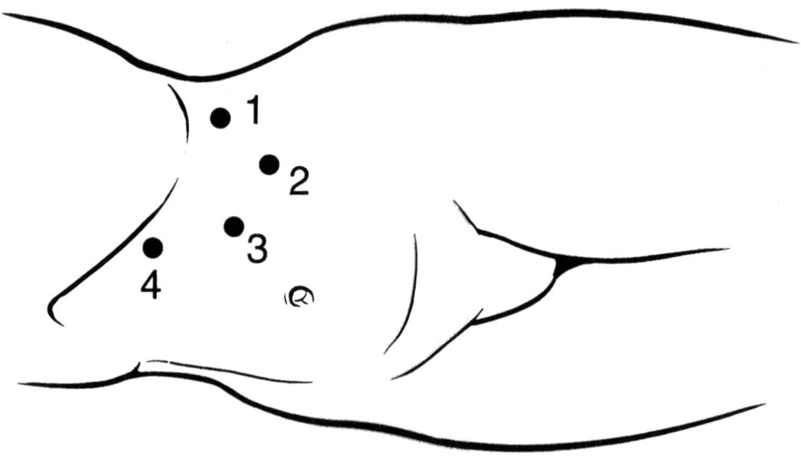


**Fig. 8.** Port placement for left transperitoneal laparoscopic adrenalectomy.

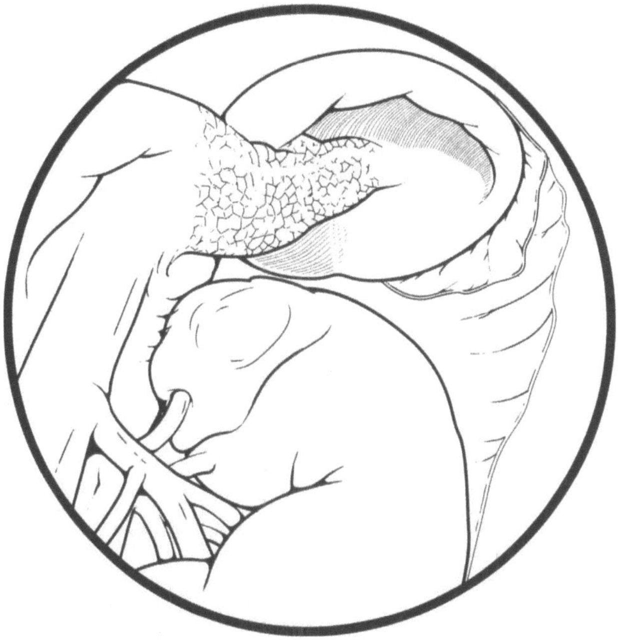

**Fig. 9.** Schematic shows spleen and tail of pancreas mobilized. Note renal vein anatomy on left.

clinical evaluation of patients *(28)*. The incidence of adrenal masses detected by CT scanning has ranged from .4 to 4.4% *(29–33)*. The incidence of adrenal masses at autopsy ranges from 1.4 to 9% *(34,35)*. Adrenal masses increase in frequency with advancing age and are seen with relatively equal frequency in both sexes *(36)*.

Clinicians are frequently asked to evaluate the incidentally detected adrenal mass. This is the most common adrenal disorder encountered by clinicians. Functional hormonal status and the potential of malignancy determine whether adrenalectomy is required *(33)*.

The differential diagnosis of incidentally discovered adrenal masses includes nonfunctioning cortical adenoma, cortisol-producing adenoma, aldosteronoma, adrenal cortical carcinoma, pheochromocytoma, metastatic tumors from other sites, cysts, myelolipoma, hematoma, ganglioneuroma, and neuroblastoma. Nonfunctioning adenomas are the most common lesions, accounting for between 36 and 94% of cases. Hormonally active tumors are much less common. The chance that an incidentally detected adrenal mass is a metastasis ranges from 0 to 21% in patients with no history of cancer, and from 32 to 73% in patients with a history of cancer *(33)*.

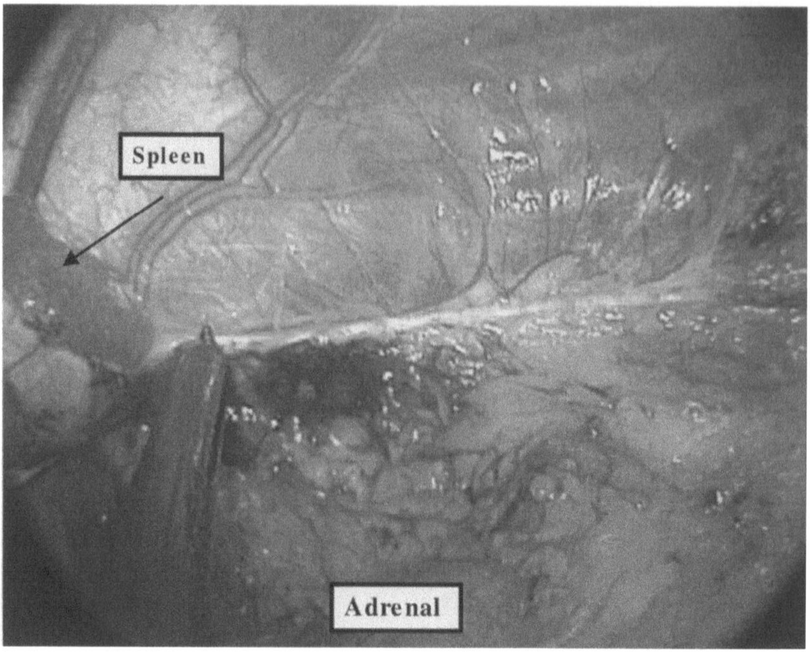


**Fig. 10.** Left adrenalectomy: Full mobilization of lateral attachments of spleen provides optional exposure of the adrenal gland.

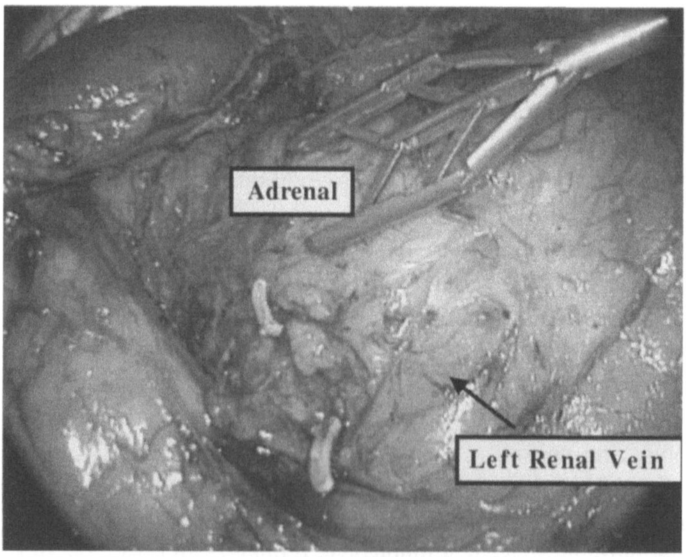


**Fig. 11.** Left adrenalectomy: After division of the left adrenal vein, the adrenal gland is retracted laterally to aid in medial and superior dissection.

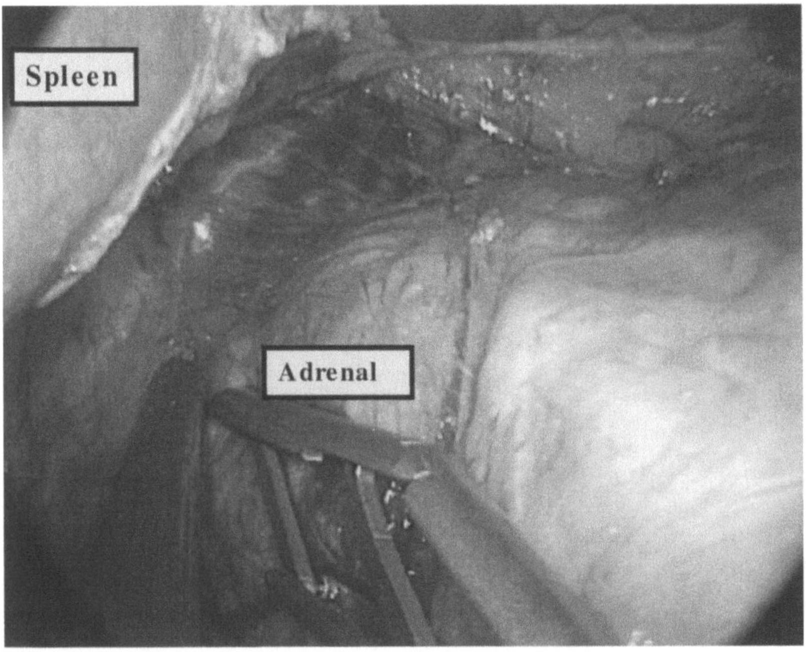


**Fig. 12.** Left adrenalectomy: Dissection superior to the adrenal gland is continued to separate the tail of the pancreas and divide the small vessels and superior attachments.

Although CT and MRI are able to identify a large number of tumors, only simple cysts, myelolipoma, adrenal hemorrhage, and tumors with obvious malignant invasion can be adequately diagnosed based on radiologic criteria alone *(33,36)*. Benign adrenal adenomas are usually homogeneous lesions with smooth regular, encapsulated margins that do not increase in size over time *(37,38)*. Most benign adenomas have low attenuation values (<10 Hounsfeld units) on unenhanced CT scans, whereas carcinomas have a much higher attenuation (>18 Hounsfeld units) on unenhanced CT scan *(39)*. Unenhanced CT has a 100% positive predictive value and a 77% negative predicting value in diagnosing adenoma *(40)*.

MRI avoids the risk of radiation to the patient, but increases cost. Adenomas exhibit low signal intensity on a T2-weighted image, whereas pheochromocytomas and adrenal metastases have a bright signal intensity on T2-weighted images *(41)*.

MRI in-phase/opposed-phase chemical shift imaging can differentiate adrenal tumors based on the amount of lipid contained. Adenomas, which have a high lipid content, show a loss of signal intensity on

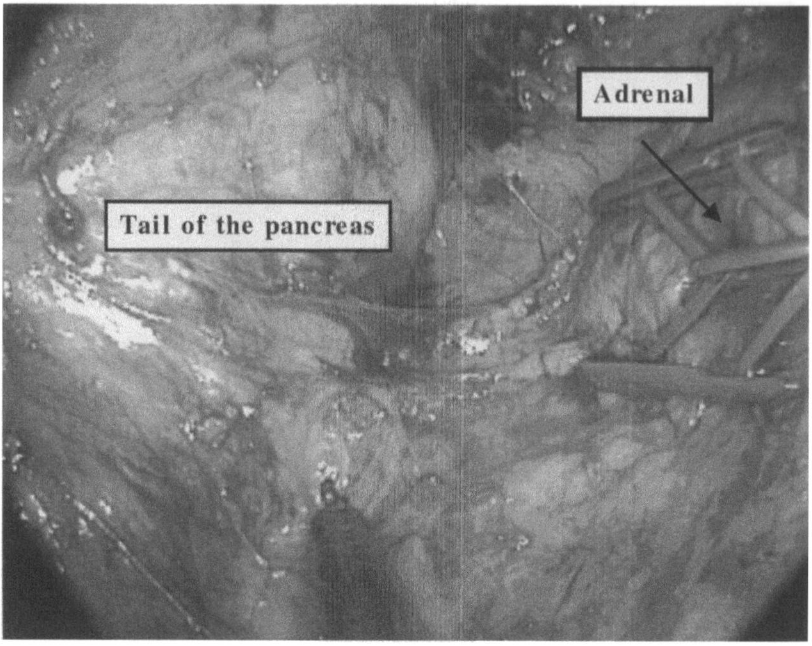


**Fig. 13.** Left adrenalectomy: Dissection of the tail of the pancreas and spleen is continued to expose the posterior body wall. Gentle inferior retraction on the adrenal aids in exposure.

opposed-phase chemical shift sequences; whereas malignant lesions fail to show any appreciable loss of signal intensity *(42,43)*.

The radionuclide agent NP-59 ($^{131}$I-6*B*-iodomethyl-norcholesterol) can also characterize the nature of adrenal lesions *(44,45)*. Benign adrenal tumors typically show uptake of NP-59, whereas malignant lesions and other nonadenomatous lesions fail to demonstrate uptake. NP-59 has not gained widespread utilization in the United States due to complexity in performing the test, need for thyroid blockade, and difficulty in obtaining the radionuclide *(36)*.

An adrenal mass in a patient with a known malignancy may undergo fine needle aspiration (FNA) to determine whether the lesion is a metastatic or a primary tumor. FNA is a minimally invasive method to confirm metastatic disease although it does possess a small risk of complications including bleeding, pneumothorax, and tract seeding *(10,46)*. FNA is often not adequate to distinguish a benign adenoma from a primary adrenocortical carcinoma and hence should only be used to diagnose possible metastatic disease when tissue diagnosis is necessary to guide treatment but complete excision is not indicated *(33)*. The

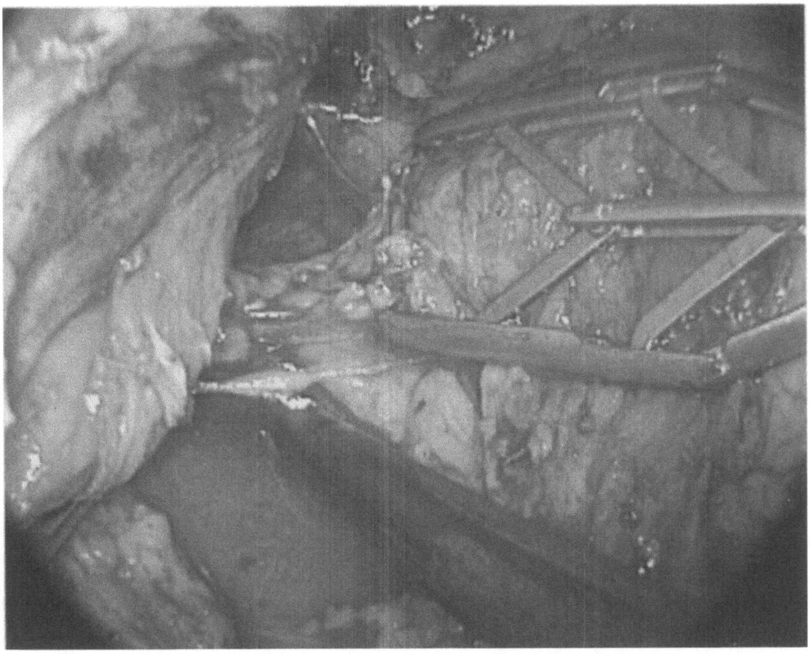

**Fig. 14.** Left adrenalectomy: After medial dissection, superior and posterior attachments are taken down until the body wall musculature is encountered. Continued inferior retraction on the adrenal gland assists in the direction.

positive predictive value of FNA biopsy and cytology in the setting of adrenal metastasis is close to 100% *(36)*.

Patients who have adrenal masses in the setting of obvious incurable widespread metastatic diseases elsewhere require no further diagnostic evaluation of the adrenal gland as this will not affect treatment. Asymptomatic patients with cysts, myelolipomas, or adrenal hemorrhages also require no further testing as these diagnoses can be established using radiologic criteria. All other patients should undergo a limited hormonal evaluation including a 24-h urine for catecholamines and metanephrines to exclude pheochromocytoma. A plasma morning cortisol and low-dose dexamethasone suppression test should be performed to exclude hypercortisolism and subclinical Cushing's. If the low-dose dexamethasone test fails to suppress cortisol production, then urine-free cortisol, serum cortisol diurnal rhythm, and plasma adrenocorticotropic hormone (ACTH) should be performed. In the presence of hypertension or hypokalemia, patients should undergo a plasma aldosterone and plasma renin activity to rule out hyperaldosteronism. Patients with hormonally active tumors should undergo adrenalectomy.

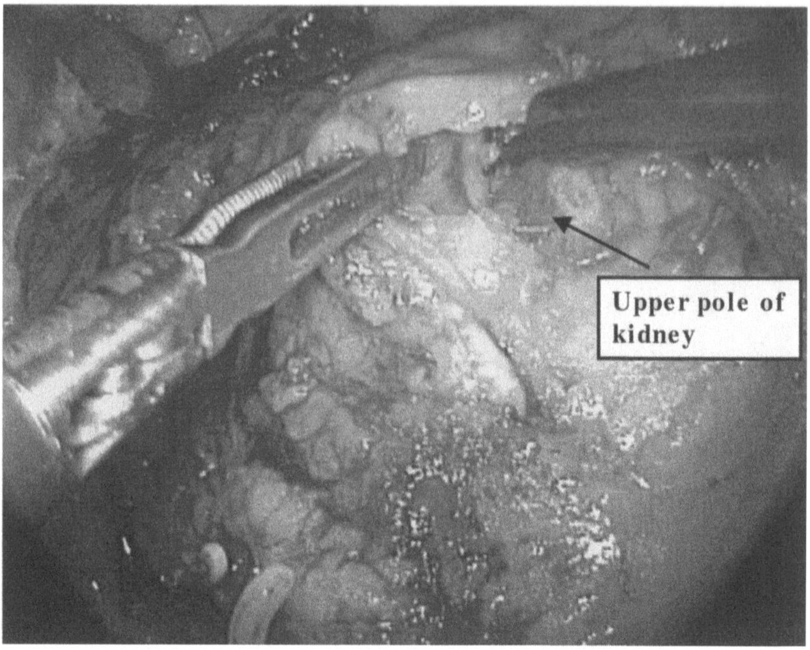


**Fig. 15.** Left adrenalectomy: After full medial, superior, and lateral mobilization; Gerota's fascia is entered to expose the upper pole of the kidney and separate the adrenal from the kidney.

The size criterion at which surgical removal of a nonfunctional adrenal mass is indicated is controversial. With the decreased morbidity of the laparoscopic approach, it is tempting to lower the size criteria for removal of an incidentally discovered adrenal mass. In a 5-yr review of more than 60,000 CT scans from the Mayo Clinic, Herrera and colleagues found that one in eight tumors resected greater than 4 cm in size were malignant. Based on this finding, they recommended removal of all adrenal glands 4 cm or larger *(32)*. Belldegrun and colleagues recommended that tumors larger than 3.5 cm should be explored *(31)*. At a 6 cm cutoff, one study suggested that nearly 60 benign adrenals would be removed for every tumor with cancer *(37)*, however adrenal cancers smaller than 6 cm have been reported *(32,47–49)*. It should be kept in mind that CT may underestimate the size of adrenal lesions less than 6 cm by 47% and tumors larger than 6 cm by 32% compared with the actual pathologic tumor measurements *(50)*. Gill recommends that patients younger than 50 yr with a 3–5 cm adrenal mass may be better served with laparoscopic adrenalectomy than conservative management

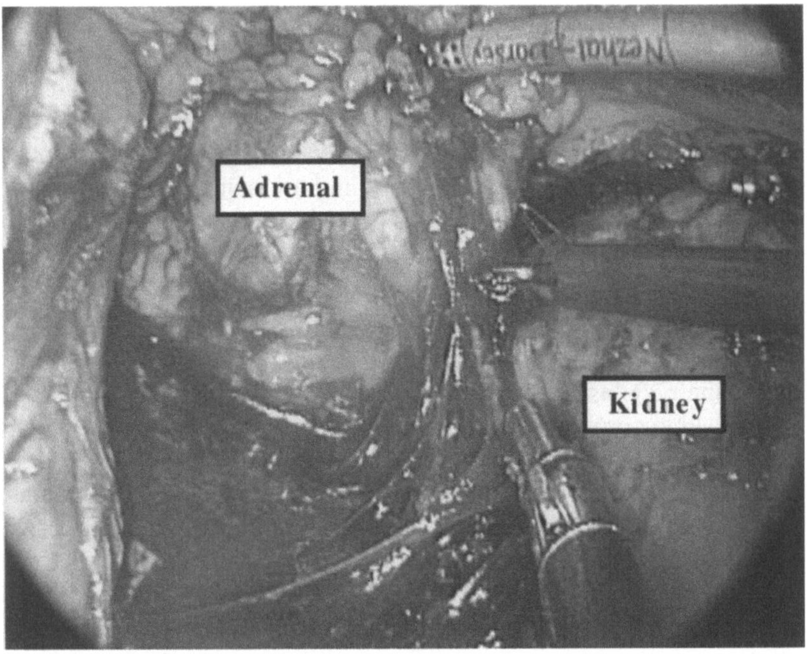


**Fig. 16.** Left adrenalectomy: The left adrenal is mobilized off the posterior body wall and upper pole of the kidney.

based on the long potential for increased size in these lesions. Using this approach, the annual imaging and hormonal work-up may be avoided *(12)*.

Most authors agree that nonfunctional tumors larger than 4–5 cm should be removed. Also, those patients with isolated adrenal metastasis should be considered for adrenalectomy *(33)*. If a unilateral adrenal lesion is noted in a patient with a prior history of malignancy who is otherwise disease-free, this should be considered for prompt resection if detailed evaluation reveals no other metastatic sites. An FNA may be considered to establish the diagnosis after biochemical studies show the absence of pheochromocytoma *(33,51)*.

Those lesions with an unenhanced CT attenuation value of 0 or less, negative biochemical evaluation, and small size less than 4–5 cm may be safely followed *(36)*. The majority of these lesions will remain hormonally inactive although isolated reports of these tumors progressing to functional state have been reported *(33)*. In one study of 251 patients followed for a minimum of 1 yr at the Mayo Clinic, no tumor that was originally hormonally inactive became active *(32)*.

## PHEOCHROMOCYTOMA

Pheochromocytomas comprise between 0 and 11% of incidentally detected adrenal lesions in most reported series *(33)*. The mean patient age at discovery is 42.3 yr *(52)*. Most pheochromocytomas occur spontaneously with no recognizable cause and are considered "sporadic." Goldstein and colleagues found that sporadic cases accounted for 84% of cases of pheochromocytomas *(52)*. In contrast, "inherited" autosomal dominant pattern pheochromocytomas are associated with different genetic syndromes and are often bilateral *(53)*.

The syndromes associated with pheochromocytoma include multiple endocrine neoplasia type 2 (MEN 2) and von Hippel-Lindau disease (VHL). Pheochromocytoma occurs rarely in families affected with neurofibromatosis type 1 *(54)*. In MEN 2, 95% have C-cell hyperplasia or medullary carcinoma of the thyroid, 50% have pheochromocytomas, and 15–20% have hyperparathyroidism *(55)*. Patients with MEN 2b have additional developmental abnormalities like marfanoid habitus or mucosal ganglioneuromas. Not all patients with MEN 2 are symptomatic, but by the age of 70 yr the rate of symptoms is 70% *(56)*. VHL disease manifestations include angioma of the retina, hemangioblastoma of the central nervous system, renal cell carcinoma (RCC), pancreatic cysts, and epididymal cystadenoma *(57)*. VHL patients presenting with pheochromocytomas rarely have pancreatic cysts or RCCs *(58)*.

The most common symptom of pheochromocytoma is hypertension (82%) followed by headache (49%), palpitations (40%), and sweating (37%). Other symptoms may include tremor, pallor, and anxiety *(33)*. Occasionally, patients may present with heart attack, stroke, or other complications related to the hemodynamic changes associated with pheochromocytoma *(33,52)*. Due to the effects of chronic vasoconstriction, these patients are often volume contracted and may have reversible catecholamine-induced cardiomyopathy *(12)*.

Open surgical resection of pheochromocytoma was originally associated with a high complication rate due to severe hemodynamic instability. Mortality occurred in up to 80% in patients with unsuspected pheochromocytoma *(36,59)*.

Originally, concern existed that the increased abdominal pressure of laparoscopy might result in significant catecholamine release *(60–64)*. Experience with laparoscopic resection of pheochromocytoma has shown no increased risk of hypertension or hypotension intraoperatively compared with open surgery *(65)*. A small percentage of appropriately blocked patients, similar to the rate at the time of induction, may demonstrate hypertension at the time of insufflation *(60)*. Some authors suggest that the laparoscopic approach allows a superior "no-touch" dissection and direct access to the adrenal vein resulting in less catecholamine release *(66)*. In a comparison of laparoscopic and open adrenalectomy for pheochromocytoma, laparoscopy resulted in similar blood pressure elevations and fewer and less severe hypotensive episodes than the open approach *(67)*. Fernandez-Cruz and colleagues showed that laparoscopy for pheochromocytoma was associated with a smaller increase in serum catecholamine than with open surgery *(64)*.

### *Diagnosis*

Urinary metanephrines may be the single best test for diagnosing pheochromocytoma as they establish the diagnosis in 92% of patients tested. The combination of urinary metanephrines and vanillylmandelic acid (VMA) has a diagnostic sensitivity in detecting pheochromocytoma of 98% *(68,69)*. Lenders and colleagues found that the sensitivity of plasma-free metanephrines was 99% (95% confidence interval [CI], 96–100%) and felt that this was the single best test to establish the diagnosis of pheochromocytoma *(70)*. Others have recommended two sets of 24-h urine collections for total and fractionated catecholamines, metanephrines, and VMA *(52,53)*. Occasionally, in indeterminate cases, a clonidine suppression test may be indicated *(71)*.

The bright signal seen on T2-weighted MRI images is highly specific for pheochromocytomas. MRI, like CT, is less reliable in patients with multicentric or extra-adrenal lesions *(53)*. At Vanderbilt, CT had a sensitivity of 94%, and a specificity of 97%, whereas MRI had a sensitivity of 83% but a specificity of 100% in diagnosing pheochromocytoma *(52)*. Use of 131 I metaiodobenzylguanidine (MIBG) scintigraphy may be useful in locating extra-adrenal tumors in hereditary cases where bilateral and extra-adrenal tumors are more likely to be encountered *(72)*.

### *Preoperative Management*

Phenoxybenzamine, a nonspecific alpha blocker, is the most frequently utilized medication to accomplish blockade prior to surgery. Doses of phenoxybenzamine begin with low levels that are gradually increased to a maximum of 250 mg per day. These agents may be administered for a period of 1–4 wk prior to surgery. The efficacy of preoperative control should be judged by the improvement of symptoms, the stabilization of arterial blood pressure, and the presence of mild orthostatic hypotension *(53)*. The use of prazosin, which is selective for $\alpha$-1 receptors has also been described for preoperative blockade *(73)*. Some authors have recommend $\beta$ blockade either alone or in combination with $\alpha$ blockade, but this may be unnecessary unless cardiac arrhythmia is present *(12,66)*. More recently, use of calcium channel blockers (verapamil-SR and nifedipine-XL), which may be started as late as 24 h prior to surgery, have been utilized. They have been shown to be as effective and possibly safer than α-blockers *(12,33,74)*.

At Vanderbilt University, 69% of patients treated without preoperative α blockade had hemodynamic instability, whereas 85% of those with blockade had a smooth operative course *(52)*. Similarly, the Cleveland Clinic reported on a series of 63 patients with pheochromocytoma, nearly half of whom had no preoperative blockade. They concluded that a skilled anesthesiologist administering sodium nitroprusside and/or nitroglycerin, alone or in combination, allowed safe surgical resection without preoperative blockade *(73)*. Although surgical resection may be accomplished without preoperative blockade, the anesthetic course is greatly simplified and there is little morbidity associated with a preoperative blockade.

### *Surgical Technique*

Both transperitoneal and retroperitoneal techniques have been safely utilized to perform laparoscopic adrenalectomy for pheochromocytoma *(27,66,75)*. The transperitoneal approach has the advantage of allowing early control of the adrenal vein using a no-touch technique, whereas the retroperitoneal approach has the advantage of causing only a small increase in intra-abdominal pressure and less stimulation of the peritoneum, which could potentially result in less catecholamine release at insufflation *(76)*. Despite this fact, the laparoscopic retroperitoneal approach is also associated with acute blood pressure elevations at the time of insufflation *(66)*.

Larger pheochromocytomas (>5 cm) may require more manipulation and may be associated with more hypertensive episodes *(75)*, although other authors have found that size does not predict hemodynamic instability *(66)*. Laparoscopic surgery for pheochromocytoma may be associated with longer operative times, greater blood loss, a longer hospitalization, and a higher conversion rate compared with laparoscopic adrenalectomy for other etiologies *(9,77)*.

### *Pathology*

The percentage of pheochromocytomas that demonstrate malignant behavior has been reported to be 8.3–47% *(52,68,78)*. Cellular hyperchromatism, bizarre mitotic figures, vascular invasion, and capsular invasion were features of both biologically benign and malignant tumors. Hence, true malignancy is defined as the occurrence of spread of tumor cells in or to anatomic areas where there is no known embryologic residue of paraganglionic tissue *(79)*. Even with no gross or histopathologic features of malignancy, the tumor will ultimately demonstrate malignant behavior in 8–9% of patients; hence, long-term followup is essential *(52,80)*.

### *Results*

The results of the laparoscopic treatment of pheochromocytoma have provided cure rates equal to open surgery with a dramatic reduction in patient morbidity. Janetschek reported a series of 24 patients managed laparoscopically and postoperatively found that blood pressure and urinary catecholamines were normal in all patients *(53)*. Walz and colleagues found normalization of all hormonal levels in 27 of 28 patients undergoing laparoscopic adrenalectomy. Brunt and colleagues found that all 34 of their patients were cured of biochemical signs of adrenal hyperfunction with a mean followup of 46 mo *(9)*. Gill found that hypertension was cured in 88.5% of patients *(12)*.

One concern in familial cases of pheochromocytoma is the propensity for tumor formation in the contralateral adrenal gland. Partial adrenalectomy is recommended in patients with bilateral pheochromocytoma and should be considered in patients with unilateral pheochromocytoma who have MEN 2 or VHL due to the risk of later development of contralateral lesions *(53)*. Partial adrenalectomy may avoid the long-term risks of steroid substitution *(9)*, but the risk of ipsilateral recurrence (8%) must be considered *(81)*.

Pheochromocytoma at the time of pregnancy can cause maternal and fetal mortality rates of 40–56% if not diagnosed prior to delivery. Antenatal diagnosis improves maternal and fetal mortality rates to 0 and 15%, respectively. Successful laparoscopic resection of pheochromocytoma during pregnancy has been reported *(82,83)*. Surgical intervention should be undertaken before 20 wk gestation *(84)*.

## ALDOSTERONOMA

Primary hyperaldosteronism is the most common cause of secondary hypertension. It is estimated to account for .7–2% of the hypertensive population *(85,86)*. The most common subtype of hyperaldosteronism is the aldosterone-producing adenoma, accounting for 70–80% of cases. Twenty to 30% of cases are due to bilateral cortical hyperplasia (idiopathic hyperaldosteronism), for which adrenalectomy is not indicated *(87)*. The aldosterone-producing adenoma (Conn's adenoma) is an ideal indication for laparoscopic adrenalectomy. These tumors are often small and technically easy to dissect *(2)*.

The clinical syndrome of hyperaldosteronism is characterized by hypertension and hypokalemia, although up to 20% of patients may not be hypokalemic *(87,88)*. If these two findings are present then patients should be further evaluated with a plasma aldosterone concentration and plasma renin activity after being upright for at least 2 h *(33)*.

Further testing to determine which subtype of aldosterone-producing adrenal tumor is present may be required. Imaging of the adrenals with CT or MRI may reveal a solitary unilateral macroadenoma larger than 1 cm in size and no contralateral adrenal abnormality. In these instances, proceeding with laparoscopic adrenalectomy is the treatment of choice *(89)*. However, in cases where the CT findings are ambiguous (no lesions on either side or bilateral lesions), adrenal venous sampling may determine the site of aldosterone overproduction *(89)*. Walz and colleagues recommend administration of oral potassium-sparing diuretics and potassium prior to surgery in patients with Conn's syndrome *(77)*.

In a series of 29 patients (mean followup 27.9 mo) undergoing laparoscopic adrenalectomy for aldosteronoma, Brunt and colleagues found clinical and biochemical resolution of symptoms in all patients. Of these patients, 92% had improved blood pressure control, although 72% still had hypertension *(9)*. Siren and colleagues, in a prospective study of 12 consecutive patients, found correction of serum potassium and improvement of blood pressure control in each case *(90)*.

The likely cause of continued elevated blood pressure in many patients may be co-existent essential hypertension. There is also evidence that a long period of hypertension prior to undergoing surgery may be associated with refractory hypertension *(9)*.

## EXCESS CORTISOL PRODUCTION

Cushing's syndrome is rare with an incidence of 1 in 100,000 to 1 in 500,000 *(91,92)*. Signs and symptoms of Cushing's syndrome include weight gain, hypertension, bruisability, diabetes mellitus, amenorrhea, hirsutism, purplish abdominal striae, edema, and a characteristic body habitus with centripetal obesity pattern *(93–95)*. The most common cause of Cushing's syndrome is iatrogenic administration of steroids for other reasons. All cases of endogenous Cushing's syndrome are due to increased production of cortisol by the adrenal gland. The cause of increased cortisol production may vary. The most frequent etiology of increased cortisol production by the adrenal glands is bilateral adrenal hyperplasia secondary to adrenocortical stimulation by excess production of ACTH. This excess production of ACTH may be due to autonomous overproduction of ACTH by a pituitary adenoma or due to a failure in the corticotropic-releasing hormone (CRH)-ACTH pathway. These patients have traditionally been considered to have Cushing's disease.

Nonendocrine tumors may also secrete polypeptides that are biologically, chemically, and immunologically indistinguishable from either ACTH or CRH that act on the adrenal and result in bilateral hyperplasia. Patients with the syndrome of ectopic ACTH secretion often have an unresectable or occult source of ACTH secretion. The metabolic manifestations of cortisol excess appear suddenly and progress rapidly. The typical Cushing's habitus may be absent, and hypokalemic alkalosis and glucose intolerance may be the prominent manifestations. Small-cell lung cancer is the malignancy most frequently associated with ectopic ACTH. Other causes include bronchial or thymic carcinoid tumors, islet cell tumors, or medullary carcinoma of the thyroid *(96)*.

Another cause of bilateral adrenal hyperplasia, is ACTH-independent nodular hyperplasia *(97)*. These patients present with the features of Cushing's syndrome and endocrinologically reveal autonomous adrenal cortisol production with suppressed ACTH and a loss in the diurnal circadian rhythm of plasma cortisol. Imaging with abdominal CT demonstrates bilateral enlargement of the adrenal glands with multiple nodules *(97)*. The biochemical findings in ACTH-independent macronodular hyperplasia include elevated plasma cortisol, low plasma adrenocorticotropic hormone, loss of diurnal rhythm of plasma cortisol and ACTH, lack of plasma cortisol suppression after a high dose (8 mg) dexamethasone suppression test, and a normal response of plasma cortisol or plasma ACTH to exogenous CRH stimulation.

Only 20% of cases of Cushing's syndrome are due to a cortisol-producing adenoma *(33)*. Five to 20% of hormonally active incidentalomas produce glucocorticoids *(92)*.

### *Diagnosis*

Diagnosis of the causes of excess cortisol production is complex and in those who lack experience may be best diagnosed with the assistance of an endocrinologist. The first step in diagnosis is to determine whether Cushing's syndrome is present, and the second step is to determine the cause of excess hypercortisolism. The presence of Cushing's syndrome may be established by collecting 24-h urine-free cortisol levels.

Once Cushing's syndrome is confirmed with elevated urine-free cortisol, plasma ACTH, CRH, and the high-dose dexamethasone test may assist in determining the etiology of cortisol excess. The high-dose dexamethasone test will suppress cortisol production by Cushing's disease, but not those with ectopic ACTH secretion or adrenal tumors *(9)*.

Imaging may also be helpful in establishing the diagnosis. A CT or MRI of the head may reveal a pituitary macroadenoma. Also US, CT, or MRI may demonstrate the adrenal adenoma, or other mass responsible for ectopic ACTH production.

All patients with an adrenal mass should be screened biochemically for hypercortisolism. The best method of screening is the test for cortisol suppressibility in response to the low-dose dexamethasone test *(36,95)*. This test is performed by giving a single 1–3 mg dose of dexamethasone at 11 PM, and a plasma cortisol level is obtained at 8 AM the following morning. Normal subjects will have a suppression of the plasma cortisol to less than 3 μg/dL. A serum cortisol level greater than 3 μg/dL on the low-dose dexamethasone test requires further investigation, including confirmation by high-dose dexamethasone (8 mg) suppression testing, a CRH test, and analysis of diurnal rhythm. Elevated plasma ACTH levels suggest a corticotropin-dependent source for the elevated cortisol. Patients with adrenal hypercortisolism should have low or normal ACTH levels *(33)*. Patients who demonstrate a suppressed plasma ACTH in response to CRH stimulation generally have adrenal insufficiency after surgery and require adequate perioperative and postoperative substitution therapy *(92)*. For a complete discussion of the evaluation of patients with hypercortisolism and subclinical hypercortisolism, the interested reader is referred to a textbook of medicine or endocrinology.

### *Treatment*

The goals of treatment in patients with Cushing's syndrome include lowering of cortisol secretion, excision of the tumor without producing permanent endocrine deficiency, and the avoidance of lifelong adrenal replacement therapy. The management of Cushing's syndrome is directed toward the cause of cortisol elevation.

If radiologic localization with a CT or MRI confirms a pituitary tumor, transsphenoidal microsurgical hypophysectomy is the primary line of treatment with a cure rate of 85–95%. Although transphenoidal surgery is the standard of care for Cushing's syndrome, some tumors invade contiguous structures precluding resection, whereas others may be so small they escape detection and are not resected at the time of surgery. Transphenoidal surgery is associated with a 20–40% failure rate even for experienced surgeons *(98–100)*. Residual hypercortisolism may be managed with radiation treatments, repeat microadenectomy, stereotactic radiosurgery, medical management, or bilateral adrenalectomy *(12)*.

Ectopic production of ACTH is best treated by resection of the primary tumor. In unresectable cases, medical therapy with amino-glutethimide, metyrapone, or ketoconazole may achieve temporary lowering of serum cortisol *(12)*. In cases of unresectable ACTH-producing tumors, or radiologically occult ACTH-producing tumors such as carcinoid tumors, laparoscopic bilateral adrenalectomy is a viable treatment option and may offer long-term relief of symptoms *(101)*.

If the source of elevated cortisol comes from a primary adrenal source, CT scan will differentiate the potential causes of elevated cortisol. If the CT demonstrates a small, less then 2 cm unilateral nodule in the adrenal gland with contralateral adrenal atrophy, the cause is likely a unilateral functional adrenal adenoma best treated with laparoscopic surgical excision. If the CT demonstrates a large unilateral mass greater than 4–6 cm in size, this may indicate adrenal cortical carcinoma, best treated with wide surgical excision via an open approach if venous or local invasion is suspected.

In instances of ACTH-independent bilateral macronodular, adrenocortical hyperplasia bilateral laparoscopic adrenalectomy is the treatment of choice *(97)*. Patients undergoing bilateral adrenalectomy must be maintained on chronic steroid supplementation.

### *Results*

Open bilateral adrenalectomy has been associated with a 7–83% perioperative morbidity and up to 19% mortality with persistent or recurrent hypercortisolism in 1–24% of patients *(12)*. The high morbidity in this population stems from the immunosuppression, compromised wound healing and high infection rate, bleeding tendency, and other complications resulting from prolonged cortisol hypersecretion *(12)*.

The open incisions associated with adrenalectomy often require rib resection, nerve retraction, and muscle transection and have been associated with incisional and musculoskeletal problems that may persist long after the operation *(102)*. These incisional problems are especially pronounced in patients with Cushing's syndrome due to poor wound healing and musculoskeletal complaints associated with the condition *(101,103)*.

A benign Cushing's adrenal adenoma is one of the ideal indications for laparoscopic surgery. These tumors are frequently small and easy to dissect *(2)*. Incisional and wound complications are infrequently reported using a laparoscopic approach *(101)*. Kollmorgen and colleagues, working in the porcine model, noted that animals undergoing adrenalectomy with a laparoscopic approach were less catabolic and had less wound complications *(104)*.

In a review of five patients with cortisol-producing adenomas, Brunt found that all were cured following laparoscopic adrenalectomy. At a mean followup of 27 mo (range 3–74 mo) all patients were normotensive and had no signs or symptoms of Cushing's syndrome *(9)*.

Vella and colleagues reported on a single center series of 19 patients from the Mayo Clinic in which 16 completed a bilateral laparoscopic adrenalectomy. Twelve patients with pituitary-dependent Cushing's syndrome and four patients with ectopic ACTH syndrome underwent successful bilateral laparoscopic adrenalectomy. The median duration of disease was 3 yr. Medical therapy with ketoconazole was attempted in four patients and with aminoglutethimide in two. Only one patient was able to tolerate medical therapy for longer than 1 mo, and adequate control of cortisol secretion was not achieved in this patient. With a mean followup of 32 mo, all patients experienced resolution of the signs and symptoms within 6 mo of adrenalectomy *(101)*.

Guazzoni and colleagues reported on a series of 161 laparoscopic adrenalectomies, of which 10 patients underwent bilateral adrenalectomy for bilateral adrenal hyperplasia following failed transsphenoidal surgery in 9 cases, and bilateral macronodular hyperplasia in 1 patient. They had no complications, no conversions, and the patients had a mean of 14 d until return to normal activity. All patients had persistently undetectable urine-free cortisol and none had evidence of pituitary adenoma regrowth on MRI imaging *(25)*.

In a literature review of patients treated with laparoscopic adrenalectomy for Cushing's syndrome, Gill reported that in 64 patients there were 5 conversions (7.9%) and a complication rate of 9.5% *(12)*.

In cases of ACTH-dependent Cushing's syndrome it is especially critical that all adrenal tissue be removed to avoid leaving residual tissue that could hypertrophy under the effects of chronic ACTH stimulation. Isolated cases of cortisol responsiveness following bilateral adrenalectomy have been reported *(105)*. Bilateral procedures do require repositioning on the surgical field unless performed through an anterior transperitoneal approach, and are associated with longer operative times and increased blood loss but may be safely performed *(12,25,101)*.

## ADRENOCORTICAL CARCINOMA

Adrenocortical carcinomas are rare tumors with an estimated incidence of 1 per 1.7 million population *(37)*. Of incidentally detected adrenal masses, adrenocortical carcinoma makes up from 0 to 25% of tumors (average 4%) *(33,106)*. The incidence of adrenocortical carcinoma in adrenal masses larger than 6 cm has ranged from 35 to 98% *(33,107)*. Although more than 90% of adrenocortical carcinomas are likely to be greater than 6 cm in diameter *(37)*, all cancers were presumably small at one time and reports of carcinomas of 2–3 cm in size have been reported *(12,36)*. In one series, 16% of adrenocortical carcinomas were less than 5 cm in diameter *(108)*.

Radiologic imaging studies may demonstrate an irregular heterogenous configuration. Unenhanced CT images with attenuation values greater than 10 HU and enhanced values greater than 30 may suggest risk of malignancy. On MRI, they often demonstrate increased signal intensity with T2-weighted images. They frequently invade adjacent structures and may metastasize to lymph nodes, lung, bone, liver, and kidney *(33)*.

Adrenocortical carcinomas may be hypersecretory, whereas one-half of patients will have no recognizable endocrine syndrome *(109)*. Plasma dehydroepiandrostenedione (DHEA) sulfate levels may serve as a useful marker to identify malignant adrenocortical carcinoma *(93,94,110)*.

CT and MRI may not demonstrate local invasion even when present. For this reason, patients with large primary adrenal cortical carcinoma are probably best managed with an open approach *(12)*. In small adrenal cortical carcinomas, evidence of resectability should be sought on imaging. Factors supporting laparoscopic resectability include visualization of fat planes between the adrenal gland and the great vessels, absence of local invasion into peri-adrenal fat or adjacent organs, and the absence of venous thrombus *(12,111)*. Guazzoni and colleagues recommend the transperitoneal laparoscopic approach for adrenal malignancy 6 cm or less in size and confined to the adrenal gland *(25)*.

The local recurrence rate with adrenocortical carcinoma is 18% and 5-yr survival is 50% or less *(12,112)*. Caution should be exercised in the application of laparoscopic adrenalectomy to suspicious lesions. There have been reports of local recurrences and intraperitoneal seeding following laparoscopic adrenalectomy for malignant lesions *(113–115, 116)*. For tumors larger than 6 cm with findings suspicious for malignancy on imaging, an open removal may provide the best curative surgery *(33)*.

## METASTATIC ADRENAL TUMORS

Adrenal metastasis may be found in autopsy series in 8–38% of patients with extra-adrenal malignancies *(33,36,117,118)*. The incidence of adrenal metastases in patients with a history of nonadrenal cancer who present with a unilateral adrenal mass has ranged from 32 to 73% *(33,36,117,118)*. Those lesions less than 3 cm in size are less likely to be malignant than those larger than 3 cm in size. Adrenal metastases are frequently bilateral *(33)*. The most common primary tumors seen with metastasis to the adrenal gland are breast, lung, lymphoma, renal cell, and melanoma *(33,117)*.

Metastatic adrenal tumors are often small and confined within the adrenal gland. The laparoscopic approach is attractive for these lesions *(12)*. Wade and colleagues found a 13%, 5-yr survival in patients with surgically resected adrenal metastasis *(51)*. In rare patients with a solitary adrenal metastasis, complete excision may confer a 5-yr survival in the 20–45% range *(119)*. Resection of solitary adrenal lesions may provide longer survival than chemotherapy *(120)*, may allow long periods of progression-free survival for metastatic RCC *(112)* and adenocarcinoma, and has been shown to provide symptom relief in patients with painful metastasis *(46)*. If feasible, the laparoscopic approach provides lower morbidity in these patients.

## NEEDLESCOPIC ADRENALECTOMY

As the experience with laparoscopic adrenalectomy has increased there has been a gradual shift toward minimizing the invasiveness of the technique. By definition, needlescopic instruments have an outer diameter of 2 mm which is similar to a 14-gauge angiocatheter needle. Due to the small size of this instrumentation, the functionality is also somewhat decreased. For this reason, most strategies utilize a 5- or 10-mm camera that may be placed at the umbilicus to minimize the cosmetic impact. An additional 5-mm port for use of clip applier and hook electrode is also inserted. The remainder of the ports may be 2-mm instruments *(121)*.

## PEDIATRIC ADRENALECTOMY

Laparoscopic adrenalectomy has been reported in children. Mirallie and colleagues reported on six children undergoing laparoscopic adrenalectomy for ganglioneuroma, neuroblastoma, and pheochromocytoma. The age of the children ranged from 2–16 yr and there were no complications associated with the technique. There were two open conversions. Laparoscopic partial adrenalectomy has also been successfully performed in children *(122)*.

## LAPAROSCOPIC PARTIAL ADRENALECTOMY

The technique of partial adrenalectomy is mainly indicated in patients suffering from bilateral adrenal disease such as is seen in patients with MEN 2a or VHL, but has also been reported for aldosteronoma *(25,123–126)*. The advantage of partial adrenalectomy in patients with bilateral adrenal disease is that the patient may avoid the long-term risks of steroid substitution including osteoporosis, hypoandrogenism, and other effects of steroid replacement *(9)*.

Imai and colleagues have reported their successful technique for partial adrenalectomy using the vascular stapler and resecting of a 5-mm cuff of normal adrenal gland adjacent to the adenoma. Using this technique in five patients, all patients with functional tumors had biochemical normalization and hemostasis was excellent in each instance *(125)*. Walz and colleagues used simple monopolar electrocautery to perform the partial resections and also noted no significant problems with bleeding *(77)*. In a series of 39 patients who underwent partial adrenalectomy reported by Walz and colleagues, there was biochemical and clinical normalization in all patients and no local recurrence was seen in the study with a median followup of 27 mo *(77)*.

A particular concern with partial adrenalectomy in patients with familial forms of pheochromocytoma is the handling of the adrenal vein. Walz and colleagues determined that the main adrenal vein could be sacrificed along with the tumor and no replacement cortisol therapy was required *(77)*. Janetschek reported laparoscopic partial adrenalectomy leaving the adrenal vein patent. A dramatic increase in pressure could be safely controlled intraoperatively by the experienced anesthesiologist or alternatively, a bulldog clamp placed across the adrenal vein while resecting the adrenal tumor *(53)*.

Enthusiasm for partial adrenalectomy must be tempered against the 8% ipsilateral adrenal recurrence rate reported by Walter and colleagues in patients with familial pheochromocytoma *(81)*. In general, laparoscopic partial adrenalectomy techniques are early in their development. Until long-term followup is available, partial adrenalectomy should be utilized in experienced centers *(25)*.

## MORBIDITY AND RECOVERY

One of the principle forces behind the acceptance of the laparoscopic approach in the treatment of most adrenal tumors has been the lower morbidity and faster recovery seen with this approach. In a comparison of laparoscopic and open surgery, Guazzoni and colleagues found a decreased blood loss, hospitalization, transfusion, and analgesia requirement, and more rapid return to work in patients treated with laparoscopy *(127)*. Guazzoni and colleagues found a mean time to normal activity of 7 d following discharge to home in unilateral cases and 14 d in patients undergoing bilateral adrenalectomy *(25)*.

Brunt and colleagues found that laparoscopic adrenalectomy patients were able to resume 100% activity an average of 10.6 +/– 4.9 d after laparoscopic adrenalectomy and returned to work a mean of 16.0 +/– 6.1 d postoperatively *(4)*.

Thompson and colleagues, in a matched case-control study, found that the mean time for return to normal activity was faster in patients undergoing laparoscopic adrenalectomy compared with those undergoing open adrenalectomy (3.8 vs 7 wk), and that the laparoscopic patients had a higher overall patient satisfaction score *(128)*. Walz and colleagues, in a series of 142 retroperitoneoscopic adrenalectomies, reported 71 patients required no postoperative analgesia and only 5 patients required pain medication for more than 24 h *(77)*. Using strict inclusion criteria, Gill and colleagues performed laparoscopic adrenalectomy as an outpatient *(129)*.

Open conversion rates have been reported ranging from 0 to 17%. No significant differences have been noted between the retroperitoneal or transperitoneal approach *(5,9,25,130,131)*. Those centers with larger experience usually report open conversion rates of 3% or less *(14,25)*. A higher rate of open conversion (50%) may be seen in cases of malignant tumors *(10)*. A conversion should not be viewed as a failure of the procedure, and should be performed in a timely fashion when indicated *(2)*.

Complication rates vary widely depending on surgical experience. Complication rates from 5.5 to 28% have been reported *(12,14,25,33,132–135)*. In a prospective study, intraoperative complications were seen in 5% and postoperative complications were seen in 13% of 142 adrenalectomies. All of the complications were minor in nature in the study *(77)*.

Brunt and colleagues reviewed all large series reported in the English literature from 1980 to 2000. A total of 1522 laparoscopic patients were compared to 2273 patients treated with open adrenalectomy. The total reported laparoscopic complication rate was 25.2% vs 10.9% with open surgery (*p* 0.0001). Laparoscopy had an increased incidence of bleeding complications (4.7% vs 3.7%; *p* 0.0001). However, the laparoscopic approach had a lower incidence of associated organ injury (0.7% vs 2.4%), wound infection (1.4% vs 6.9%), pulmonary complications (0.9% vs 5.5%), cardiac (0.3% vs 1.6%), and infectious complications (1.6% vs 5.8%) (all *p* 0.0001). There were no significant differences in gastrointestinal, thromboembolic, and neurologic complications or mortality *(136)*.

Many studies have demonstrated a reduced rate of respiratory complications and a dramatic decrease in wound complications advantages with the laparoscopic approach *(5,128,137,138)*. Patients requiring adrenalectomy for Cushing's syndrome may benefit particularly from the laparoscopic approach due to less risk of infections, hematomas, dehiscence, and slow healing frequently observed with large open incisions *(104,139)*.

Other authors have also found a decreased incidence of complications associated with the laparoscopic approach *(1)*. In a retrospective study, Brunt and colleagues demonstrated that patients undergoing laparoscopic adrenalectomy had significantly fewer complications than those who undergo the open posterior technique *(4)*. In a prospective case-control study comparing laparoscopic adrenalectomy to conventional open posterior adrenalectomy, Thompson and colleagues demonstrated that early morbidity (6% vs 18%) and late morbidity (0% vs 54%) were significantly decreased in the laparoscopic group *(128)*.

Both open conversion rate and complication rate tend to be much higher early in the learning curve, and these rates drop as a center gains experience with the technique *(132)*. Henry and colleagues reported that the early complications in their series with laparoscopic adrenalectomy were from lack of experience and bleeding *(139)*. Suzuki and colleagues reported a high complication rate (28%) and found that most of the complications occurred in their first 25 cases *(134)*.

## COST

Although the laparoscopic approach to adrenal removal has demonstrated clear advantages in patient morbidity and a faster recovery, critics have cited increased cost for intraoperative supplies and increased operative time. Thompson and colleagues found that the median hospital charges were slightly higher ($7000 vs $6000) in a group of patients undergoing laparoscopic adrenalectomy compared with those undergoing an adrenalectomy with an open posterior approach ($p = 0.05$).

With increased experience, surgical times may be equal to or shorter than open adrenalectomy. Also, reusable laparoscopic instrumentation and shorter hospitalization have resulted in a decrease in the cost of laparoscopic surgery. Korman reported that laparoscopic adrenalectomy was less expensive when comparing direct costs ($3645 vs $5752) and total costs ($8188 vs $12,840) *(140)*. Similarly, Hobart and colleagues at the Cleveland Clinic compared costs in 15 patients treated with a needlescopic approach to 15 contemporary patients treated with open surgery. They noted an 18% higher intraoperative cost but a 63% decrease in postoperative costs. Overall, the laparoscopic approach was 18% less expensive than open surgery *(141)*.

## CONTRAINDICATIONS TO THE LAPAROSCOPIC APPROACH

Only very large tumor size, local invasion, or large suspected adrenal cortical carcinoma are now considered contraindications to a laparoscopic approach *(33)*. Some authors set the size limit for a laparoscopic approach at 7–9 cm due to the increased risk of malignancy in larger tumors *(4,137,142,143)*. Henry and colleagues determined that tumors larger than 12 cm should be removed with open surgery *(10)*. The actual size cutoff will depend on a surgeon's experience with laparoscopic techniques and the anatomic variables of the particular patient.

Using a purely laparoscopic approach, margin status may not be obtained in the morcellated specimen. This may be of little consequence in the majority of benign adrenal lesions, and would only be of significance in cases of malignant pheochromocytoma or adrenal cortical carcinoma. In the case of malignancy a concern of port-site metastasis exists. Obvious malignancy with local invasion is best managed with an open operation at the present time *(2,10)*. Feminizing and masculinizing tumors are often malignant and hence should be removed with open surgery *(2)*.

Pheochromocytomas are effectively treated laparoscopically but due to their increased vasculature, capsular friability, larger size and hemodynamic effects, these tumors should be treated by surgeons experienced with laparoscopy *(53)*.

Patients with morbid obesity were once considered a contraindication for laparoscopic adrenalectomy. Fazeli-Marten and colleagues found that obese patients undergoing laparoscopic adrenalectomy had shorter hospital stays, lower pain medication requirement, and similar outcomes compared to open surgery. All obese patients (open or laparoscopic) were at an increased risk of complications but the incidence of complications was no greater in the laparoscopic group *(144)*. The procedure is certainly more challenging and may increase the risk of open conversion *(25)*.

Previous upper abdominal surgery such as partial or total nephrectomy, hepatic resection on the right side, and distal pancreatectomy or splenectomy on the left side, are relative contraindications to a laparoscopic approach. Patients who have undergone prior partial adrenalectomy are significantly more difficult *(10)*. Although prior abdominal surgery complicates the laparoscopic approach, Gill and colleagues reported successful laparoscopic right adrenalectomy even following liver transplantation *(145)*.

## SUMMARY

The laparoscopic approach to adrenal tumors has demonstrated equal efficacy to open surgery in the treatment of incidentally detected adrenal masses, pheochromocytomas, aldosteronomas, patients with cortisol excess, and in patients with isolated or painful adrenal metastases. Only extremely large tumors (> 8–12 cm), and primary adrenocortical carcinomas are best treated with open surgery. The laparoscopic approach has also resulted in dramatic reductions in hospital stay, analgesia requirement, recovery time, and complication rates. As experience with laparoscopic adrenalectomy increases, the surgical times and hospital costs are comparable to open surgery. For these reasons, the laparoscopic approach is the treatment of choice for most adrenal tumors.

## REFERENCES


1. McCallum RW, Connell JM. Laparoscopic adrenalectomy. Clin Endocrinol (Oxf), 2001; 55(4): 435–436.
2. Marescaux J, Mutter D, Vix M, Leroy J. Endoscopic surgery: ideal for endocrine surgery? World J Surg 1999; 23(8): 825–834.
3. Gagner M, Lacroix A, Bolte E. Laparoscopic adrenalectomy in Cushing's syndrome and pheochromocytoma. N Engl J Med 1992; 327(14): 1033.
4. Brunt LM, Doherty GM, Norton JA, et al. Laparoscopic adrenalectomy compared to open adrenalectomy for benign adrenal neoplasms. J Am Coll Surg 1996; 183(1): 1–10.
5. Gagner M, Pomp A, Heniford BT, Pharand D, Lacroix A. Laparoscopic adrenalectomy: lessons learned from 100 consecutive procedures. Ann Surg 1997; 226(3): 238–246; discussion 246–247.
6. Rutherford JC, Stowasser M, Tunny TJ, Klemm SA, Gordon RA. Laparoscopic adrenalectomy. World J Surg 1996; 20(7): 758–760; discussion 761.
7. Terachi T, Matsuda T, Terai A, et al. Transperitoneal laparoscopic adrenalectomy: experience in 100 patients. J Endourol 1997; 11(5): 361–365.
8. Lezoche E, Guerrieri M, Paganni AM, et al. Laparoscopic adrenalectomy by the anterior transperitoneal approach: results of 108 operations in unselected cases. Surg Endosc 2000; 14(10): 920–925.
9. Brunt LM, Moley JF, Doherty GM, et al. Outcomes analysis in patients undergoing laparoscopic adrenalectomy for hormonally active adrenal tumors. Surgery 2001; 130(4): 629–634; discussion 634–635.
10. Henry JF, Defechereux T, Gramatica L, Raffaelli M. Should laparoscopic approach be proposed for large and/or potentially malignant adrenal tumors? Langenbecks Arch Surg 1999; 384(4): 366–369.
11. Fernandez-Cruz L, Saenz A, Benarroch G, Torres E, Astudillo E. Technical aspects of adrenalectomy via operative laparoscopy. Surg Endosc 1994; 8(11): 1348–1351.
12. Gill IS. The case for laparoscopic adrenalectomy. J Urol 2001: 166(2): 429–436.
13. Kuriansky J, Saenz A, Astudillo E, et al. Laparoscopic adrenalectomy in the elderly. J Laparoendosc Adv Surg Tech A 1999: 9(4): 317–320.
14. Salomon L, Soulie M, Mouly P, et al. Experience with retroperitoneal laparoscopic adrenalectomy in 115 procedures. J Urol 2001; 166(1): 38–41.

15. Duh QY, Siperstein AE, Clark OH, et al. Laparoscopic adrenalectomy. Comparison of the lateral and posterior approaches. Arch Surg 1996; 131(8): 870–875; discussion 875–876.
16. Bonjer HJ, Lange JF, Kazemier G, et al. Comparison of three techniques for adrenalectomy. Br J Surg 1997; 84(5): 679–682.
17. Fernandez-Cruz L, Saenz A, Benarroch G, et al. Laparoscopic unilateral and bilateral adrenalectomy for Cushing's syndrome. Transperitoneal and retroperitoneal approaches. Ann Surg 1996; 224(6): 727–734; discussion 734–736.
18. Miyake O, Yoshimura K, Yoshioka T, et al. Laparoscopic adrenalectomy. Comparison of the transperitoneal and retroperitoneal approach. Eur Urol 1998; 33(3): 303–307.
19. Ng CS, Gill IS, Sung GT, et al. Retroperitoneoscopic surgery is not associated with increased carbon dioxide absorption. J Urol 1999; 162(4): 1268–1272.
20. Suzuki K, Kageyama S, Hirano Y, et al. Comparison of 3 surgical approaches to laparoscopic adrenalectomy: a nonrandomized, background matched analysis. J Urol 2001; 166(2): 437–443.
21. Takeda M. Laparoscopic adrenalectomy: transperitoneal vs retroperitoneal approaches. Biomed Pharmacother 2000; 54(Suppl 1): 207s–210s.
22. Fernandez-Cruz L, Saenz A, Taura P, Benarroch G, Astudillo E, Sabater L. Retroperitoneal approach in laparoscopic adrenalectomy: is it advantageous? Surg Endosc 1999; 13(1): 86–90.
23. Fletcher DR, Beiles CB, Hardy KJ. Laparoscopic adrenalectomy. Aust N Z J Surg 1994; 64(6): 427–430.
24. Shekarriz B, Gholami SS, Rudnick DM, Duh QY, Stoller ML. Radially expanding laparoscopic access for renal/adrenal surgery. Urology 2001; 58(5): 683–687.
25. Guazzoni G, Cestari A, Montorsi F, et al. Eight-year experience with transperitoneal laparoscopic adrenal surgery. J Urol 2001; 166(3): 820–824.
26. Heniford BT, Iannitti DA, Hale J, Gagner M. The role of intraoperative ultrasonography during laparoscopic adrenalectomy. Surgery 1997; 122(6): 1068–1073; discussion 1073–1074.
27. Salomon L, Rabii R, Soulie M, et al. Experience with retroperitoneal laparoscopic adrenalectomy for pheochromocytoma. J Urol 2001; 165(6 Pt 1): 1871–1874.
28. Griffing GT. A-I-D-S: the new endocrine epidemic. J Clin Endocrinol Metab 1994; 79(6): 1530–1531.
29. Glazer HS, Weyman PJ, Sagel SS, Levitt RG, McClennan BL. Nonfunctioning adrenal masses: incidental discovery on computed tomography. AJR Am J Roentgenol 1982; 139(1): 81–85.
30. Prinz RA, Brooks MH, Churchill R, et al. Incidental asymptomatic adrenal masses detected by computed tomographic scanning. Is operation required? JAMA 1982; 248(6): 701–704.
31. Belldegrun A, Hussain S, Seltzer SE, et al. Incidentally discovered mass of the adrenal gland. Surg Gynecol Obstet 1986; 163(3): 203–208.
32. Herrera MF, Grant CS, van Heerden JA, Sheedy PF, Ilstrup DM. Incidentally discovered adrenal tumors: an institutional perspective. Surgery 1991; 110(6): 1014–1021.
33. Brunt LM, Moley JF. Adrenal incidentaloma. World J Surg 2001; 25(7): 905–913.
34. Hedeland H, Ostberg G, Hokfelt B. On the prevalence of adrenocortical adenomas in an autopsy material in relation to hypertension and diabetes. Acta Med Scand 1968; 184(3): 211–214.

35. Abecassis M, McLoughlen MJ, Langer B, Kudlow JE. Serendipitous adrenal masses: prevalence, significance, and management. Am J Surg 1985; 149(6): 783–788.
36. Kloos RT, Korobkin M, Thompson NW, et al. Incidentally discovered adrenal masses. Endocr Rev 1995; 16(4): 460–484.
37. Copeland PM. The incidentally discovered adrenal mass. Ann Intern Med 1983; 98(6): 940–945.
38. Francis IR, Gross MD, Shapiro B, Korobkin M, Quint LE. Integrated imaging of adrenal disease. Radiology 1992; 184(1): 1–13.
39. Lee MJ, Hahn PF, Papanicolaou N, et al. Benign and malignant adrenal masses: CT distinction with attenuation coefficients, size, and observer analysis. Radiology, 1991; 179(2): 415–418.
40. Korobkin M, Brodeur FJ, Yutzy GG, et al. Differentiation of adrenal adenomas from nonadenomas using CT attenuation values. AJR Am J Roentgenol 1996; 166(3): 531–536.
41. Dunnick NR, Korobkin M, Francis I. Adrenal radiology: distinguishing benign from malignant adrenal masses. AJR Am J Roentgenol 1996; 167(4): 861–867.
42. Korobkin M, Lombardi TJ, Aisen AM, et al. Characterization of adrenal masses with chemical shift and gadolinium-enhanced MR imaging. Radiology 1995; 197(2): 411–418.
43. Mayo-Smith WW, Lee MJ, McNicholas MM, et al. Characterization of adrenal masses (< 5 cm.) by use of chemical shift MR imaging: observer performance versus quantitative measures. AJR Am J Roentgenol 1995; 165(1): 91–95.
44. Gross MD, Wilton GP, Shapiro B, et al. Functional and scintigraphic evaluation of the silent adrenal mass. J Nucl Med 1987; 28(9): 1401–1407.
45. Gross MD, Shapiro B. Scintigraphic studies in adrenal hypertension. Semin Nucl Med 1989; 19(2): 122–143.
46. Lo CY, van Heerden JA, Soreide JA, et al. Adrenalectomy for metastatic disease to the adrenal glands. Br J Surg 1996; 83(4): 528–531.
47. Hofle G, Gasser RW, Lhotta K, et al. Adrenocortical carcinoma evolving after diagnosis of preclinical Cushing's syndrome in an adrenal incidentaloma. A case report. Horm Res 1998; 50(4): 237–242.
48. Gross MD, Shapiro B, Francis IR, et al. Scintigraphy of incidentally discovered bilateral adrenal masses. Eur J Nucl Med 1995; 22(4): 315–321.
49. van Erkel AR, van Gils AP, Lequin M, et al. CT and MR distinction of adenomas and nonadenomas of the adrenal gland. J Comput Assist Tomogr 1994; 18(3): 432–438.
50. Cerfolio RJ, Vaughan ED Jr, Brennan TG Jr, Hirvela ER. Accuracy of computed tomography in predicting adrenal tumor size. Surg Gynecol Obstet 1993; 176(4): 307–309.
51. Wade TP, Longo WE, Virgo KS, Johnson FE. A comparison of adrenalectomy with other resections for metastatic cancers. Am J Surg 1998; 175(3): 183–186.
52. Goldstein RE, O'Neill JA Jr, Holcomb GW III, et al. Clinical experience over 48 years with pheochromocytoma. Ann Surg 1999; 229(6): 755–764; discussion 764–766.
53. Janetschek G, Neumann HP. Laparoscopic surgery for pheochromocytoma. Urol Clin North Am 2001; 28(1): 97–105.
54. Riccardi VM. Von Recklinghausen neurofibromatosis. N Engl J Med 1981; 305(27): 1617–1627.

55. Eng C. Seminars in medicine of the Beth Israel Hospital, Boston. The RET proto-oncogene in multiple endocrine neoplasia type 2 and Hirschsprung's disease. N Engl J Med 1996; 335(13): 943–951.
56. Easton DF, Ponder MA, Cummings T, et al. The clinical and screening age-at-onset distribution for the MEN-2 syndrome. Am J Hum Genet 1989; 44(2): 208–215.
57. Neumann HP, Berger DP, Sigmund G, et al. Pheochromocytomas, multiple endocrine neoplasia type 2, and von Hippel-Lindau disease. N Engl J Med 1993; 329(21): 1531–1538.
58. Neumann HP, Wiestler OD. Clustering of features of von Hippel-Lindau syndrome: evidence for a complex genetic locus. Lancet 1991; 337(8749): 1052–1054.
59. Sutton MG, Sheps SG, Lie JT. Prevalence of clinically unsuspected pheochromocytoma. Review of a 50-year autopsy series. Mayo Clin Proc 1981; 56(6): 354–360.
60. Joris JL, Hamoir EE, Hartstein GM, et al. Hemodynamic changes and catecholamine release during laparoscopic adrenalectomy for pheochromocytoma. Anesth Analg 1999; 88(1): 16–21.
61. Mann C, Millat B, Boccara G, Atger J, Colson P. Tolerance of laparoscopy for resection of phaeochromocytoma. Br J Anaesth 1996; 77(6): 795–797.
62. Rose CE Jr, Althaus JR, Kaiser DL, Miller ED, Carey RM. Acute hypoxemia and hypercapnia: increase in plasma catecholamines in conscious dogs. Am J Physiol 1983; 245(6): H924–H929.
63. Mobius E, Nies C, Rothmund M. Surgical treatment of pheochromocytomas: laparoscopic or conventional? Surg Endosc 1999; 13(1): 35–39.
64. Fernandez-Cruz L, Taura P, Saenz A, Benarroch G, Sabater L. Laparoscopic approach to pheochromocytoma: hemodynamic changes and catecholamine secretion. World J Surg 1996; 20(7): 762–768; discussion 768.
65. Col V, de Canniere L, Collard E, Michel L, Donckier J. Laparoscopic adrenalectomy for phaeochromocytoma: endocrinological and surgical aspects of a new therapeutic approach. Clin Endocrinol (Oxf) 1999; 50(1): 121–125.
66. Atallah F, Bastide-Heulin T, Soulie M, et al. Haemodynamic changes during retroperitoneoscopic adrenalectomy for phaeochromocytoma. Br J Anaesth 2001; 86(5): 731–733.
67. Sprung J, O'Hara JF Jr, Gill IS, et al. Anesthetic aspects of laparoscopic and open adrenalectomy for pheochromocytoma. Urology 2000; 55(3): 339–343.
68. Remine WH, Chong GC, van Heerden JA, Sheps SG, Harrison EG. Current management of pheochromocytoma. Ann Surg 1974; 179(5): 740–748.
69. Orchard T, Grant CS, van Heerden JA, Weaver A. Pheochromocytoma—continuing evolution of surgical therapy. Surgery 1993; 114(6): 1153–1158; discussion 1158–1159.
70. Lenders JW, Pacak K, Walther MM, et al. Biochemical diagnosis of pheochromocytoma: which test is best? JAMA 2002; 287(11): 1427–1434.
71. Sjoberg RJ, Simcic KJ, Kidd GS. The clonidine suppression test for pheochromocytoma. A review of its utility and pitfalls. Arch Intern Med 1992; 152(6): 1193–1197.
72. Pattou FN, Combemale FP, Poirett JF, et al. Questionability of the benefits of routine laparotomy as the surgical approach for pheochromocytomas and abdominal paragangliomas. Surgery 1996; 120(6): 1006–1011; discussion 1012.
73. Boutros AR, Bravo EL, Zanettin G, Straffon RA. Perioperative management of 63 patients with pheochromocytoma. Cleve Clin J Med 1990; 57(7): 613–617.
74. Ulchaker JC, Goldfarb DA, Bravo EL, Novick AC. Successful outcomes in pheochromocytoma surgery in the modern era. J Urol 1999; 161(3): 764–767..
75. Brunaud L, Cormier L, Ayav A, et al. [Does the size of pheochromocytoma influence the results of its laparoscopic excision?] Ann Chir 2002; 127(5): 362–369.

76. Chiu AW, Chang LS, Birkett DH, Babayan RK. The impact of pneumoperitoneum, pneumoretroperitoneum, and gasless laparoscopy on the systemic and renal hemodynamics. J Am Coll Surg 1995; 181(5): 397–406.
77. Walz MK, Peitgen K, Walz MV, et al. Posterior retroperitoneoscopic adrenalectomy: lessons learned within five years. World J Surg 2001; 25(6): 728–734.
78. O'Riordain DS, Young WF Jr, Grant CS, Carney JA, van Heerden JA. Clinical spectrum and outcome of functional extraadrenal paraganglioma. World J Surg 1996; 20(7): 916–921; discussion 922.
79. Scott HW Jr, Halter SA. Oncologic aspects of pheochromocytoma: the importance of follow-up. Surgery 1984; 96(6): 1061–1066.
80. van Heerden JA, Roland CF, Carney JA, Sheps GS, Grant CS. Long-term evaluation following resection of apparently benign pheochromocytoma(s)/paraganglioma(s). World J Surg 1990; 14(3): 325–329.
81. Walther MM, Keiser HR, Choyke PL, et al. Management of hereditary pheochromocytoma in von Hippel-Lindau kindreds with partial adrenalectomy. J Urol 1999; 161(2): 395–398.
82. Finkenstedt G, Gasser RW, Hofle G, et al. Pheochromocytoma and sub-clinical Cushing's syndrome during pregnancy: diagnosis, medical pre-treatment and cure by laparoscopic unilateral adrenalectomy. J Endocrinol Invest 1999; 22(7): 551–557.
83. Janetschek G, Finkenstedt G, Gasser R, et al. Laparoscopic surgery for pheochromocytoma: adrenalectomy, partial resection, excision of paragangliomas. J Urol 1998; 160(2): 330–334.
84. Hadden DR. Adrenal disorders of pregnancy. Endocrinol Metab Clin North Am 1995; 24(1): 139–151.
85. Brunaud L, Duh QY. Aldosteronoma. Curr Treat Options Oncol 2002; 3(4): 327–333.
86. Melby JC. Diagnosis and treatment of primary aldosteronism and isolated hypoaldosteronism. Clin Endocrinol Metab 1985; 14(4): 977–995.
87. Ganguly A. Primary aldosteronism. N Engl J Med 1998; 339(25): 1828–1834.
88. Weinberger MH, Grim CE, Hollifield JW, et al. Primary aldosteronism: diagnosis, localization, and treatment. Ann Intern Med 1979; 90(3): 386–395.
89. Young WF Jr. Primary aldosteronism: A common and curable form of hypertension. Cardiol Rev 1999; 7(4): 207–214.
90. Siren J, Haglund C, Huikuri K, Sivula A, Hoapiainer R. Laparoscopic adrenalectomy for primary aldosteronism: clinical experience in 12 patients. Surg Laparosc Endosc 1999; 9(1): 9–13.
91. Zeiger MA, Nieman LK, Cutler GB, et al. Primary bilateral adrenocortical causes of Cushing's syndrome. Surgery 1991; 110(6): 1106–1115.
92. Reincke M. Subclinical Cushing's syndrome. Endocrinol Metab Clin North Am 2000; 29(1): 43–56.
93. Osella G, Terzolo M, Borretta G, et al. Endocrine evaluation of incidentally discovered adrenal masses (incidentalomas). J Clin Endocrinol Metab 1994; 79(6): 1532–1539.
94. Mantero F, Masini AM, Opocher GM, Giovagnetti M, Arnaldi G. Adrenal incidentaloma: an overview of hormonal data from the National Italian Study Group. Horm Res 1997; 47(4–6): 284–289.
95. Reincke M, Nieke J, Krestin GP, et al. Preclinical Cushing's syndrome in adrenal "incidentalomas": comparison with adrenal Cushing's syndrome. J Clin Endocrinol Metab, 1992; 75(3): 826–832.
96. Aniszewski JP, Young WF Jr, Thompson GB, Grant CS, van Heerden JA. Cushing syndrome due to ectopic adrenocorticotropic hormone secretion. World J Surg 2001; 25(7): 934–940.

97. Shinojima H, Kakizaki H, Usuki T, et al. Clinical and endocrinological features of adrenocorticotropic hormone- independent bilateral macronodular adrenocortical hyperplasia. J Urol 2001; 166(5): 1639–1642.
098. Invitti C, Giraldi FP, de Martin M, Cavognini F. Diagnosis and management of Cushing's syndrome: results of an Italian multicentre study. Study Group of the Italian Society of Endocrinology on the Pathophysiology of the Hypothalamic-Pituitary-Adrenal Axis. J Clin Endocrinol Metab 1999; 84(2): 440–448.
99. Toms GC, McCarthy MI, Niven MJ, et al. Predicting relapse after transsphenoidal surgery for Cushing's disease. J Clin Endocrinol Metab 1993; 76(2): 291–294.
100. McCance DR, Russell CF, Kennedy TL, et al. Bilateral adrenalectomy: low mortality and morbidity in Cushing's disease. Clin Endocrinol (Oxf) 1993; 39(3): 315–321.
101. Vella A, Thompson GB, Grant CS, et al. Laparoscopic adrenalectomy for adrenocorticotropin-dependent Cushing's syndrome. J Clin Endocrinol Metab 2001; 86(4): 1596–1599.
102. Buell JF, Alexander HR, Norton JA, Yu KC, Fraker DL. Bilateral adrenalectomy for Cushing's syndrome. Anterior versus posterior surgical approach. Ann Surg 1997; 225(1): 63–68.
103. van Heerden JA, Young WF Jr, Grant CS, Carpenter PC. Adrenal surgery for hypercortisolism—surgical aspects. Surgery 1995; 117(4): 466–472.
104. Kollmorgen CF, Thompson GB, Grant CS, et al. Laparoscopic versus open posterior adrenalectomy: comparison of acute-phase response and wound healing in the cushingoid porcine model. World J Surg 1998; 22(6): 613–619; discussion 619–620.
105. Chapuis Y, Chastanet S, Dousset B, Luton JP. Bilateral laparoscopic adrenalectomy for Cushing's disease. Br J Surg 1997; 84(7): 1009.
106. Siren JE, Haapiainen RK, Huikuri KT, Sivula AH. Incidentalomas of the adrenal gland: 36 operated patients and review of literature. World J Surg 1993; 17(5): 634–639.
107. Ross NS, Aron DC. Hormonal evaluation of the patient with an incidentally discovered adrenal mass. N Engl J Med 1990; 323(20): 1401–1405.
108. Fishman EK, Deutch BM, Hartman DS, et al. Primary adrenocortical carcinoma: CT evaluation with clinical correlation. AJR Am J Roentgenol 1987; 148(3): 531–535.
109. Latronico AC, Chrousos GP. Extensive personal experience: adrenocortical tumors. J Clin Endocrinol Metab 1997; 82(5): 1317–1324.
110. Bornstein SR, Stratakis CA, Chrousos GP. Adrenocortical tumors: recent advances in basic concepts and clinical management. Ann Intern Med 1999; 130(9): 759–771.
111. Hobart MG, Gill IS, Schweizer D, Surg GT, Brava EL. Laparoscopic adrenalectomy for large-volume (> or = 5 cm.) adrenal masses. J Endourol 2000; 14(2): 149–154.
112. Heniford BT, Arca MJ, Walsh RM, Gill IS. Laparoscopic adrenalectomy for cancer. Semin Surg Oncol 1999; 16(4): 293–306.
113. Ushiyama T, Suzuki K, Kageyama S, et al. A case of Cushing's syndrome due to adrenocortical carcinoma with recurrence 19 months after laparoscopic adrenalectomy. J Urol 1997; 157(6): 2239.
114. Foxius A, Ramboux A, Lefebvre Y, et al. Hazards of laparoscopic adrenalectomy for Conn's adenoma. When enthusiasm turns to tragedy. Surg Endosc 1999; 13(7): 715–717.

115. Iacconi P, Bendinelli C, Miccoli P, Bernini, GP. Re: A case of Cushing's syndrome due to adrenocortical carcinoma with recurrence 19 months after laparoscopic adrenalectomy. Re: Re: A case of Cushing's syndrome due to adrenocortical carcinoma with recurrence 19 months after laparoscopic adrenalectomy. J Urol 1999; 161(5): 1580–1581.
116. de Canniere L, Michel L, Hamoire E, et al. Multicentric experience of the Belgian Group for Endoscopic Surgery (BGES) with endoscopic adrenalectomy. Surg Endosc 1997; 11(11): 1065–1067.
117. Siekavizza JL, Bernardino ME, Samaan NA. Suprarenal mass and its differential diagnosis. Urology 1981; 18(6): 625–632.
118. Hussain S, Belldegrun A, Seltzer SE, et al. Differentiation of malignant from benign adrenal masses: predictive indices on computed tomography. AJR Am J Roentgenol 1985; 144(1): 61–65.
119. Elashry OM, Clayman RV, Soble JJ, McDougall EM. Laparoscopic adrenalectomy for solitary metachronous contralateral adrenal metastasis from renal cell carcinoma. J Urol 1997; 157(4): 1217–1222.
120. Luketich JD, Burt ME. Does resection of adrenal metastases from non-small cell lung cancer improve survival? Ann Thorac Surg 1996. 62(6): 1614–1616.
121. Gill IS. Needlescopic urology: current status. Urol Clin North Am 2001; 28(1): 71–83.
122. Mirallie E, Leclair MD, de Lagausie P, et al. Laparoscopic adrenalectomy in children. Surg Endosc 2001; 15(2): 156–160.
123. Al-Sobhi S, Peschel R, Zihak C, et al. Laparoscopic partial adrenalectomy for recurrent pheochromocytoma after open partial adrenalectomy in von Hippel-Lindau disease. J Endourol 2002; 16(3): 171–174.
124. Al-Sobhi S, Peschel R, Bartsch G, et al. Partial laparoscopic adrenalectomy for aldosterone-producing adenoma: short-and long-term results. J Endourol 2000; 14(6): 497–499.
125. Imai T, Tanaka Y, Kikumor T, et al. Laparoscopic partial adrenalectomy. Surg Endosc 1999; 13(4): 343–345.
126. Walz MK, Peitgen K. Laparoscopic partial adrenalectomy. Surg Endosc 2000; 14(11): 1089–1090.
127. Guazzoni G, Montorsi F, Bocciardi A, et al. Transperitoneal laparoscopic versus open adrenalectomy for benign hyperfunctioning adrenal tumors: a comparative study. J Urol 1995; 153(5): 1597–1600.
128. Thompson GB, Grant CS, van Heerden JA, et al. Laparoscopic versus open posterior adrenalectomy: a case-control study of 100 patients. Surgery 1997; 122(6): 1132–1136.
129. Gill IS, Hobart MG, Schweizer D, Bravo EL. Outpatient adrenalectomy. J Urol 2000; 163(3): 717–720.
130. Gill IS, Clayman RV, McDougall EM. Advances in urological laparoscopy. J Urol 1995; 154(4): 1275–1294.
131. Higashihara E, Baba S, Nakagawa K, et al. Learning curve and conversion to open surgery in cases of laparoscopic adrenalectomy and nephrectomy. J Urol 1998; 159(3): 650–653.
132. Soulie M, Salomon L, Seguin P, et al. Multi-institutional study of complications in 1085 laparoscopic urologic procedures. Urology 2001; 58(6): 899–903.
133. Soulie M, Seguin P, Richeux L, et al. Urological complications of laparoscopic surgery: experience with 350 procedures at a single center. J Urol 2001; 165(6 Pt 1): 1960–1963.

134. Suzuki K, Ushiyama T, Ihara H, et al. Complications of laparoscopic adrenalectomy in 75 patients treated by the same surgeon. Eur Urol 1999; 36(1): 40–47.
135. Yoshida O, Terachi T, Matsuda T, et al. Complications in 369 laparoscopic adrenalectomies: a multi-institutional study in Japan. J Urol 1997; 161(21): abstract 70.
136. Brunt LM. The positive impact of laparoscopic adrenalectomy on complications of adrenal surgery. Surg Endosc 2002; 16(2): 252–257.
137. Prinz RA. A comparison of laparoscopic and open adrenalectomies. Arch Surg 1995; 130(5): 489–492; discussion 492–494.
138. Chapuis Y, Maignien B, Abboud B. [Adrenalectomy under celioscopy. Experience of 25 operations]. Presse Med 1995; 24(18): 845–848.
139. Henry JF, Defechereux T, Raffaelli M, Lubrano D, Gramatica L. Complications of laparoscopic adrenalectomy: results of 169 consecutive procedures. World J Surg 2000; 24(11): 1342–1346.
140. Korman JE, Ho T, Hiatt JR, Phillips EH. Comparison of laparoscopic and open adrenalectomy. Am Surg 1997; 63(10): 908–912.
141. Hobart MG, Gill IS, Schweizer D, Bravo EL. Financial analysis of needlescopic versus open adrenalectomy. J Urol 1999; 162(4): 1264–1267.
142. Gagner M. Laparoscopic adrenalectomy. Surg Clin North Am 1996; 76(3): 523–537.
143. Stoker ME, Patwardhan N, Maini BS. Laparoscopic adrenal surgery. Surg Endosc 1995; 9(4): 387–390; discussion 391.
144. Fazeli-Matin S, Gill IS, Hsu TH, Sung GT, Novick AC. Laparoscopic renal and adrenal surgery in obese patients: comparison to open surgery. J Urol 1999; 162(3 Pt 1): 665–669.
145. Gill IS, Meraney AM, Mayes JT, Bravo EL. Laparoscopic right adrenalectomy after liver transplantation. Transplantation 2001; 71(9): 1350–1351.

# 12 Laparoscopic Adrenalectomy for Carcinoma

*Paul K. Pietrow,* MD
*and David M. Albala,* MD

*CONTENTS*

INTRODUCTION
CONTRAINDICATIONS
OVERVIEW OF SURGICAL TECHNIQUE
RESULTS
CONTROVERSY
REFERENCES

## INTRODUCTION

The role of laparoscopy for the treatment of adrenal carcinoma remains controversial. The lack of a capsule around the adrenal gland and the propensity of primary tumors to invade the surrounding fat, make it difficult to ensure a wide surgical margin. When coupled with the technical challenges of operating in this small space with ill-defined planes, it is hard for laparoscopic surgeons to adhere to strict oncologic principles. Unfortunately, for many of these patients, these same difficulties also apply to open surgery, leading to very poor 5-yr survival rates for patients with primary adrenal carcinoma *(1,2)*.

Meanwhile, laparoscopy is commonly employed in the surgical management of benign adrenal lesions. Multiple authors have demonstrated that perioperative morbidity, complications, and recovery times are all improved with this technique *(3–8)*. The control of the endocrine disorders associated with many of these lesions remains excellent and laparoscopy has become the standard of care for benign disease in many

From: *Laparoscopic Urologic Oncology*
Edited by: J. A. Cadeddu © Humana Press Inc., Totowa, NJ

institutions *(9)*. The literature supporting this application are reviewed more fully in Chapter 11.

There is a growing body of evidence that supports a laparoscopic approach for isolated metastases to the adrenal gland. Reasonable survival rates have been reported if the patient can be rendered free of obvious disease. Other authors have attempted to create size limitations and guidelines when addressing carcinoma within the adrenal gland (both primary and metastatic). The existing literature surrounding these issues are addressed later in this chapter.

The future of laparoscopy for adrenal carcinoma remains to be determined. As experience grows and followup is lengthened, the true role of this technique will be better defined. As such, the realistic indications remain to be determined.

## CONTRAINDICATIONS

Despite the desire to provide surgical care in a minimally invasive fashion, there are clear contraindications. Tumors with obvious extension into the peri-adrenal fat or neighboring structures should not be approached laparoscopically. Obvious or suspicious adrenal vein thrombus should also be approached with an open technique with proper vascular control and adequate margins. Some researchers have argued that no primary adrenocortical carcinomas should be excised via a laparoscopic approach because of the propensity of the tumor to extend outside of the gland or to recur diffusely within the abdomen *(3,5,10)*.

Pheochromocytomas in general should be approached with great respect, although not necessarily with trepidation. Carcinoma is infrequently encountered in these lesions (10% or less) and is often suspected based on preoperative imaging. The risk of adrenergic storm should always be anticipated, and patients should get adequate preoperative $\alpha$-adrenergic blockade. Despite these risks, most pheochromocytomas can be approached with this technique, perhaps avoiding only those patients with significant endocrine storm and multisystem crisis. The transperitoneal laparoscopic approach can also allow for a complete intraperitoneal survey in the event that the patient is suspected of harboring extra-adrenal sites of this lesion.

Certain patient characteristics can also serve as a contraindication to laparoscopy. Although uncommonly encountered, an uncontrolled coagulopathy is an absolute contraindication to a laparoscopic approach, as is active peritonitis. A prior history of multiple abdominal procedures may suggest adhesions, which can make transperitoneal laparoscopy difficult. This would not preclude a retroperitoneal approach, however.

Obesity has been suggested to be a relative contraindication of a laparoscopic approach to the adrenal gland. Indeed, early series have shown a higher rate of complications (especially minor) in patients with an elevated body mass index. Although more recent investigators have noted that obesity is associated with longer operating room times and slight increases in complication rates, most authors feel that obese patients are easily managed as the surgeon gains operative experience and advances along the learning curve *(11)*.

Perhaps the most important reason not to perform a laparoscopic resection of a suspected adrenal malignancy is surgeon inexperience. Many authors have stressed that this procedure is technically challenging and should be reserved for experienced surgeons at tertiary centers of excellence *(4,8,12)*.

## OVERVIEW OF SURGICAL TECHNIQUE

### *Technical Steps*

#### Access/Trocars

Once the patient has been adequately placed in the flank position, prepped and draped, the operation begins with the creation of the pneumoperitoneum. A Veress needle can be used or an open Hasson technique may be applied depending on surgeon experience and preference. In either case, we have typically placed our first trocar in the anterior axillary line, two finger-breadth's below the costal margin.

After adequate insufflation of the abdomen to 15 mm Hg, a 10/12-mm trocar is inserted in the subcostal area at the level of the anterior axillary line. A 30° angled laparoscope is then inserted through this trocar. One additional 10/12-mm trocar is inserted under direct vision in the midclavicular line while flanking 5-mm trocars are placed in the posterior axillary line and the midline of the abdomen (Fig. 1). Using endoscopic scissors, the white line of Toldt is divided near the splenic/hepatic flexure of the colon to open the retroperitoneal space between the colon and the lateral abdominal wall. This incision is continued superiorly to further release the spleen/liver as well.

#### Left Adrenalectomy

The upper pole of the left kidney is identified and exposed by freeing the posterolateral attachments of the spleen in the direction of the diaphragm (Fig. 2). Using a fan or blunt retractor, the spleen is retracted medially and superiorly. This maneuver exposes the adrenal gland and will allow the dissection to begin in the correct plane.

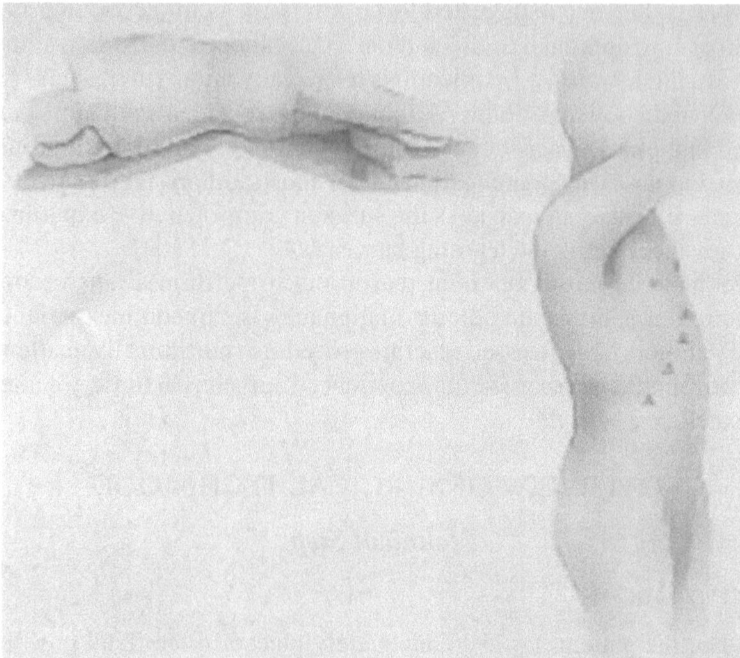

**Fig. 1.** The patient is placed in a true flank position. Trocar sites are indicated.

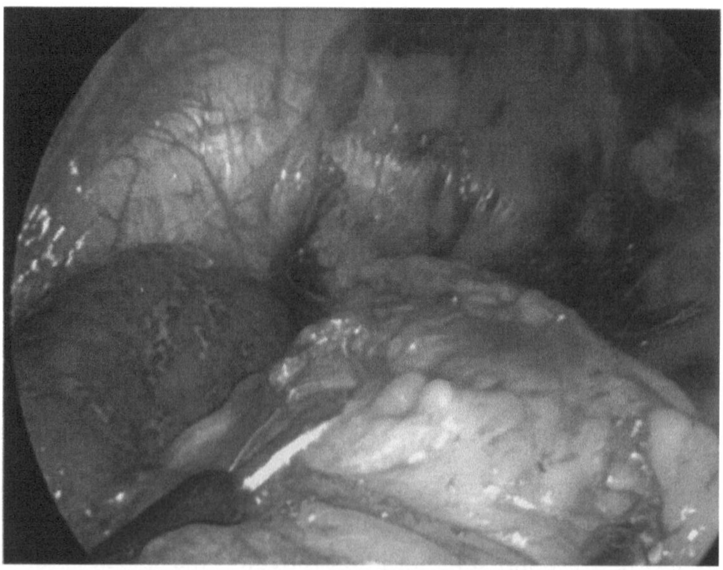

**Fig. 2.** The white line of Toldt has been divided and the spleen has been allowed to fall cephalad.

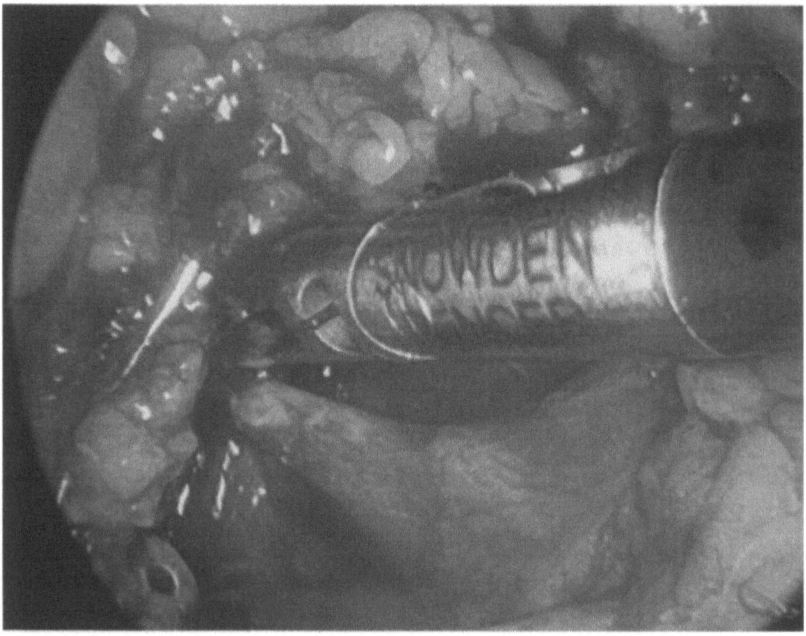

**Fig. 3.** The left adrenal vein can be seen arising from the larger main renal vein.

After entering Gerota's fascia, the superior aspect of the adrenal gland is exposed and the dissection is carried medially. The dissection of the inferior portion of the gland should be performed last, as starting here will lead to superior gland retraction and unnecessary bleeding. The inferior phrenic arterial branches are ligated with titanium clips after mobilization of the superior pole of the gland. The left adrenal vein is then visualized (Fig. 3), dissected free, and ligated with two laparoscopic clips (Fig. 4). The inferior portion of the adrenal gland is dissected last and the gland is separated from the surrounding tissue (Fig. 5). Hemostasis is obtained by using a suction/irrigation device in concert with electrocautery.

### Right Adrenalectomy

The liver is retracted in a cephalad direction and the posterior peritoneum is then divided close to the liver edge. This incision is carried from the line of Toldt to the inferior vena cava (IVC). The hepatic flexure of the colon does not need aggressive mobilization if this incision is carried far enough laterally. The upper pole of the kidney is identified and the perinephric fat is dissected superiorly and close to the IVC to expose the adrenal gland. The dissection begins at the superior

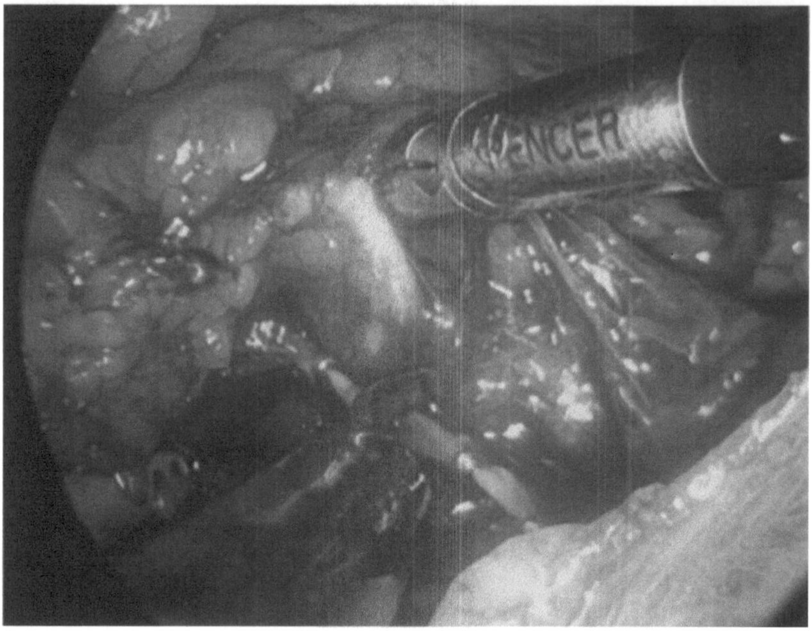

**Fig. 4.** Clips have been applied to adrenal vein and scissors are being used to divide the vessel.

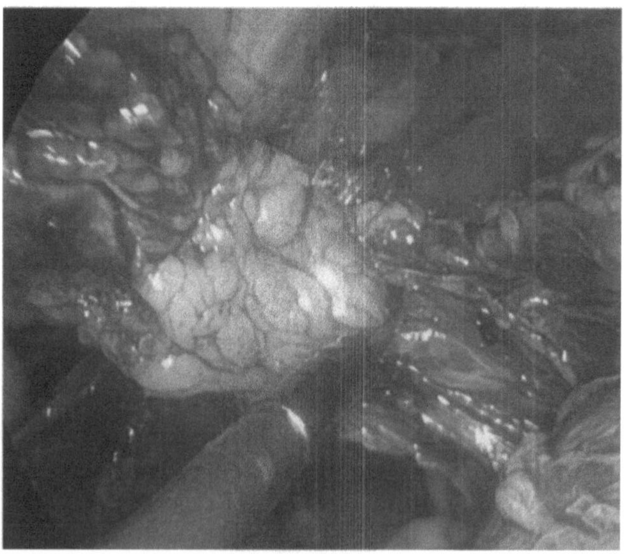

**Fig 5.** The adrenal gland and its investing fat is lifted away from body and the fatty attachments are divided with electrocautery.

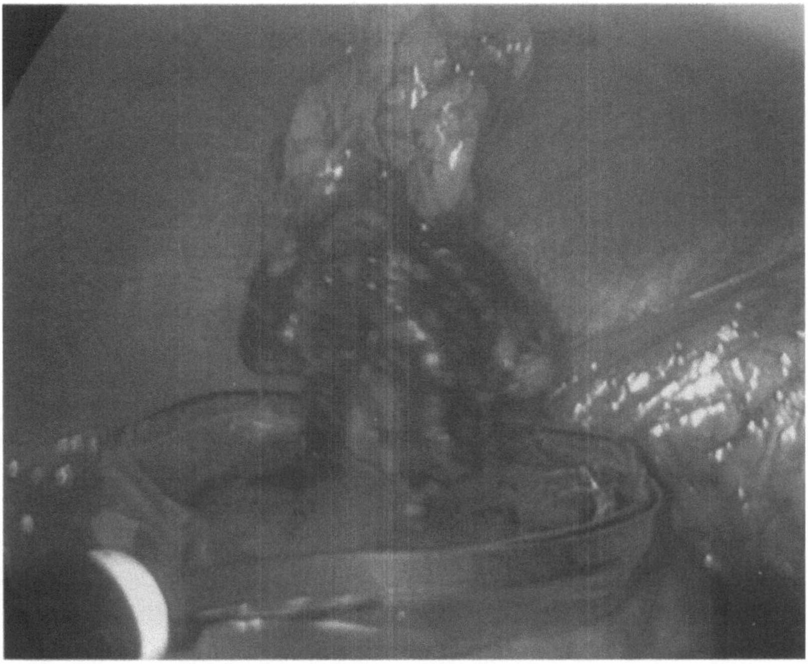

**Fig. 6.** The specimen is placed into an impervious entrapment sack.

and anterior aspect of the right adrenal gland. Small vessels are secured with laparoscopic clips or electrocautery and a laparoscopic kittner dissector is used to retract the adrenal gland in a lateral direction. Meticulous dissection in this area will prevent tears from the lateral vascular branches of the IVC and to the body of the adrenal gland itself, which can lead to tiresome oozing.

The adrenal vein is identified, isolated, and laparoscopic clips are placed, leaving two clips on the patient side. The vein is then divided between the clips. Extreme care must be taken when mobilizing the right adrenal vein as it is short and has a direct entry into the IVC.

### Specimen Retrieval/Closure

A small, impervious entrapment sack is then placed through the medial trocar, the bag is opened, and the adrenal gland is placed into the entrapment sack under laparoscopic control (Fig. 6). The bag is removed through the most inferior trocar site with minimal spreading of the oblique muscles using a Kelly clamp. Prior to exiting the abdomen, the insufflation is typically lowered to 5 mm Hg and the operative site is searched for bleeding. Persistent bleeding can be addressed with elec-

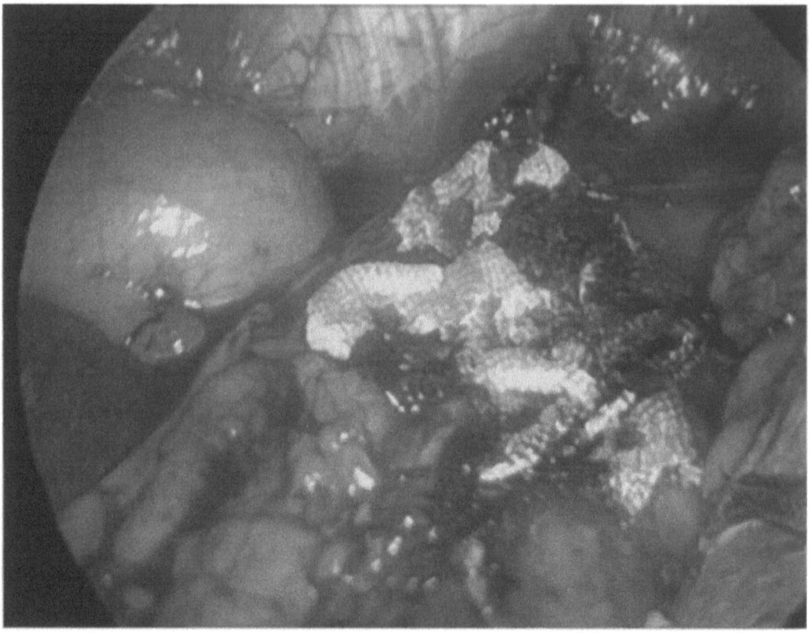

**Fig. 7.** Hemostatic agents may be placed into the empty surgical fossa to aid in the control of small bleeders.

trocautery or with Surgicel that is introduced through a larger trocar (Fig. 7). All trocar sites 10 mm or larger require a facial closure using 2-0 absorbable suture, while the skin is reapproximated using 4-0 suture. A fascial closure device, such as the Puncture Closure Device (ConMed Corp., Utica, NY) can be very helpful and avoids difficult and often blind suturing of the abdominal fascia.

### *Variations in Technique*

The respective merits of a transperitoneal vs a retroperitoneal laparoscopic approach to the adrenal gland have been greatly discussed in the literature *(13–15)*. Most surgeons recognize the inherent difficulties of the reduced operating space with a retroperitoneal route, but espouse the advantages that come with avoidance of the peritoneal cavity and its risk of adhesions and port-site hernias. Importantly, retroperitoneal access allows for the rapid mobilization and early ligation of the adrenal vein (especially on the left side). This is particularly important for pheochromocytomas and malignant masses.

Published series have reported the need for increased surgeon experience with retroperitoneoscopy, but have not necessarily noted differences in overall complication rates *(13,15)*. It is important to note, however, that the retroperitoneal portions of some of these series were performed after the transperitoneal cases, making it difficult to differentiate between the importance of surgeon experience vs the importance of operative approach.

Nevertheless, there are currently no series that specifically address the benefits of one approach over the other when applied to laparoscopy for cancer of the adrenal gland. It does seem intuitive to recommend that each case should be planned on an individual basis, accounting for the size of the lesion, the side of the pathology, the patient's past surgical history, and the experience of the surgeon.

## RESULTS

### *Primary Adrenal Carcinoma*

It is important to note that at the time of this writing there are no published series of laparoscopic cases performed purely for primary adrenal carcinoma. Many of the cancers that have been resected are reported in larger series describing the surgeon's overall experience with the technique for all lesions. Additionally, individual cases have been reported, some with good results and others with catastrophic followup.

Iino et al. reported the *en bloc* resection of a 5-cm adrenocortical carcinoma via a transperitoneal laparoscopic approach *(10)*. No complications were reported and the patient was initially presumed to have had a benign functioning adenoma. The authors specify that pathologic examination demonstrated an intact capsule around the gland. Unfortunately, the patient developed diffuse peritoneal carcinomatosis 15 mo following surgery. Although she responded to carboplatin, etoposide, and mitotane, she ultimately succumbed to neurological impairment from the neurotoxic chemotherapeutic agents. The authors, therefore, warned against a laparoscopic approach for tumors suspected of harboring a malignancy, regardless of size.

Suzuki and colleagues describe the local and diffuse abdominal recurrence of a primary adrenocortical carcinoma 19 mo after resection *(16)*. Additionally, two patients from the same series with metastatic adrenocortical carcinoma to the contralateral gland were converted to open procedures secondary to major hemorrhage and extensive adhesions. Similar results with intraperitoneal dissemination have also been experienced by Li et al. *(17)*, in which three patients suffered from diffuse pheochromacytosis following lapascopic adrenalectomy of presumed benign lesions. Furthermore, Deckers et al. reported the diffuse peritoneal recurrence of an aldosterone- and cortisol-producing tumor 6 mo after complete laparoscopic resection *(18)*.

Henry et al. concluded that laparoscopy can be applied to tumors up to 12 cm in size or for potentially malignant tumors if there is no evidence of local invasion on preoperative imaging *(19)*. Despite such enthusiasm, the authors also report that of three patients with primary adrenocortical tumors, only one was suspected of having carcinoma prior to the start of the case, and this patient required open conversion due to dense adhesions and tumor-feeding vessels. The other tumors, a leiomyosarcoma (4 cm) and an androgen-producing carcinoma (3.5 cm) had not recurred at a maximum of 4 yr followup. It is promising to note that as the authors expanded their criteria for this approach, they did not notice an increase in complications. Early in their series, only patients with benign tumors smaller than 4 cm in size were considered candidates. Total complications for these patients were 7.8%, with a 4.9% conversion rate. The second group of patients with tumors as large as 12 cm and potentially malignant had an 8.3% rate of complications, with 6.2% requiring open conversion. These authors reiterate the necessity for experienced surgeons to manage tumors larger than 6 cm.

Guazzoni and colleagues reported their experience with laparoscopic adrenalectomy spanning over 8 yr *(20)*. Of 161 patients, 2 had a primary malignancy within the adrenal gland. One of these patients had a 5-cm tumor, but required open conversion due to dense adhesions and a significant adrenal vein tumor thrombus. The second patient underwent successful resection of tumor less than 3 cm in size. Length of survival for this patient was not specifically reported. Based on this experience and with their results managing two metastatic lesions, the authors are willing to laparoscopically approach potentially malignant masses up to 6 cm in size provided there is no preoperative evidence of local invasion.

Gagner and colleagues described their results with 100 consecutive laparoscopic adrenalectomies, where they found carcinoma in eight patients *(21)*. Two patients had metastatic involvement of the adrenal gland, three had malignant pheochromocytomas, and three had nonfunctioning tumors with microscopic features of carcinoma. Although difficult to extract from the text, the authors appeared to have better results with the pheochromocytomas than with the primary malignancies. Two of the three total conversions for the entire series involved these cancers. One was required to allow an *en bloc* resection of the gland and of surrounding muscle for a sarcoma, whereas the second was converted due to direct vascular invasion into the IVC. The authors make special notice to emphasize the helpful role of intraoperative ultrasound for all of these cases, and especially for those suspected of harboring malignancy. Despite the difficulties with the locally invasive tumors, the investigators conclude that masses as large as 15 cm can be approached laparoscopically, albeit with the realization that visualization around these large masses may be challenging. Additionally, extra attention is required to manage all of the parasitic vessels that arise out of the retroperitoneum to support these tumors. Survival was not reported for these patients, although the authors state that no tumors have recurred locally during an unspecified amount of followup.

Finally, Porpiglia et al. reported on 72 consecutive laparoscopic adrenalectomies performed over a 4-yr period *(5)*. Only one patient was found to have carcinoma in her 10-cm specimen. This patient was alive and without evidence of disease after 40 mo of followup. Despite this encouraging outcome, the authors still caution against the use of this technique for known adrenal malignancy, calling it "an absolute contraindication."

### *Metastatic Cancer to the Adrenal*

The adrenal gland is a common site for metastatic foci. Indeed, autopsy studies have revealed that the gland may be involved as often as 10–36% of the time in the case of renal cell carcinoma (RCC) alone *(8)*. The role of surgical resection of adrenal metastatic disease by any technique is not completely clear. Certainly, the overall health of the patient and the volume of metastatic disease should be the most important decision factors. Nevertheless, there have been encouraging reports of patient benefit from open resection of metastatic tumors of multiple origins *(22)*. Indeed, from a large series of 52 patients, 11 of 12 patients with symptomatic lesions achieved pain relief following resection. Overall survival was 73% at 1 yr and 40% at 2 yr. Not surprisingly, those patients with adenocarcinoma and those who underwent a potentially curative resection fared better than those treated for palliation.

These results are generally supported by Kim et al., who reported the outcomes of 37 patients who underwent open resection of clinically isolated adrenal metastases *(23)*. The median survival for the entire cohort was 21 mo with an actuarial 5-yr survival rate of 24%. Buried within these statistics are three patients (12.5%) with survival greater than 5 yr. The authors also found that patients with a longer disease-free interval before the appearance of their adrenal metastasis tended to fare better than patients with synchronous lesions discovered at the time of their initial diagnosis.

The role of a laparoscopic approach to the resection of metastatic adrenal lesions seems more secure than for primary tumors. Although there are no head-to-head comparison studies with open surgery, the results seem promising when compared to previous retrospective reviews. Tsuji et al. reported on the 18-mo (and counting) disease-free followup of a 69-yr-old male with metastatic squamous cell lung cancer *(24)*. Although the total operative time was long at 4 h, 30 min, the specimen had negative margins and total blood loss was only 50 cc. The patient recovered well without apparent complications.

Elashry and colleagues described positive results in the laparoscopic management of late, solitary metastases from contralateral sources of RCC *(25)*. Both patients in the series successfully underwent complete resection of the adrenal gland revealing RCC with negative surgical margins. Blood loss was minimal for both cases (50 cc and 75 cc), whereas operative times varied (2.5 and 4.5 h). Notably, one patient had a permanent elevation in his serum creatinine following the surgery, possibly caused by injury to a segmental renal arterial branch.

Valeri et al. reported their results following a laparoscopic approach to eight patients with presumed isolated adrenal metastases *(26)*. The average surgical time for these patients was 160 min, mean blood loss was 262 ml and average hospital stay was 4 d (range 3–11). The average specimen size was 4.5 cm (range 2.5–6 cm). There were no complications or mortalities. Five patients were found to have metastatic lung cancer in their specimen and one patient had metastatic RCC. Two patients with primary lung cancers had simple adenomas in the adrenal specimen. Three of the five patients with metastatic lung cancer were still alive at 3, 5, and 16 mo of followup, whereas two were dead at 18 and 36 mo. The one patient with RCC died at 36 mo. The authors stressed that there were no local or port-site recurrences, and that all deaths were related to distant metastatic disease.

The largest reported series to date is from Heniford et al. *(27)*. These surgeons performed 12 laparoscopic adrenalectomies for cancer in 11 patients (1 of whom had a primary adrenocortical neoplasm). Using a mix of transperitoneal and retroperitoneal approaches, the surgical times averaged 181 min (range 100–315), blood loss averaged 138 mL (range 20–1300), and the specimens were a mean of 5.9 cm (1.8–12). There was one epigastric artery laceration that was repaired laparoscopically. There were no perioperative deaths. One patient with metastatic adrenal carcinoma to the contralateral gland required open conversion due to extensive vena cava invasion that was identified with intraoperative ultrasound (this was the same patient with the 1300 mL blood loss). From an oncologic perspective, the results appear promising, although it should be noted that the followup was relatively short. At a mean of 8 mo (range 0.5–19 mo), 10 patients are still alive. All specimens had negative margins and there have been no port-site or local recurrences. Two have undergone additional resections of previously identified metastases, and one patient has developed a new hepatic nodule. One patient with aggressive melanoma died 4.5 mo after his adrenal resection. Based on these results, the authors conclude that laparoscopic adrenalectomy for cancer is a safe and feasible endeavor in the hands of experienced surgeons.

## CONTROVERSY

It should come as no surprise that the greatest controversy surrounding laparoscopy for adrenal cancer is not which anatomic route to take, but rather whether it should be applied at all. The literature is replete with case reports and small series, but lacks direct comparison to open, oncolgic surgery. Despite this obvious shortcoming, it is also apparent that patients fare better when spared the morbidity of an open procedure. The published followup that does exist for laparoscopy is at least as good as that for open techniques with these aggressive tumors. It is because of these reasons that laparoscopy is gaining a foot-hold in the realm of adrenal malignancy at centers of excellence. Following some obvious caveats concerning evidence of local invasion on preoperative imaging, even tumors as large as 10–15 cm in diameter may be excised. Nagging concerns about the risk of peritoneal dissemination remain and need to be compared to this risk from open techniques. The final decision over the relevance of laparoscopy for adrenal cancer will be determined by time and increasing experience, but it appears highly likely that it will grow to replace open surgery at many centers.

## REFERENCES


1. Vaughan EDJ, Blumenfeld JD. The adrenals. In: *Campbell's Urology*. (Walsh PC, Retik A, Vaughan D, Wein A., eds.), W.B. Saunders, Philadelphia, PA, 1998, pp. 2915–2972.
2. Luton J-P, Cerdas S, Billaud L, et al., Clinical features of adrenocortical carcinoma, prognostic factors, and the effect of mitotane therapy. N Engl J Med 1990; 322: 1195.
3. Winfield HN, Hamilton BD, Bravo EL, Novick AC. Laparoscopic adrenalectomy: the preferred choice? A comparison to open adrenalectomy. J Urol 1998; 160(2): 325–329.
4. Valeri A, Borrelli A, Presenti L, et al. Laparoscopic adrenalectomy. Personal experience in 78 patients. G Chir 2001; 22(5): 185–189.
5. Porpiglia F, Garrone C, Giraudo G, et al. Transperitoneal laparoscopic adrenalectomy: experience in 72 procedures. J Endourol 2001; 15(3): 275–279.
6. Lezoche E, Guerrieri M, Paganini AM, et al. Laparoscopic adrenalectomy by the anterior transperitoneal approach: results of 108 operations in unselected cases. Surg Endosc 2000; 14(10): 920–925.
7. Henry JF. Minimally invasive adrenal surgery. Best Pract Res Clin Endocrinol Metab 2001; 15(2): 149–160.

8. Gill IS. The case for laparoscopic adrenalectomy. J Urol 2001; 166(2): 429–436.
9. Kok KY, Yapp SK. Laparoscopic adrenal-sparing surgery for primary hyperaldosteronism due to aldosterone-producing adenoma. Surg Endosc 2002; 16(1): 108–111.
10. Iino K, Oki Y, Sasano H. A case of adrenocortical carcinoma associated with recurrence after laparoscopic surgery. Clin Endocrinol (Oxf) 2000; 53(2): 243–248.
11. Fazeli-Matin S, Gill IS, Hsu TH, Sung GT, Novick AC. Laparoscopic renal and adrenal surgery in obese patients: comparison to open surgery. J Urol 1999; 162(3 Pt 1): 665–669.
12. Hobart MG, Gill IS, Schweizer D, Sung GT, Bravo EL. Laparoscopic adrenalectomy for large-volume (> or = 5 cm) adrenal masses. J Endourol 2000; 14(2): 149–154.
13. Terachi T, Yoshida O, Matsuda T, et al. Complications of laparoscopic and retroperitoneoscopic adrenalectomies in 370 cases in Japan: a multi-institutional study. Biomed Pharmacother 2000; 54(Suppl 1): 211s–214s.
14. Salomon L, Soulie M, Mouly P, et al. Experience with retroperitoneal laparoscopic adrenalectomy in 115 procedures. J Urol 2001; 166(1): 38–41.
15. Bonjer HJ, Sorm V, Berends FJ, et al. Endoscopic retroperitoneal adrenalectomy: lessons learned from 111 consecutive cases. Ann Surg 2000; 232(6): 796–803.
16. Suzuki K, Ushiyama T, Ihara H, et al. Complications of laparoscopic adrenalectomy in 75 patients treated by the same surgeon. Eur Urol 1999; 36(1): 40–47.
17. Li ML, Fitzgerald PA, Price DC, Norton JA. Iatrogenic pheochromocytomatosis: A previously unreported result of laparoscopic adrenalectomy. Surgery 2001; 130(6): 1072–1077.
18. Deckers S, Derdelinckx L, Cd V, Hamels J, Maiter D. Peritoneal carcinomatosis following laparoscopic resection of an adrenocortical tumor causing primary hyperaldosteronism. Horm Res 1999; 52(2): 97–100.
19. Henry JF, Defechereux T, Gramatica L, Raffaelli M. Should laparoscopic approach be proposed for large and/or potentially malignant adrenal tumors? Langenbecks Arch Surg 1999; 384(4): 366–369.
20. Guazzoni G, Cestari A, Montorsi F, et al. Eight-year experience with transperitoneal laparoscopic adrenal surgery. J Urol 2001; 166(3): 820–824.
21. Gagner M, Pomp A, Heniford BT, Pharand D, Lacroix, A. Laparoscopic adrenalectomy: lessons learned from 100 consecutive procedures. Ann Surg 1997; 226(3): 238–246; discussion 246–247.
22. Lo CY, van Heerden JA, Soreide JA, et al. Adrenalectomy for metastatic disease to the adrenal glands. Brit J of Surg 1996; 83(4): 528–531.
23. Kim SH, et al. The role of surgery in the treatment of clinically isolated adrenal metastases. Cancer 1998; 82(2): 389–394.
24. Tsuji Y, Yasuhuku M, Haryu T, et al. Laparoscopic adrenalectomy for solitary metachronous adrenal metastasis from lung cancer: report of a case. Surg Today 1999; 29(12): 1277–1279.
25. Elashry OM, Clayman RV, Soble JJ, et al. Laparoscopic adrenalectomy for solitary metachronous contralateral adrenal metastasis from renal cell carcinoma. J Urol 1997; 157(4): 1217–1222.
26. Valeri A, Borrelli A, Presenti L, et al. Adrenal masses in neoplastic patients: the role of laparoscopic procedure. Surg Endosc 2001; 15(1): 90–93.
27. Heniford BT, Arca MJ, Walsh RM, Gill IS. Laparoscopic adrenalectomy for cancer. Semin Surg Oncol 1999; 16: 293–306.

# V PROSTATE CANCER

# 13 Role of Laparoscopic Pelvic Lymph Node Dissection in Adenocarcinoma of the Prostate

*Matthew T. Gettman,* MD

*CONTENTS*

INTRODUCTION
INDICATIONS AND CONTRAINDICATIONS
SURGICAL TECHNIQUE
RESULTS
CONTROVERSIES
SHORTCOMINGS OF PROCEDURE
CONCLUSION
REFERENCES

## INTRODUCTION

With the introduction of urologic laparoscopy in the early 1990s, laparoscopic pelvic lymph node dissection (L-PLND) was a popular, minimally invasive technique for staging patients with prostatic adenocarcinoma *(1,2)*. L-PLND was introduced early in the era of prostate-specific antigen (PSA) testing when a higher percentage of patients had pelvic lymph node metastasis *(3)*. The laparoscopic approach offered less morbidity and a faster convalescence than the traditional approach for PLND *(4–6)*. The rationale behind utilization of a separate staging PLND was that discovery of pelvic lymph node metastasis would spare patients unnecessary morbidity associated with noncurative definitive therapy. Although L-PLND is considered an effective staging proce-

From: *Laparoscopic Urologic Oncology*
Edited by: J. A. Cadeddu © Humana Press Inc., Totowa, NJ

**Table 1**
**Indications for L-PLND**

1. Separate staging procedure for high-risk patients (PSA >20 ng/mL, Gleason score 8, clinical stage T3a) when intended definitive treatment is one of the following:
   - open RP
   - radiotherapy (external beam or interstitial)
   - cryoablation
2. In conjunction with laparoscopic RP (based on practice patterns of surgeon)
3. Staging candidates for salvage therapy (after failed radiotherapy or cryoablation)

L-PLND = laparoscopic pelvic lymph node dissection; PSA = prostate-specific antigen; RP = radical prostatectomy

dure, utilization has been decreased by advances in clinical diagnosis of prostate cancer and the introduction of less invasive open procedures. This chapter reviews the current indications, treatment efficacy, controversies, and shortcomings of L-PLND.

## INDICATIONS AND CONTRAINDICATIONS

In most clinical scenarios, the risk of pelvic lymph node metastasis can accurately be predicted from validated nomograms or artificial neural networks based on clinical stage, PSA, and biopsy Gleason score *(7–12)*. Furthermore, the incidence of lymph node metastasis for patients with newly diagnosed prostate cancer is less than 10% *(7,8,10)*. As such, most patients do not require staging L-PLND before intended definitive therapy. A separate staging L-PLND is considered only for patients exhibiting the upper extremes of clinical staging (Table 1). Indeed, the role of L-PLND may be greatest when intended therapy does not permit direct access to the pelvic lymph nodes (perineal prostatectomy, radiotherapy, cryosurgery) *(13–18)*. In most cases, staging L-PLND is not considered before intended laparoscopic radical prostatectomy (LRP). Alternatively, L-PLND would be considered for all patients during LRP. In similar fashion, open pelvic lymph node dissection (O-PLND) would be considered for all patients undergoing open retropubic RP in which a staging L-PLND was not performed. For patients failing definitive radiotherapy or cryoablation (and no previous PLND), L-PLND would also be considered for staging prior to intended salvage therapy *(19,20)*.

Patients undergoing L-PLND must be satisfactory candidates for general anesthesia. One relative contraindication to L-PLND is a history of hip and knee replacement *(21)* because these patients can develop lymph node sinus histiocytosis, which increases the difficulty and risk of complications with L-PLND. For similar reasons, a mesh inguinal hernia repair is another relative contraindication to L-PLND.

## SURGICAL TECHNIQUE

When staging patients with prostatic adenocarcinoma, a bilateral obturator lymphadenectomy is most commonly performed and the laparoscopic technique has been previously described in detail *(22,23)*. Although an extraperitoneal technique has been described, the transperitoneal technique is preferred at Mayo Clinic *(24–27)*. After establishing pneumoperitoneum, four ports are positioned in a diamond configuration, especially when a separate staging procedure is performed. In the diamond configuration, 5-mm trocars are placed bilaterally near McBurney's point at the midclavicular line and 10-mm trocars are placed at the umbilicus and 5 cm above the pubic symphysis. For obese patients or when L-PLND is being performed in conjunction with LRP, a horseshoe configuration is preferred. With the horseshoe configuration, 10-mm trocars are placed at the umbilicus and slightly below the umbilicus just lateral to the left rectus abdominis. Additionally, 5-mm trocars are placed on the right lateral to the rectus abdominis and bilaterally midway between the umbilicus and pubic symphysis *(22,23)*.

Bipolar cautery is used for the initial incision of the posterior peritoneum just lateral to the medial umbilical ligament. Additionally, bipolar cautery is used preferentially for dissection during lymphadenectomy. In some cases, traction on the ipsilateral testis facilitates identification of surgical landmarks. After dividing the vas deferens, L-PLND is performed within the following boundaries of dissection: circumflex iliac artery (inferior), external iliac vein (laterally), obturator nerve (medially), and hypogastric artery (superiorly). Large lymphatics are clipped or carefully fulgurated and resected lymph nodes are removed in a LapSac through a 10-mm port. Frozen section analysis is performed only for suspicious nodes or when definitive therapy is planned during the same anesthesia.

## RESULTS

Besides the laparoscopic approach, PLND is also performed using a traditional 9-cm midline incision (O-PLND) or 6-cm minilaparotomy incisions (minilaparotomy pelvic lymph node dissection [M-PLND]) *(4–6,28–33)*. Oncologic efficacy of L-PLND is evaluated by comparing completeness of lymphadenectomy, number of resected lymph nodes, and local recurrence rates (trocar metastasis) to O-PLND and M-PLND. Overall efficacy of L-PLND, in comparison to O-PLND and M-LND, is additionally assessed by considering operative time, length of hospitalization, perioperative complications, analgesic requirements, length of convalescence, and overall procedural costs (Tables 1–4).

### *Oncologic Efficacy*

In 21 reports published since 1992, the mean number of resected lymph nodes during extraperitoneal or transperitoneal L-PLND was 14 and 12, respectively *(4–6,24–28,30–32,34–43)*. Although these results are comparable to the mean number of resected lymph nodes for O-PLND (mean of 12 lymph nodes) or M-PLND (mean of 13 lymph nodes), the lymph node yield for L-PLND is also influenced by boundaries of dissection *(4–6,28–33)*. For example, Schuessler et al. removed an average of 45 lymph nodes from each patient undergoing L-PLND within an extended boundary of dissection (obturator and iliac lymph nodes) *(34)*. In 30% of cases, positive nodes were found only in the iliac specimens, implying that resection of only the obturator nodes was inadequate *(34)*. Stone et al. also compared the extent of dissection on the yield of resected nodes during L-PLND *(40)*. Among 150 patients undergoing an obturator dissection, an average of 9 lymph nodes were removed, but extended dissection in 39 patients yielded an average of 18 lymph nodes. Although the extended dissection was associated with a higher percentage of node positivity (23% vs 7%), differences in node positivity were not influenced by the dissected template among high-risk patients (PSA >20, Gleason >7, stage >T2b) *(40)*. As such, Stone et al. recommended an obturator lymphadenectomy when staging prostate cancer patients at high risk for pelvic lymph node metastasis.

When a staging L-PLND is performed before open retropubic RP, an opportunity exists to gauge the completeness of lymphadenectomy. Among 30 patients undergoing open retropubic RP, Guazzoni et al. removed a mean of six residual lymph nodes after staging L-PLND *(35)*. Most concerning was that in three patients the residual lymph nodes contained cancer not discovered at laparoscopy (laparoscopic false-negative rate of 10%). Maffezzini et al. similarly discovered residual lymph nodes in 33% of patients at the time of open retropubic RP that were not resected during staging L-PLND *(39)*. Furthermore, three patients also had residual lymph nodes that contained cancer (laparoscopic false-negative rate of 7%). Conversely, completeness of resection is rarely a problem for O-PLND or M-PLND because visualization and palpation of the template is easy to perform. In part, the completeness of resection may also reflect the learning curve for L-PLND as the incidence of residual nodes appears inversely proportional to surgical experience. Among 103 patients undergoing L-PLND, Rukstalis et al. evaluated the efficacy of lymphadenectomy by planned open exploration in the first 20 cases. The mean number of residual nodes was 3.6 for cases 1–5 but decreased to 0.4 lymph nodes for cases 16–20 *(37)*.

Given the differences in surgical technique between open surgery and laparoscopy, one concern with minimally invasive approaches has been the issue of local recurrence and port-site metastasis during laparoscopic applications in urologic oncology. Although the development of port-site metastasis appears multifactorial, characteristics of the primary tumor in addition to careful surgical technique appear most important in the pathogenesis of port-site metastasis *(44)*. Prostate cancer has a relatively low tumor aggressiveness when compared other tumors for which L-PLND is utilized (bladder cancer, urethral cancer, penile cancer), therefore it is not surprising that port-site recurrences are extremely uncommon among prostate cancer patients. In fact, the single case of port-site recurrence reported by Bagma et al. occurred after staging a 61-yr-old male with hormone-resistant prostate cancer for adjuvant radiotherapy *(45)*. At 6-mo followup, the patient presented with a cutaneous metastasis at a trocar site and died from metastatic disease 2 mo later. Cadeddu and colleagues also evaluated the oncologic safety of L-PLND among 52 prostate cancer patients with positive pelvic lymph nodes *(46)*. At a mean followup of 3.1 yr, no evidence of abdominal wall tumor implantation or trocar-site recurrence was recorded. Among the 45 men treated with early androgen deprivation therapy, the 5-yr biochemical and progression-free survival rates were 45% and 55%, respectively *(46)*.

Although the available data suggests L-PLND is safe from an oncologic standpoint, additional followup is warranted. The issues of local recurrence and port-site metastasis have been amplified with the introduction of laparoscopy, but cutaneous prostate cancer metastases were also reported before the advent of L-PLND *(45)*. When performing L-PLND for prostate cancer, the risks of cutaneous metastasis are likely the same as the other methods of PLND. Nonetheless, appropriate safeguards should be followed with specimen removal during L-PLND to decrease the risk of trocar-site recurrence *(47)*.

Table 2
Perioperative Data for L-PLND Performed via a Transperitoneal Approach

| *Author (reference)* | *Year* | *No. pts* | *Operative time, mean* | *Resected lymph nodes* | *Patients with positive lymph* nodes | *Residual lymph nodes* | *Length of stay, mean (d)* | *Analgesia requirement (MS equiv),* | *Convalescence, mean (d)* | *Complication rate (%) (%)* | *Open conversion (%)* | *Surgical reintervention* |
|---|---|---|---|---|---|---|---|---|---|---|---|---|
| Winfield et al. *(5)* | 1992 | 66 | 150 | 9 | 21% (14/66) (*n*=26) | Mean of 2.4 nodes/pt | 1.5 | 6.5 | 7 | 32% (21/66) | 22% (11/51) | 0 |
| Parra et al. *(4)* | 1992 | 12 | 185 | 11 (3/12) | 25% (0/9) | 0 | 1 | 0 | 3 | 0 | 0 | NR |
| Schuessler et al. *(34)* | 1993 | 147 | 150 | 45 | 23% (20/86) | NR | 2 | NR | 85% by 14 d | 31% (45/147) | NR | 7% (11/147) |
| Kerbl et al. *(6)* | 1993 | 30 | 199 | NR | 41% (12/30) | NR | 1.7 | 1.6 | 11 | 30% (9/30) | NR | 3.3% (1/30) |
| Guazzoni et al. *(35)* | 1994 | 30 | 136 | 18 | 13% (4/30) | Mean of 6 nodes/pt | 2 | NR | 7 | 23% (7/30) | 0 | NR |
| Lang et al. *(36)* | 1994 | 100 | 138 | 9 | 9% (9/100) | 12 (1/8) | 1.1 | NR | NR | 9% (9/100) | 0 | 3% (3/100) |
| Rukstalis et al. *(37)* | 1994 | 103 | 156 | 9 | 19% (20/103) | 0.4-4 node/pt (*n*=20) | 1.6 | 0.8 | NR | 15% (11/73) | 10% (3/100) | 0 |
| Doublet et al. *(38)* | 1994 | 29 | 90 | 8 | 21% (6/29) | 0 (0/16) | 2 | NR | NR | 28% (8/29) | 7% (2/29) | 7% (2/29) |
| Maffezzini et al. *(39)* | 1995 | 158 | NR | 11 | 26% (41/151) | 33 (14/42) | 2–3 | NR | NR | 21% (31/151) | 5% (7/158) | NR |
| Brant et al. *(31)* | 1996 | 60 | 120 | 10 | 13% (8/60) | NR | <1 | NR | NR | 6% (4/60) | 3% (2/60) | NR |
| Perrotti et al. *(28)* | 1996 | 20 | 190 | 9 | 35% (7/20) | NR | 1.2 | 4.5 | NR | 20% (4/20) | 5% (1/20) | 0 |

| | | | | | | | | | | | | |
|---|---|---|---|---|---|---|---|---|---|---|---|---|
| St. Lezin et al. *(32)* | 1997 | 22 | 175 | NR | 27% (6/22) | NR | 1.6 | NR | NR | 32% (7/22) | 5% (1/22) | 14% (3/22) |
| Herrell et al. *(30)* | 1997 | 19 | 210 | 8.5 | NR | NR | 1.6 | NR | NR | 0 | 0 | NR |
| Stone et al. *(41)* | 1997 | 189 | NR | 9 (mod.) 18(ext.) | 11% (23/189) | NR | 1 | NR | NR | 9% (17/189) | 0 | 0 |
| Kava et al. *(41)* | 1998 | 24 | 174 | 11 | 25% (6/24) | NR | 1.2 | NR | NR | 13% (3/24) | 0 | 0 |
| Shackley et al. *(42)* | 1999 | 27 | 55 | 7 | 7% (2/27) | NR | 1 | NR | NR | 27% (7/26) | 0 | 0 |
| Parkin et al. *(43)*[a] | 2002 | 50 | 110 | 6 | 24% (12/50) | NR | 1.8 | NR | NR | 18% (9/50) | 0 | 2% (1/50) |
| TOTALS | 1992–2002 | 1086 | 144 min[b] (55-210) | 12 (6-45) | 9–35% | — | 1.5 d (<1–3) | 0.8–6.5 mg MS equiv. | 3–14 d | 0–32% | 0–22% | 0–14% |

[a]Includes both extraperitoneal and transperitoneal approaches; [b]Weighted mean. L-PLND = laparoscopic pelvic lympsh node dissection; NR=not reported; MS=morphine sulfate.

Table 3
**Perioperative Data for L-PLND Performed via an Extraperitoneal Approach**

| *Author (reference)* | *Year* | *No. pts.* | *Operative time, mean (min)* | *Resected lymph nodes, mean* | *Patients with positive lymph nodes (n)* | *Residual lymph nodes (at open tx), (%)* | *Length of stay, mean (days)* | *Analgesia requirement (MS equiv), mean mg* | *Convalescence mean (d)* | *Complication rate (%)* | *Open conversion (%)* | *Surgical reintervention (%)* |
|---|---|---|---|---|---|---|---|---|---|---|---|---|
| Shafik *(24)* | 1992 | 9 | 106 | 20 | 22% | NR (2/9) | 0 | NR | NR | 0 | 0 | 0 |
| Villers et al. *(25)* | 1993 | 18[a] | 84 | NR (2/18) | 11% (0/7) | 0 | 2 (3/18) | NR | <7 | 17% | 0 | 0 |
| Das and Tashima *(26)* | 1994 | 9 | 50–110 | 12 (1/9) | 11% | 11 | 1 | NR (1/9) | NR | 11% (1/9) | 0 | 0 |
| Raboy et al. *(27)* | 1997 | 125 | 104 | 10 (24/125) | 19% | NR | 2.1 | 0.7 (based on 123 pts) | NR | 3% (4/125) | 2.4% (3/125) | NR |
| TOTALS | 1992–1997 | 161 | 102 min[b] | 14 (10-20) | 11–22% | — | 1.3 d (0-2.1) | — | <7 d | 0–17% | 0–2.4% | 0 |

[a]Includes three TCC patients; [b]Weighted mean. L-PLND = laparoscopic pelvic lymph node dissection; tx = ; NR=not reported, MS=morphine sulfate.

**Table 4**
**Perioperative Data for O-PLND**

| *Author (references)* | *Year* | *No. pts.* | *Operative time, mean (min)* | *Resected lymph nodes (n) mean* | *Patients with Positive lymp nodes (n)* | *Length of hospitalization, mean (d)* | *Analgesia requirement (MS equiv), mean mg* | *Convalescence mean (d)* | *Complication rate (%)* |
|---|---|---|---|---|---|---|---|---|---|
| Winfield et al. *(5)*[a] | 1992 | 27 | 124 | 11 | 100% (27/27) | 6.5 | NR | 17 | NR |
| Parra et al. *(4)* | 1992 | 12 | NR | 11 | 8% (1/12) | 4 | 15 | 14 | 0 |
| Kerbl et al. *(6)* | 1993 | 16 | 102 | NR | 44% (7/16) | 5.3 | 47 | 66 | 0 |
| Steiner and Marshall *(29)* | 1993 | 8 | NR | 15 | NR | NR | NR | NR | NR |
| Perrotti et al. *(28)* | 1996 | 7 | 90 | 12 | 14% (1/7) | 7 | NR | NR | NR |
| Herrell et al. *(30)* | 1997 | 38 | 114 | 9 | NR | 6.5 | NR | NR | 13% (5/38) |
| TOTALS | 1992–1997 | 108 | 114 min[b] (90–124) | 12 (9–15) | 8–100% | 5.9 d (4–7) | 31 mg MS equiv. | 32 d (14–66) | 0–13% |

[a]Includes patients for whom planned RP aborted with positive nodes; [b]Weighted mean. O-PLND = open pelvic lymph node dissection; NR=not reported, MS=morphine sulfate.

### *Procedural Efficacy*

Among 21 series published between 1992 and 2002, the mean operative times for L-PLND performed via a transperitoneal or extraperitoneal approach were 144 and 102 min, respectively *(4–6,24–28,30–32, 34–43)*. On the other hand, the mean operative times for O-PLND or M-PLND performed in the same era were 114 and 57 min, respectively *(4–6,28–33)*. For L-PLND, operative times from the earliest reports may reflect the learning curve of the laparoscopic pioneers developing the minimally invasive procedure. Contemporary L-PLND series have not reported dramatic improvements in mean operative time, however, this may reflect the decreased utilization of the staging procedure. Based on current data, L-PLND appears less advantageous to O-PLND or M-PLND with regard to mean operative time.

One major advantage of minimally invasive surgery has been decreased length of hospitalization. Among reports published between 1992 and 2002, the mean length of hospitalization for L-PLND was 1.4 d, whereas the mean length of hospitalization for O-PLND was 5.9 d *(4–6,24–32,34–43)*. To minimize morbidity and decrease length of hospitalization for O-PLND, Steiner and Marshall introduced the technique of M-PLND *(29)*. In seven series published between 1992 and 1998, the mean length of hospitalization for M-PLND was 1.7 d *(28–33)*. Although a paucity of information is available, mean analgesia requirements during hospitalization are lower for L-PLND (mean MS equiv. = 3 mg) than O-PLND (mean MS equiv. = 31 mg) *(4–6,28,37)*. Additionally, postoperative convalescence is improved following minimally invasive surgery. In studies published between 1992 and 2002, reported mean convalescence for L-PLND was 3–14 d, whereas the reported mean convalescence for O-PLND was 14–66 d *(4–6,24–32,34–43)*. Additionally, Idom and Steiner reported a mean convalescence of 3.3 d for a group of 24 patients undergoing M-PLND *(33)*. Regarding length of hospitalization, analgesic requirements, and convalescence, L-PLND and M-PLND appear favorable to O-PLND.

Because L-PLND is a relatively new procedure that is more difficult to perform than O-PLND or M-PLND, the incidence of complications is an important perioperative variable to consider. The overall range of complications for L-PLND, O-PLND, and M-PLND is 0–32%, 0–13%, and 0–9%, respectively *(4–6,24–43)*. In part, the complication rate of L-PLND may reflect the learning curve associated with laparoscopy. Lang et al. compared perioperative characteristics of the first 50 patients to the second 50 patients undergoing L-PLND *(36)*. Treatment groups were comparable regarding mean operative time and length of hospitalization, but perioperative complications were significantly decreased in the latter treatment group (2% vs 14%). In fact, the complication rate was 25% among the first 20 cases but only 5% for the subsequent 80 cases *(36)*.

Another factor that may influence the incidence of complications is access technique. Prior reports have suggested that the risk of complications for transperitoneal L-PLND may be higher than L-PLND performed via an extraperitoneal approach *(24–27)*. The higher prevalence of complications could also reflect the preference of urologists to perform the transperitoneal technique for L-PLND. Proponents of extraperitoneal L-PLND suggest that transperitoneal L-PLND may increase the risk of complications (e.g., bowel injury) that otherwise would not be associated with O-PLND or M-PLND *(24–27)*. In the multicenter report on complications associated with transperitoneal L-PLND, Kavoussi et al. reported an overall complication rate of 15% (55 complications) *(48)*. Analysis of the 55 complications revealed a 15% incidence of visceral injuries and a 13% incidence of gastrointestinal complications that may have been attributed to the transperitoneal approach. Nonetheless, the majority of complications in the report by Kavoussi et al. appear unrelated to the approach used for L-PLND. Additionally, initial access with the extraperitoneal approach can be more difficult than the transperitoneal approach. Furthermore, the extraperitonal approach is also associated with a higher chance of specific complications (e.g., hypercarbia) typically not observed with the corresponding transperitoneal approach *(24–27)*. In comparison, complications are rarely reported for patients undergoing O-PLND or M-PLND. As such, O-PLND and M-PLND appear favorable to L-PLND regarding perioperative complication rates, but this advantage may also reflect the learning curve for laparoscopy that is decreased with clinical experience.

Because of increased operative time, increased supplies, and use of disposable operative equipment, operating room costs of laparoscopy are traditionally higher than open surgery. Higher operating room costs, however, are counterbalanced by decreased length of hospitalization characteristically associated with minimally invasive surgery. Shortly after the introduction of L-PLND, Troxel and Winfield compared overall costs for 50 patients undergoing L-PLND to 11 patients undergoing O-PLND *(49)*. Overall, L-PLND cost $1250 more than O-PLND. Although the mean length of hospitalization was 1.6 d for L-PLND patients, operating room costs were 52% greater for L-PLND than O-PLND. The authors suggested, however, that the unmeasured value of a shorter convalescence would favor L-PLND rather than O-PLND when patient-related financial issues were considered (shorter recovery, earlier return to work) *(49)*. In another financial analysis performed by Kerbl et al., the overall cost of bilateral L-PLND was $10,277, whereas bilateral O-PLND cost $8221 *(6)*. On the other hand, Perrotti et al. reported the costs of O-PLND and L-PLND were comparable (O-PLND: $4262, L-PLND: $4245) *(28)*. Although postoperative costs of hospitalization were only $393 for L-PLND (mean length of hospitalization = 1.2 d), the operating room costs associated with the mean operating time of 190 min were $2121 *(30)*.

When the costs of L-PLND and O-PLND are compared to M-PLND, M-PLND emerges the most cost-effective procedure. Herrell et al. compared the results of L-PLND, M-PLND, and O-PLND for 68 patients with cT3 prostate cancer and noted mean operative times of 210, 102, and 114 min, respectively *(30)*. Additionally, mean length of hospitalization for L-PLND, M-PLND, and O-PLND were 2.7, 3.3, and 6.5 d, respectively. Based on decreased resource utilization and overall effectiveness of the procedure, the authors recommended M-PLND as the staging procedure of choice especially when the costs of laparoscopy or the laparoscopic learning curve could not be overcome *(30)*. In the similar report by Perrotti et al., M-PLND was also favorable to L-PLND and O-PLND from an oncologic, patient morbidity, and cost standpoint *(28)*. The overall costs for M-PLND ($2516) were approx 40% lower than O-PLND ($4262) or L-PLND ($4245), respectively. Although many clinical comparisons between M-PLND and L-PLND are equivalent (e.g., length of hospitalization), L-PLND typically requires more expensive operative equipment and longer operative time than M-PLND and these factors are responsible for the cost differences between the minimally invasive procedures *(28)*. Thus, from a standpoint of cost-effectiveness, M-PLND appears advantageous to L-PLND and O-PLND.

## CONTROVERSIES

### *Patient Selection*

Although most urologists agree that a staging PLND is indicated only for "high-risk" patients, the definition of a high-risk is formulated by a varying number of clinical factors including intended therapeutic modality, PSA, clinical stage, and prostate biopsy results. Recommendations to proceed with staging PLND can also be influenced by institutional practice patterns based on retrospective outcomes analysis of patients with or without pTxN+ prostatic adenocarcinoma. O'Dowd et al. performed a meta-analysis of 142 studies evaluating staging modalities for newly diagnosed prostatic adenocarcinoma. On the basis of the analysis, the investigators recommended a staging PLND prior to RP for the following indications: PSA greater than 20 ng/mL, biopsy Gleason score 8–10, five or more systematic biopsies, positive seminal vesical biospy, and advanced palpable tumor (cT3-4) *(50)*.

Despite the broad recommendations reported by O'Dowd et al., many centers consider the following clinical variables singularly or in combination as indications for a separate staging PLND: PSA greater than 20 ng/mL, extracapsular disease (cT3), and Gleason sum greater than 6. Maffezzini et al. reported that the yield of node positivity correlated significantly with an increasing number of high-risk clinical factors *(39)*. Additionally, Stone et al. found that node positivity was significantly higher in the presence of multiple high-risk features. As such, Stone et al. recommended L-PLND could safely be limited to only the obturator nodes when the procedure was performed on patients at high risk for metastasis *(40)*. Before intended open retropubic RP, Walsh recommended a staging L-PLND only for patients with a biopsy Gleason score of 8–10 and clinically organ-confined disease *(51)*. These recommendations were based on the findings of Sgrignoli et al., who performed a retrospective analysis of 113 cT1–T3 prostate cancer patients undergoing open retropubic RP and delayed androgen deprivation therapy for pTxN+ disease at Johns Hopkins Hospital between 1974 and 1991 *(52)*. In multivariate analysis, only biopsy Gleason grade significantly predicted cancer progression. Men with biospy Gleason scores of 7 or less had metastasis-free survival rates of 82% and 59% at 5 and 10 yr, respectively. In contrast, the 10-yr metastasis-free survival rates for men with a biopsy Gleason score of 8 or higher were 15% at 5 yr *(52)*.

The choice of intended therapeutic intervention, especially when direct access to the pelvic lymph node is not possible, can also influence the recommendations for a staging L-PLND. For instance, Kozlowski and Winfield recommended a staging L-PLND for patients with clinical stage T2b/T3a, PSA greater than 20 ng/nL, or clinical stage T1b with Gleason sum greater than 7, except when the intended definitive treatment was perineal RP *(22)*. For these patients, L-PLND was recommended regardless of the clinical variables. Wolf also recommend L-PLND on the basis of metastatic risk and intended therapeutic intervention *(53)*. For instance, patients with moderate risk (serum PSA 10 or Gleason score 7 or clinical stage T2c) would undergo staging L-PLND before intended perineal RP, however moderate-risk patients would not undergo a staging L-PLND before intended retropubic RP. Indications for a separate staging L-PLND included the following: PSA of 50 or more, PSA of 20 or more and Gleason score of 7 or more, or PSA of 10 or more and Gleason score of 8 or more *(53)*. The recommendations suggested by Wolf were based on a decision analysis performed by Wolf et al., which took into account the following treatment issues: clinical factors, patient preference, cost, and planned definitive treatment *(54)*. On the basis of the work, Wolf et al. found L-PLND was beneficial for patients with a 39% chance of lymph node metastasis if the intended surgical procedure was retropubic RP, whereas L-PLND was beneficial for patients with a 20% chance of lymph node metastasis if the intended therapy was a perineal RP *(54)*. Parkin et al. similarly recommended that a 20% probability of lymph node metastasis should be used for all intended therapies, not just perineal RP *(43)*.

Although it seems prudent that the indications for PLND are expanded when access to the lymph nodes is not possible with definitive therapy, the issue of L-PLND before planned radiotherapy remains controversial *(13–15,55)*. Based on long-term results (10 and 15 yr) of 536 patients treated with interstitial and external beam radiotherapy, status of the lymph nodes and posttreatment biospy results were the only significant multivariate predictors of cause-specific survival. On this basis, Puthawala et al. recommended that PLND should be performed prior to radiotherapy, especially in high-risk patients *(14)*. At 15-yr followup, a similar advantage for staging PLND before external beam radiotherapy was reported by Lee and Sause *(15)*. Cause-specific survival was 40% among 20 patients with confined disease, whereas node positive patients ($n$ = 36) had a cause-specific survival of 6% at 15 yr. Buskirk et al. reported knowledge of lymph node metastasis favors recommendations for adjuvant androgen-deprivation therapy, which possibly provides a survival advantage for node-positive patients treated with external beam radiotherapy *(18)*. Among 60 pTxN+ patients treated with external beam radiotherapy and androgen-deprivation therapy, Buskirk et al. reported 5-yr biochemical relapse-free and cause-specific survival rates of 82% and 80%, respectively *(18)*. On the other hand, Gerber et al. compared radiotherapy among 31 patients staged with L-PLND to 42 men undergoing treatment without L-PLND and demonstrated no differences in treatment outcome *(55)*. On this basis, the authors suggested that L-PLND did not provide acceptable accuracy in defining favorable groups of patients for radiotherapy. Also, rather than recommending a staging PLND, some radiotherapists have circumvented the issue by extending the boundaries of radiotherapy to include the pelvic lymph nodes *(53)*.

Although a consensus is present in the literature to perform a staging PLND only for patients at highest risk for pelvic lymph node metastasis, standardized recommendations are not available. Given the ongoing stage migration of prostate cancer attributed to early detection and PSA screening protocols, the indications for a separate staging PLND will most likely continue to decrease. Furthermore, a separate staging PLND may best be utilized when the planned definitive therapy does not provide direct access to the pelvic lymph nodes.

### *Utility of Procedure*

Given the significant changes in the clinical diagnosis of prostate cancer in the PSA era, the overall utility of L-PLND from an oncologic and technical standpoint may be questioned, especially when the intended therapy is open retropubic RP. From a technical standpoint, a staging L-PLND can make planned open retropubic RP more difficult. Parra et al. compared groups of patients treated with L-PLND before retropubic RP, L-PLND before perineal RP, or O-PLND before retropubic RP *(16)*. The researchers concluded the combination of L-PLND and perineal RP was associated with less morbidity. In contrast, patients staged with L-PLND before planned retropubic RP experienced greater blood loss, longer operative times, and increased morbidity *(16)*.

Additionally, the rationale behind development of PLND as a staging procedure was that discovery of positive lymph nodes would preclude an attempt with curative treatment (RP or radiation) and not subject individuals to the unacceptable risks of treatment morbidity. Increasing reports suggest that the combination of RP and early androgen-deprivation therapy is advantageous to androgen-deprivation therapy alone for node-positive prostate cancer patients *(3,52,57–59)*. As such, the concept of performing a separate staging L-PLND for high-risk patients before open retropubic RP also appears controversial. Ghavamian et al. performed a matched comparison of 79 patients with pTxN+ prostatic adenocarcinoma after retropubic RP plus early adjuvant orchiectomy to 79 patients with pTxN+ prostatic adenocarcinoma treated only with orchiectomy *(56)* At 10-yr followup, patients treated with RP plus orchiectomy had significantly higher overall (66% vs 28%) and cause-specific survival (79% vs 39%) than node-positive patients treated with orchiectomy alone *(56)*. In a prospective randomized trial of lymph node-positive patients, Messing et al. reported that the addition of androgen-deprivation therapy with radical prostatectomy provided a survival advantage in comparison to radical prostatectomy alone *(57)*. Furthermore, with the stage migration of prostate cancer, the incidence of lymph node involvement has decreased and many patients have evidence of only micrometastatic disease. In a study of 269 pTxN+ patients treated in the PSA era with RP and androgen-deprivation therapy, Cheng et al. reported that cancer volume of lymph node metastasis was the most significant multivariate predictor of disease progression *(59)*. Additionally, the morbidity of RP has progressively decreased making this argument a less compelling reason to avoid RP in light of pelvic lymph node metastasis. Because RP may provide a therapeutic benefit in the presence of pelvic lymph node metastasis, preliminary M-PLND may be the preferred approach for staging the pelvic lymph nodes in high-risk prostate cancer patients. If the resected lymph nodes were grossly uninvolved, a decision could then be made to proceed with retropubic RP during the same anesthetic.

Even for high-risk patients in which the intended therapy is not open retropubic RP, the utility of L-PLND is also debatable when compared to M-PLND. M-PLND appears equivalent to L-PLND from a standpoint of minimally invasiveness (length of stay, analgesic requirement, convalescence), but M-PLND may be advantageous with regard to operative time, cost, risk of initial complications, and the learning curve. Nonetheless, L-PLND would still have an important staging role among patients undergoing definitive therapy with laparoscopic RP. Given the increasing popularity of LRP, utilization of L-PLND may again increase when performed concurrently with this definitive treatment.

## SHORTCOMINGS OF PROCEDURE

### *Pathologic Assessment of Lymph Nodes*

The 7–28% false-negative rate associated with frozen section analysis of resected lymph nodes can limit the accuracy of a staging PLND *(60)*. To gain the most accurate staging information from PLND, results of permanent sections are required. In some instances, this issue has therefore precluded the use of one anesthesia for PLND and planned definitive therapy. Because of the false-negative rate and the added expense of frozen section analysis, many urologists refrain from obtaining routine frozen sections and alternatively wait for the results of permanent sections, especially when the resected lymph nodes are grossly benign. Frozen section analysis is helpful when grossly malignant lymph nodes are encountered during a separate staging L-PLND. In this situation, the diagnosis of metastasis can be reliably established without subjecting the patient to prolonged operative times and risks of the contralateral dissection. The issue of false-negative frozen section analysis should be addressed with the patient, especially when the results of frozen section are being used to proceed with definitive therapy during the same anesthetic.

Another issue with regard to pathologic assessment of the pelvic lymph nodes is the selection of patients for staging PLND at the time of open RP or LRP. Recently, the same nomograms that have decreased utilization of a staging PLND before planned definitive therapy have also decreased utilization of PLND during open retropubic (RP) or LRP *(7,8,12)*. In low-risk patients, PLND is increasingly omitted because the rationale is that the procedure is unnecessary and associated with increased operative time, risk of complications, and cost. Although the overall incidence of detected lymph node metastasis is low, performing staging PLND at the time of definitive RP when the lymph nodes are easily accessible can provide the individual patient with the best clinical staging that can affect adjuvant treatment recommendations (androgen-deprivation therapy). Furthermore, from a research standpoint, biological characteristics of all tumors are best defined when all patients are staged.

### *Learning Curve*

One of the biggest ongoing limitations of laparoscopy is acquisition of skills required to perform the advanced minimally invasive techniques. Because of differences in visualization and instrumentation, laparoscopy is more difficult to perform than open surgery. The learning curve for L-PLND, as well as other laparoscopic procedures, is most commonly reflected by the longer operative times and higher complication rates associated with a surgeon's initial clinical experience. A specific factor, reflective of the learning curve for L-PLND, is the number of residual lymph nodes removed during subsequent open retropubic RP. Although improvements in each of these perioperative variables have occurred with experience, the estimated learning curve for L-PLND is approx 20 cases *(35,36)*. Recent studies have not evaluated the learning curve for L-PLND, but the learning curve may be less steep given the fact that urologic laparoscopy is more commonplace and that more difficult laparoscopic procedures are routinely performed. The decreased requirements for staging prostate cancer patients, however, could adversely impact the learning curve for L-PLND, unless utilization is again increased in conjunction with LRP.

## CONCLUSION

L-PLND remains an effective staging procedure for prostate cancer patients, however, refinements in clinical diagnosis and development of alternative surgical procedures have significantly reduced the clinical indications. In fact, with the ongoing stage migration in prostatic adenocarcinoma, patient selection and the overall utility of PLND from an oncologic standpoint appear controversial. From a procedural standpoint, L-PLND and M-PLND appear advantageous to O-PLND when considering length of hospitalization, convalescence, and analgesic requirements. With regard to operative time, procedural costs, potential for perioperative complications, and the learning curve, M-PLND currently appears beneficial to L-PLND. Nonetheless, recommendations to proceed with L-PLND are influenced by characteristics of the operating surgeon and the intended therapeutic intervention. In fact, with the increased popularity of LRP or other therapies that do not provide direct access to the pelvic lymph nodes, the utilization of L-PLND may again increase.

## REFERENCES


1. Winfield HN, Ryan KJ. Laparoscopy: new urological applications. J Urol 1989; 141(Suppl): 176A.
2. Schuessler WW, Vancaillie TG, Reich H, et al. Transperitoneal endosurgical lymphadenectomy in patients with localized prostate cancer. J Urol 1991; 145: 988–991.
3. Seay TM, Blute ML, Zincke H. Long-term outcome in patients with pTxN+ adenocarcinoma of prostate treated with radical prostatectomy and early androgen ablation. J Urol 1998; 159: 357–364.
4. Parra RO, Andrus C, Boullier J, et al. Staging laparoscopic pelvic lymph node dissection: comparison of results with open pelvic lymphadenectomy. J Urol 1992; 147: 875–878.
5. Winfield HN, Donovan JF, See WA, et al. Laparoscopic pelvic lymph node dissection for genitourinary malignancies: indications, techniques, and results. J Endourol 1992; 6: 103.
6. Kerbl K, Clayman RV, Petros J, et al. Staging pelvic lymphadenectomy for prostate cancer: a comparison of laparoscopic and open techniques. J Urol 1993; 150: 396–398.
7. Bluestein DL, Bostwick DG, Bergstralh EJ, et al. Eliminating the need for bilateral pelvic lymphadenectomy in select patients with prostate cancer. J Urol 1994; 151: 1315–1320.
8. Partin AW, Kattan MW, Subong MS, et al. Combination of prostate-specific antigen, clinical stage and Gleason score to predict pathological stage of localized prostate cancer: a multi-institutional update. JAMA 1999; 277: 1445–1451.
9. Crawford ED, Batuello JT, Snow P, et al. The use of artificial intelligence technology to predict lymph node spread in men with clinically localized prostate cancer. Cancer 2000; 88: 2105–2109.
10. Blute ML, Bergstralh EJ, Partin AW, et al. Validation of Partin tables for predicting pathological stage of clinically localized prostate cancer. J Urol 2000; 164: 1591–1595.
11. Penson DF, Grossfeld GD, Li Y, et al. How well does the Partin nomogram predict pathological stage after radical prostatectomy in a community based population? Results of the cancer of the prostate strategic urological research endeavor. J Urol 2002; 167: 1653–1657.
12. Partin AW, Mangold LA, Lamm DM, et al. Contemporary update of prostate cancer staging nomograms (Partin tables) for the new millennium. Urology 2001; 58: 843–848.
13. Gray CL, Powell CR, Riffenburgh RH, et al. 20-year outcome of patients with T1-3N0 surgically staged prostate cancer treated with external beam radiation therapy. J Urol 2001; 166: 116–118.

14. Puthawala AA, Syed AMN, Austin PA, et al. Long-term results of treatment for prostate carcinoma by staging pelvic lymph node dissection and definitive irradiation using low-dose rate temporary iridium-192 interstitial implant and external beam radiotherapy. Cancer 2001; 92: 2084–2094.
15. Lee RJ, Sause WT. Surgically staged patients with prostatic carcinoma treated with definitive radiotherapy: fifteen-year results. Urology 1994; 43: 640–644.
16. Parra RO, Boullier JA, Rauscher JA, et al. The value of laparoscopic lymphadenectomy in conjunction with radical perineal or retropubic prostatectomy. J Urol 1994; 151: 1599–1602.
17. Zisman A, Pantuck AJ, Cohen JK, et al. Prostate cryoablation using direct transperineal placement of ultrathin probes through a 17-gauge brachytherapy template-technique and preliminary results. Urology 2001; 58: 988–993.
18. Buskirk SJ, Pisansky TM, Atkinson EJ, et al. Lymph-node positive prostate cancer: evaluation of the result of the combination of androgen deprivation therapy and radiation therapy. Mayo Clin Proc 2001; 76: 702–706.
19. Lund GO, Winfield HN, Donovan JF, et al. Laparoscopic pelvic lymph node dissection following definitive radiotherapy for carcinoma of the prostate. J Urol 1997; 157: 548–551.
20. Jarrard DF, Chodak, GW. Prostate cancer staging after radiation utilizing laparoscopic pelvic lymphadenectomy. Urology 1995; 46: 538–541.
21. Cooper CS, Donovan JF, Terrell RB, et al. Hip and knee replacement as a relative contraindication to laparoscopic pelvic lymph node dissection. J Urol 1997; 158: 128–130.
22. Kozlowski PM, Winfield HN. Laparoscopic lymph node dissection: pelvic and retroperitoneal. Semin Laparosc Surg 2000; 7: 150–159.
23. West DA, Moore RG. Laparoscopic pelvic lymphadenectomy. In *Atlas of Laparoscopic Retroperitoneal Surgery*. (Bischoff JT, Kavoussi LR, eds.), J.B.Saunders, Philadelphia, PA, 2000, pp. 225–236.
24. Shafik A. Extraperitoneal laparoscopic lymphadenectomy in prostate cancer: preliminary report of a new approach. J Endourol 1992; 6: 113–117.
25. Villers A, Vannier J, Abecassis R, et al. Extraperitoneal endosurgical lymphadenectomy with insufflation in the staging of bladder and prostate cancer. J Endourol 1993; 7: 229–235.
26. Das S, Tashima M. Extraperitoneal laparoscopic staging pelvic lymph node dissection. J Urol 1994; 151: 1321–1323.
27. Raboy A, Adler H, Albert P. Extraperitoneal endoscopic pelvic lymph node dissection: a review of 125 patients. J Urol 1997; 158: 2202–2204.
28. Perrotti M, Gentle DL, Barada JH, et al. Mini-laparotomy pelvic lymph node dissection minimizes morbidity, hospitalization and cost of pelvic lymph node dissection. J Urol 1996; 155: 986–988.
29. Steiner MS, Marshall FF. Mini-laparotomy staging pelvic lymphadenectomy (MINILAP). Urology 1993; 41: 201–206.
30. Herrell SD, Trachtenberg J, Theodorescu D. Staging pelvic lymphadenectomy for localized carcinoma of the prostate: a comparison of 3 surgical techniques. J Urol 1997; 157: 1337–1339.
31. Brandt LA, Brandt WO, Brown MH, et al. A new minimally invasive open pelvic lymphadenectomy surgical technique for the staging of prostate cancer. Urology 1996; 47: 416–421.
32. Lezin MS, Cherrie R, Cattolica EV. Comparison of laparoscopic and mini-laparotomy pelvic lymphadenectomy for prostate cancer staging in a community practive. Urology 1997; 49: 60–63.

33. Idom CB, Jr, Steiner MS. Minilaparotomy staging pelvic lymphadenectomy follow-up: a safe alternative to standard and laparoscopic pelvic lymphadenectomy. World J Urol 1998; 16: 396–399.
34. Schuessler WW, Pharand D, Vancaillie TG. Laparoscopic standard pelvic node dissection for carcinoma of the prostate: it it accurate? J Urol 1993; 150: 898–901.
35. Guazzoni G, Montorsi F, Bergamaschi F, et al. Open surgical revision of laparoscopic pelvic lymphadenectomy for staging of prostate cancer: the impact of the laparoscopic learning curve. J Urol 1994; 151: 930–933.
36. Lang GS, Ruckle HC, Hadley HR, et al. One hundred consecutive laparoscopic pelvic lymph node dissections: comparing complications of the first 50 cases to the second 50 cases. Urology 1994; 44: 221–225.
37. Rukstalis DB, Gerber GS, Vogelzang NJ, et al. Laparoscopic pelvic lymph node dissection: a review of 103 consecutive cases. J Urol 1994; 151: 670–674.
38. Doublet JD, Gattegno B, Thibault P. Laparoscopic pelvic lymph node dissection for staging of prostate cancer. Eur Urol 1994; 25: 194–198.
39. Maffezzini M, Carmignani G, Perachino M, et al. Benefits and complications of laparoscopic pelvic lymphadenectomy for detection of stage D1 prostate cancer: a multicenter experience. Eur Urol 1995; 27 135–137.
40. Stone NN, Stock RG, Unger P. Laparoscopic pelvic lymph node dissection for prostate cancer: comparison of the extended and modified techniques. J Urol 1997; 158: 1891–1894.
41. Kava BR, Dalbagni G, Conlon KC, et al. Results of laparoscopic pelvic lymphadenectomy in patients at high risk for nodal metastases from prostate cancer. Ann Surg Oncol 1998; 5: 173–180.
42. Shackley DC, Irving SO, Brough WA, et al. Staging laparoscopic pelvic lymphadenectomy in prostate cancer. BJU Int 1999; 83: 260–264.
43. Parkin J, Keeley FX Jr, Timoney AG. Laparoscopic lymph node sampling in locally advanced prostate cancer. BJU Int 2002; 89: 14–17.
44. Reymond MA, Schneider C, Kastl S, Hohenberger W, Kockerling F. The pathogenesis of port-site recurrences. J Gastrointest Surg 1998; 2: 406–414.
45. Bangma CH, Kirkels WJ, Chadha S, et al. Cutaneous metastasis following laparoscopic pelvic lymphadenectomy for prostate carcinoma. J Urol 1995; 153: 1635–1636.
46. Cadeddu JA, Elashry OM, Snyder O, et al. Effect of laparoscopic pelvic lymph node dissection on the natural history of D1 (T1-3, N1-3, M0) prostate cancer. Urology 1997; 50: 391–394.
47. Elbahnasy AM, Hoenig DM, Shalhav A, McDougall EM, and Clayman RV. Laparoscopic staging of bladder tumor: concerns about port site metastases. J Endourol 1998; 12: 55–59.
48. Kavoussi LR, Sosa E, Chandhoke P, et al. Complications of laparoscopic pelvic lymph node dissection. J Urol 1993; 149: 322–325.
49. Troxel S, Winfield HN. Comparative financial analysis of laparoscopic versus open pelvic lymph node dissection for men with cancer of the prostate. J Urol 1994; 151: 675–680.
50. O'Dowd GJ, Veltri RW, Orozco R, et al. Update on the appropriate staging evaluation for newly diagnosed prostate cancer. J Urol 1997; 158: 687–698.
51. Walsh PC. Minimally invasive treatment of prostate cancer. (editorial) J Endourol 2001; 15: 447.
52. Sgrignoli AR, Walsh PC, Steinberg GD, et al. Prognostic factors in men with stage D1 prostate cancer: identification of patients less likely to have prolonged survival after radical prostatectomy. J Urol 1994; 152: 1077–1081.

53. Wolf JS Jr. Indications, technique and results of laparoscopic pelvic lymphadenectomy. J Endourol 2001; 15: 427–435.
54. Wolf JS Jr. Shinihara K, Kerlikowske KM, et al. Selection of patients for laparoscopic pelvic lymphadenctomy prior to radical prostatectomy: a decision analysis. Urology 1993; 42: 680–688.
55. Gerber GS, Bales GT, Gornick HL, et al. Treatment of prostate cancer using external beam radiotherapy after laparoscopic pelvic lymph node dissection. Br J Urol 1996; 77: 870–875.
56. Ghavamian R, Bergstralh EJ, Blute ML, et al. Radical retropubic prostatectomy plus orchiectomy versus orchiectomy alone for pTxN+ prostate cancer: a matched comparison. J Urol 1999; 161: 1223–1227.
57. Messing EM, Manola J, Sarosdy M, et al. Immediate hormonal therapy compared with observation after radical prostatectomy and pelvic lymphadenectomy in men with node-positive prostate cancer. N Engl J Med 1999; 341: 1781–1788.
58. Cadeddu JA, Partin AW, Epstein JI, et al. Stage D1 (T1-3, N1-3, M0) prostate cancer: a case-controlled comparison of conservative treatment versus radical prostatectomy. Urology 1997; 50: 251–255.
59. Cheng L, Bergstralh EJ, Cheville JC, et al. Cancer volume of lymph node metastasis predicts progression in prostate cancer. Am J Surg Pathol 1998; 22: 1491–1500.
60. Link RE, Morton RA. Indications for pelvic lymphadenectomy in prostate cancer. Urol Clin N Am 2001; 28: 491–498.

# 14 Laparoscopic Radical Prostatectomy

*Michael D. Fabrizio*, MD,
*Douglas Soderdahl*, MD,
*and Paul F. Schellhammer*, MD

*CONTENTS*

INTRODUCTION
INDICATIONS
CONTRAINDICATIONS
SURGICAL TECHNIQUE
OPERATIVE RESULTS
ONCOLOGICAL RESULTS
PERIOPERATIVE OUTCOMES
CONTROVERSIAL ISSUES AND SHORTCOMINGS

## INTRODUCTION

Among the various treatment alternatives, radical prostatectomy (RP) offers the most definitive pathological staging and prognostic information while removing the affected organ. This surgical procedure has been shown to provide excellent long-term cancer control in those patients with pathologically confirmed, organ-confined prostate cancer *(1,2)*.

From: *Laparoscopic Urologic Oncology*
Edited by: J. A. Cadeddu © Humana Press Inc., Totowa, NJ

Surgical removal has been traditionally accomplished by the retropubic or perineal approach. Following the progression of many other open urological procedures, the laparoscopic approach is being explored as a surgical alternative for RP. In fact, laparoscopy has evolved from limited use in benign conditions to becoming a standard of care for such operations as radical nephrectomy, nephroureterectomy, and adrenalectomy. These procedures have the benefits of traditional open approaches (i.e., efficacy and proven safety) while providing the well-established benefits laparoscopy (i.e., shorter recovery, less postoperative pain, improved cosmesis). The retropubic or perineal RP have proven records in oncological control, functional results (i.e., continence and potency), and reproducibility as well. It is against this well-established procedure that all novel curative interventions for prostate cancer including the laparoscopic radical prostatectomy (LRP) must be compared.

Schuessler et al. performed the first LRP in 1991 and reported their series in 1997 *(3)*. The average operative time was more than 9 h, and they concluded that "laparoscopy is not an efficacious surgical alternative to open prostatectomy for malignancy." This comment illustrates the technical challenges behind the LRP. In 1998, two French groups—Abbou et al. at Henri Mondor Hospital and Guillonneau and Vallancien at Montsouris Hospital—refined the LRP *(4,5)*. Schuessler and colleagues demonstrated the feasibility in their original series; however, more recent series have demonstrated the efficacy of this procedure. This chapter describes the surgical technique of the LRP, reviews current operative data, and perhaps more importantly reviews the early postoperative oncological and functional results. It also addresses current controversies that surround the procedure.

## INDICATIONS

LRP is indicated in patients who would have a life expectancy of at least 10 yr *(6)*. The same indications apply to the laparoscopic, open, and perineal approaches. Patients should have organ-confined prostate cancer at the time of presentation. The choice of a nerve-sparing or a non-nerve-sparing approach should be mutually agreed on by the surgeon and patient. In general, contraindications to the nerve-sparing approach include palpable disease at the apex, Gleason grade 5 disease, markedly elevated prostate-specific antigen (PSA) (i.e., greater than 20 ng/mL), and a preoperative impotence *(7)*. Although unable to palpate induration at the time of the LRP, any intraoperative difficulties with mobilization of the neurovascular bundle including fixation should be a relative contraindication to a nerve-sparing approach. Those patients with prostate volumes of greater than 100 g may be more difficult; however, the authors have removed a 179-g prostate using the LRP. Laparoscopic pelvic lymph node dissection (L-PLND) is reserved for those patients with Gleason grade 4 or 5 disease, high-volume disease, or a PSA greater than 10 ng/mL.

## CONTRAINDICATIONS

Previous abdominal surgery is no longer a contraindication to LRP. The type of previous abdominal procedure, however, may change the approach. The authors have performed LRPs on patients with previous colon resections and a history of elective abdominal procedures, but caution should be used when there is a history of peritonitis. Additionally, pelvic lipomatosis is an absolute contraindication to the LRP based on the authors' experience. Finally, due to the extreme Trendelenburg position typically employed during the procedure, any known intracranial pathology such as arteriovenous malformations, cerebral aneurysms, or a history of cerebral vascular accidents should serve as a contraindication to the LRP.

## SURGICAL TECHNIQUE

In addition to the normal preoperative laboratory and radiographic studies, the patient receives a mechanical bowel preparation the day before surgery. On the morning of surgery, the patient is typed and screened, undergoes a 500 cc neomycin enema, and receives a cephalosporin antibiotic. We use sequential pneumatic compression devices throughout the procedure.

LRP is performed with the patient in the supine position with the arms tucked and the table slightly flexed. A rectal bougie is placed and the abdomen/genitalia are prepped and draped in the usual sterile fashion. A 20 French Foley catheter is inserted into the urinary bladder after the sterile field has been established. At this point, a Veress needle is used to insufflate the abdominal cavity to 20 cm$^{h20}$ pressure. After a pneumoperitoneum has been established, five trocars are placed. The first 12-mm trocar is placed at the level of the umbilicus (Fig. 1). This can be placed using an optical port, employing an open technique, or by gently applying pressure to the 12-mm trocar and introducing it into the abdomen. We use a 0° lens throughout the procedure and inspect the abdominal cavity after placement of our first trocar. Our next two 12-mm trocars are placed just lateral to the rectus on the right- and left-hand side, respectively. These 12-mm trocars are placed 2–4 cm inferior to the umbilicus. Finally, two 5-mm trocars are placed off the anterior iliac

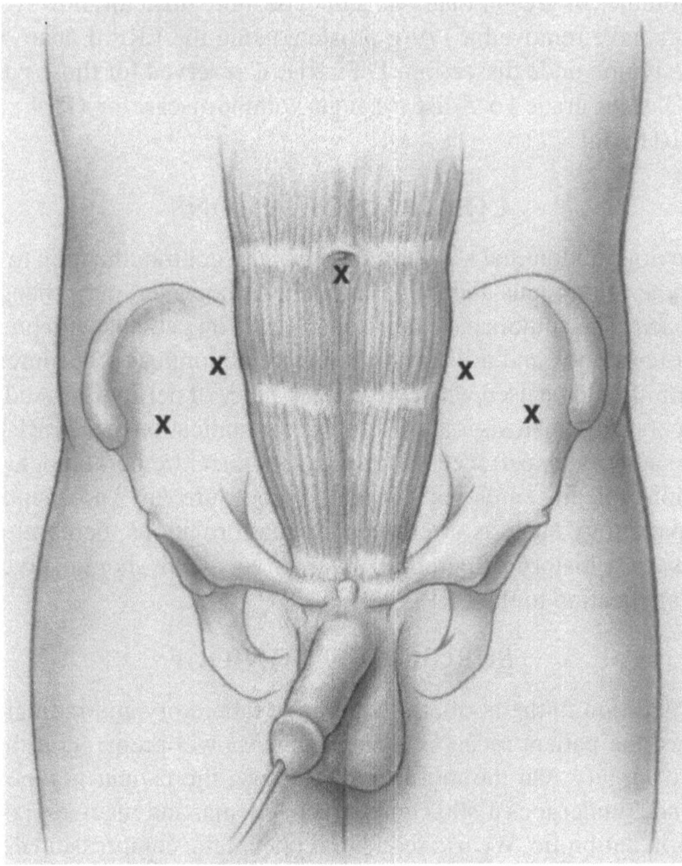


**Fig. 1.** Port placement.

spine on the right- and left-hand sides, respectively. Thus, a total of five ports are utilized throughout the procedure (Fig. 1). The patient is now placed into extreme Trendelenburg position. At this point, an L-PLND can be performed if warranted.

If available, the Aesop (Computer Motion, Inc., Goleta, CA) is placed on the patient's right-hand side of the table and used to control the 0° laparoscope through the umbilical port. The assistant stands on the patient's right side and the surgeon stands on the patient's left side throughout the procedure. A fan retractor is used through the right 12-mm port to provide retraction of the bowel. Once the cul-de-sac is clearly identified and any sigmoid attachments are incised, the vas deferens is identified on both the right- and left-hand sides at the level of the internal ring. The peritoneum is scored in a line along the vas deferens

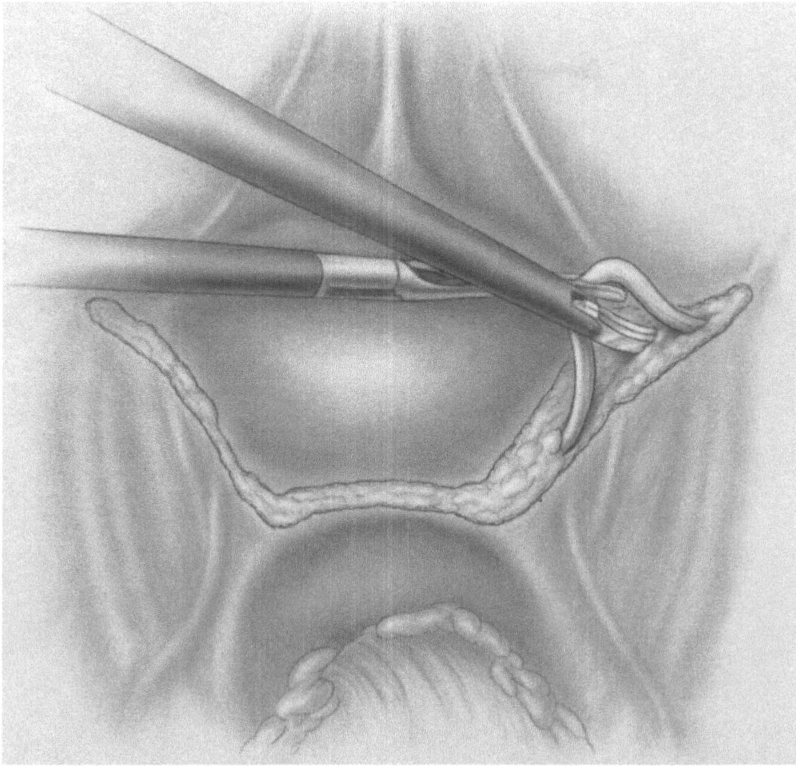

**Fig. 2.** Incising the vas deferens and peritoneum into the cul-de-sac.

down to the cul-de-sac (Fig. 2). This incision is carried down to the second peritoneal fold in the cul-de-sac. The vas deferens is skeletonized on the right- and the left-hand sides. The vas deferens is dissected down to the level of the seminal vesicles on both right- and the left-hand sides. Hemostasis is maintained with the bipolar cautery. Once the seminal vesicles are identified, the assistant retracts the vas deferens anteriorly using a grasper through the 5-mm right-sided port and assist using the irrigator-aspirator through the 12-mm right-sided port. The surgeon now proceeds to dissect the seminal vesicles using a combination of sharp and blunt dissection with the bipolar cautery and scissors. The seminal vesicles are completely mobilized to their tips. In the next step, the surgeon and assistant retract the seminal vesicles and Denonvillier's fascia is incised, which creates a plane between the posterior surface of the prostate and the rectum. The peri-rectal adipose tissue should be clearly identified. If necessary, a rectal bougie can be manipulated by an assistant in order to confirm the exact location of the rectum.

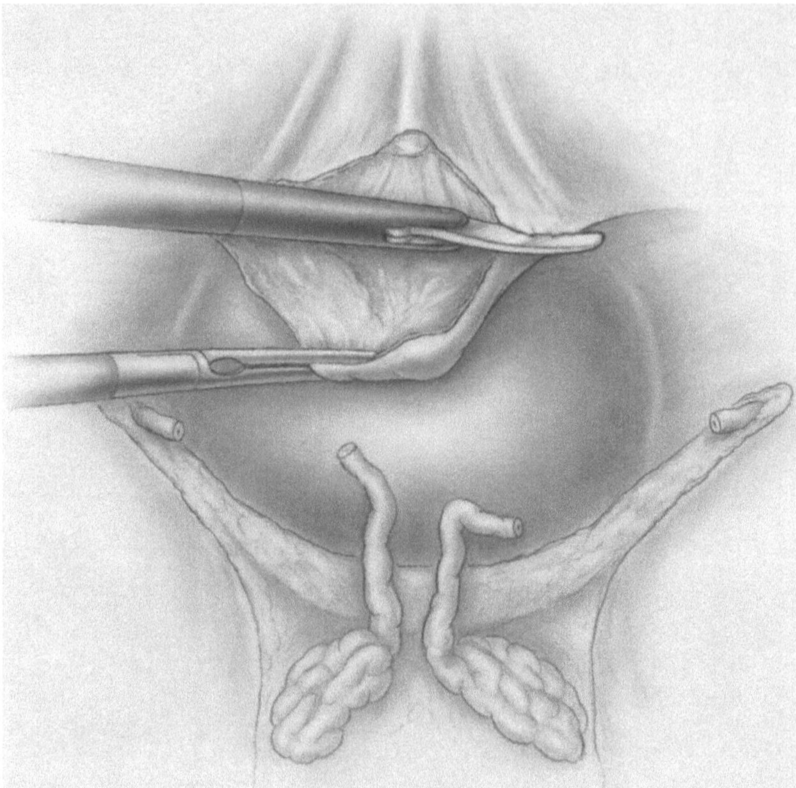

**Fig. 3.** Freeing the bladder off the anterior abdominal wall.

Attention is now focused at the level of the bladder. The bladder is filled with 200 cc of saline and, using the bipolar cautery and laparoscopic scissors through the left-sided ports, the lateral aspect of the bladder is dissected off the anterior abdominal wall by connecting the points between the incised median and umbilical ligaments and the lateral peritoneal reflection (Fig. 3). The bladder is emptied and now has been mobilized. The endopelvic fascia can be seen on both the left- and right-hand sides without difficulty. The surgeon incises the endopelvic fascia bilaterally and the fatty tissue overlying the prostate is carefully dissected away using the bipolar cautery. The superficial dorsal vein is cauterized using the bipolar forceps. Thus, the anterior surface of the prostate is exposed, and the pubo-prostatic ligaments on the right- and left-hand side are sharply divided with the laparoscopic scissors. The deep dorsal venous complex runs parallel to the urethra at the level of the prostatic apex and is now ligated with a 0-Vicryl suture ligature on

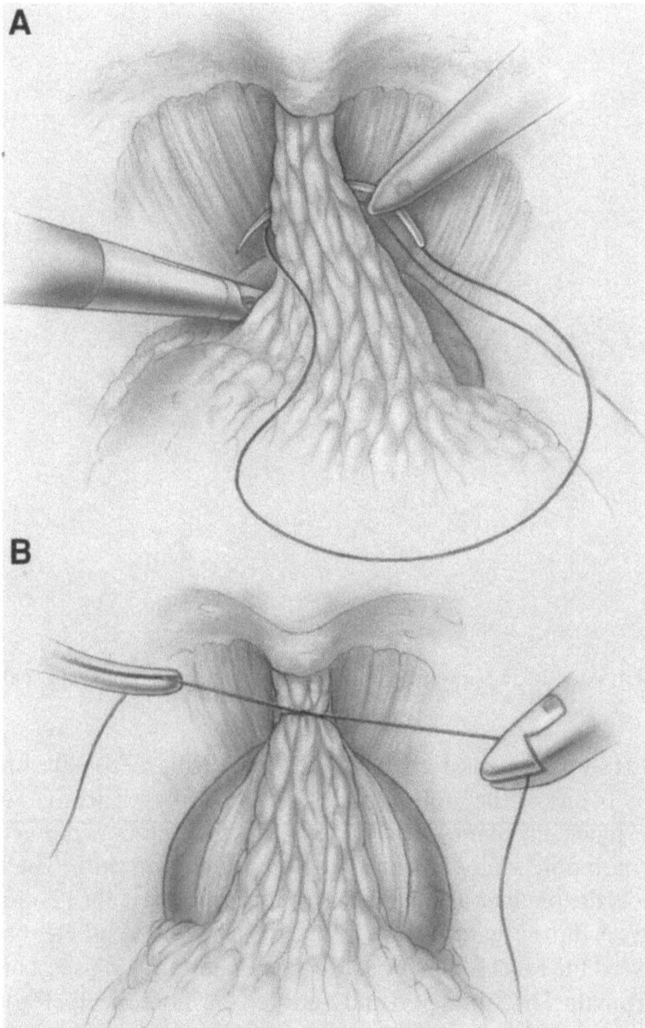


**Fig. 4.** Ligation of the dorsal vein complex.

a CT-1 needle. The needle is slightly straightened and passed through the right 12-mm port using a laparoscopic needle driver. A laparoscopic grasper is used from the left 12-mm port site. The assistant uses a 5-mm irrigator-aspirator through the right 5-mm port for retraction. Using the 0-Vicryl, the dorsal vein complex is ligated with a figure-of-8 suture passed anterior to the urethra and posterior to this deep venous dorsal complex (Fig. 4). The suture is tied intracorporeally and the dorsal vein complex is secured but not divided at this point.

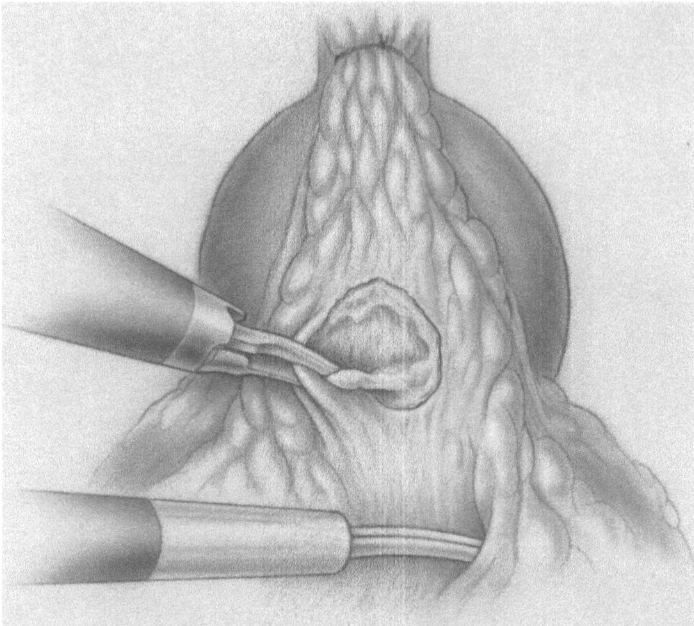

**Fig. 5.** Division of the anterior bladder neck using the harmonic scalpel.

The next step involves division of the prostatic base from the bladder neck. This is one of the more difficult portions of the LRP. However, with experience, the plane is easily visualized. The authors prefer to use a curved harmonic scalpel for this portion of the procedure. The assistant retracts the bladder using a fan retractor from the right 12-mm port and using a 5-mm irrigator-aspirator outlines the Foley catheter balloon down toward the level of the prostatic base. The surgeon uses a bipolar cautery from the left 5-mm port and a curved harmonic scalpel from the left 12-mm port to begin division of the prostatic base from the bladder neck (Fig. 5). The detrusor fibers are often seen at this point and the prostatic base is developed anteriorly. The bladder is entered and the Foley catheter is identified. The balloon is deflated and the assistant retracts the Foley catheter cephalad using a grasper from the right 5-mm port site. The posterior bladder mucosa is scored with the harmonic scalpel, and this is carried through the posterior surface of the prostate (Fig. 6). The seminal vesicles and accompanying vas deferens, which have been dissected posteriorly, are now brought anteriorly and grasped by the assistant using the laparoscopic 5-mm grasper.

The next sequence of maneuvers is determined by the decision to perform a nerve-sparing approach. If a nerve-sparing approach is

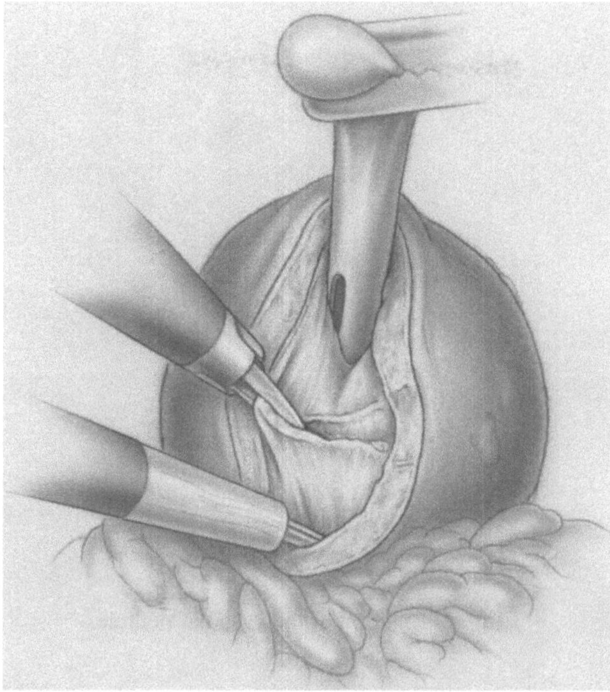

**Fig. 6.** Division of the posterior bladder mucosa.

attempted, a right-angled dissector can be utilized through the right 12-mm port site to free the neurovascular bundle on the lateral surface of the prostate. Apically, the neurovascular bundle can be sharply dissected from the apex of the prostate prior to division of the dorsal venous complex and at the base, the neurovascular bundle can be dissected free with a combination of right-angle dissection and laparoscopic scissors. With the assistant lifting the seminal vesicle anteriorly, the vascular pedicle can be divided using the harmonic scalpel. Sharp dissection can be used to free the remaining reflection of endopelvic fascia off the lateral surface of the prostate. The rectum is gently pushed posteriorly while working toward the apex of the prostate. A rectal bougie can be utilized to identify the rectum if necessary. Small perforating blood vessels may be encountered and are best left alone.

If a non-nerve-sparing approach is performed, the assistant grasps the seminal vesicle lifting anteriorly and the surgeon divides the entire vascular pedicle and neurovascular bundle with the harmonic scalpel working toward the apex of the prostate (Fig. 7). At this point, the prostate is attached posteriorly by the rectrourethralis muscle and the

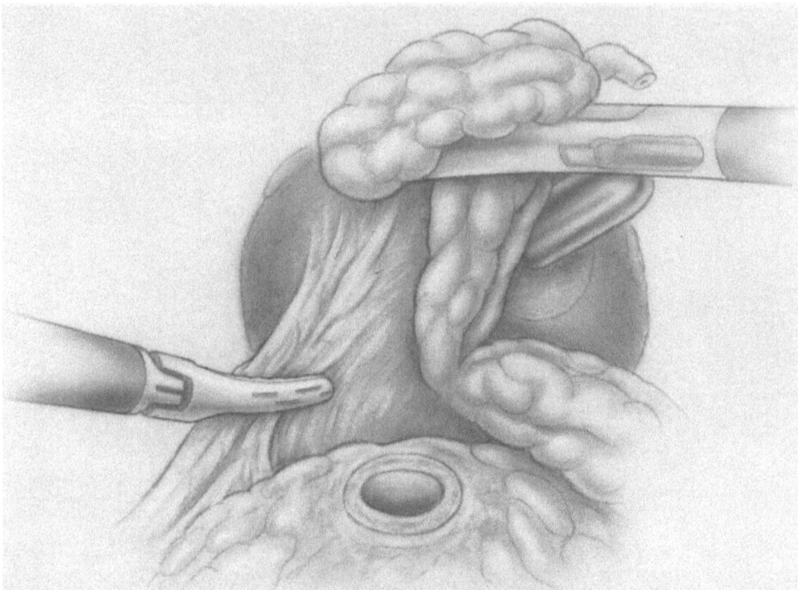

**Fig. 7.** Ligation of the vascular pedicle.

urethra. The dorsal vein complex is sharply incised, and the apical notch of the prostate developed. The anterior urethra is now sharply divided, exposing the catheter, which is gently retracted, and the posterior urethra is subsequently divided (Fig. 8). The assistant provides gentle cephalad retraction by grasping the base of the prostate in order to allow maximum exposure of the urethra. The rectrourethralis muscle is sharply incised with either the harmonic scalpel or scissors and the prostate can be rolled to both the left- and right-hand side to facilitate this maneuver. Once again, a rectal bougie can facilitate visualization of the rectum. The prostate with the accompanying seminal vesicles and vas deferens is now placed into the left lower quadrant, and the pelvis is copiously irrigated. Any bleeding is addressed with the bipolar cautery.

The rectal bougie is used to manipulate the rectum to inspect the anterior surface of the rectum, and if necessary a 20 French Foley catheter can be gently placed in the rectum and the pelvis filled with saline. Air is injected into the Foley catheter. If there is no evidence of leak, it can be assumed that there is no immediate rectal injury.

Next, the bladder neck is identified and the ureteral orifices are observed for efflux of urine. A urethral sound is placed. Urethral or bladder neck margins may be sent for frozen section if necessary. Once the ureteral orifices are identified, the ureterovesical anastomosis is

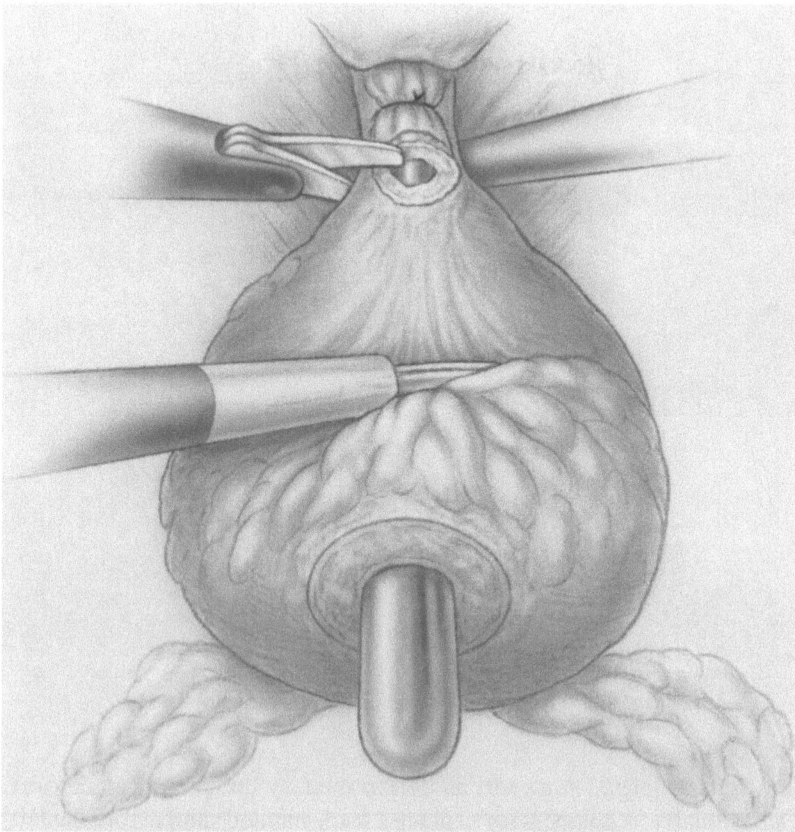

**Fig. 8.** Division of the anterior urethra.

begun (Fig. 9). Using a 2/0-Vicryl on a UR-6 needle through the right 12-mm port, the anastomosis is begun by placing a stitch through the posterior bladder neck from outside the bladder. The needle is grasped and using the right 12-mm port, the posterior stitch on the right side of the urethra is placed. Next, a second suture is introduced through the left 12-mm port, and in similar fashion, the posterior bladder neck is sutured outside-in followed by the posterior urethra inside-out. Thus, the knots are tied on the outside of the bladder (Fig. 9). The table is reflexed and the bladder is reapproximated to the urethra. The assistant may facilitate this maneuver by grasping the posterior bladder from the right side and holding it in place while the sutures are tied intracorporeally. At this point, the remaining portion of the anastomosis is completed. Using the 2/0-Vicryl suture, the sutures are placed circumferentially from either

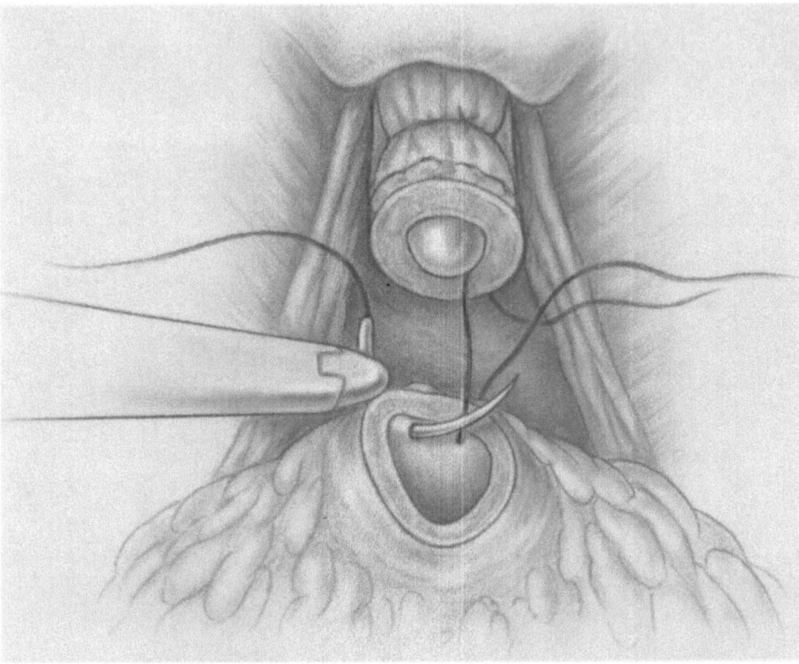

**Fig. 9.** Completing the ureterovesical anastomosis.

the right or left 12-mm port as determined by the patient's anatomy. Occasionally, it is necessary to place a back-handed suture from the left-sided 12-mm port.

If necessary, bladder neck reconstruction can be performed anteriorly using a 2/0-Vicryl on a UR-6 needle, the bladder neck can be reconstructed by placing a suture through the anterior portion of the bladder neck in interrupted fashion. The sutures are tied intracorporeally. The remaining anterior sutures can be placed. A new 20 French Foley catheter is placed under direct visualization prior to completing the anastomosis and the final anterior sutures are tied intracorporeally. The bladder is tested by instilling 60 cc of saline, and if a leak is detected another suture can be placed. Generally seven to eight sutures are used for the ureterovesical anastomosis. Next, the right 5-mm port site incision is extended to accompany a 10-mm Endocatch device (Tyco, Inc. Norwalk, CT). Once the endocatch is deployed, the accompanying needles and prostate with accompanying seminal vesicles and vas deference are delivered into the bag. The bag is closed and brought through the right 5-mm port site. The external oblique fascia and muscle are incised with electrocautery and the bag removed. This small incision is closed using a two-layer technique of 0 Vicryl for the muscle followed by the oblique fascia. The abdomen is reinsufflated, and then a Jackson Pratt drain is placed through the left 5-mm port. It is secured in place with a 3/0 Nylon suture. The remaining port sites are closed in standard fashion using 0-Vicryl. The authors prefer to use a Carter-Thomason (Inlet Medical, MN) instrument. All wounds are copiously irrigated and a 4/0 Monocryl is used for the skin. The Foley catheter is left to gravity drainage and the Jackson-Pratt drain left to bulb suction.

The extraperitoneal technique has also been described for LRP *(8,9)*. Results appear to be equivalent to the transperitoneal route. Bollens et al. described 42 such procedures with an operative time of 317. Although operative time is long, potential advantages include potentially less risk of intraperitoneal organ injury, complications of urinary extravasation, and possibly less complications from subsequent radiotherapy. Disadvantages are related to less working space and perhaps longer operative times.

## OPERATIVE RESULTS

### *Operative Time*

When assessing the efficacy and feasibility of the LRP, operative data must be compared with the gold standard retropubic and perineal RP approaches. Operative times for the retropubic and perineal RP are routinely under 3 h. Mean operative time in the first reported series of LRPs was 9.4 h *(3)*. Guillonneau et al. reported a mean operative time of 270 min in their initial 40 procedures and Abbou et al. reported similar results *(5,10)*. More recently, the operative time has dropped to 170 min for the last 350 patients in Guillonneau's series *(11)*. Similarly, Turk et al. reported a reduction to 200 min in their last 40 patients *(12)*. Interestingly, Menon has adopted a robotically assisted LRP and compared this approach to his first 40 LRPs. There was no statistically significant difference in mean operative time (258 min for the laparoscopic vs 274 min for the robot assisted; $p = 0.40$) *(13)*. It is clear that as the learning curve for the LRP is achieved, operative times become comparable to their open counterpart. However, it is the learning curve that seems to be one of the most challenging aspects of this operation and perhaps one of its limiting steps to widespread acceptance. At least 30 to 50 procedures are necessary to achieve surgical proficiency. Mentor-initiated programs may reduce this learning curve substantially. We found no statistically significant difference between the trainee and mentor's operative times when the mentor's first 12 cases were compared to the trainee's subsequent 18 cases *(14)*.

### *Blood Loss*

Historically, RP has been associated with significant blood loss often requiring transfusion and contributing to the morbidity of the procedure. Before 1988, RP was associated with median estimated blood loss (EBL) in the range of 1500 cc *(15,16)*. Recent series have reported EBL in the ranges of 530 cc up to 1500 cc *(15–17)*. In Lepor's recent review of complications in 1000 cases, 9.7% required allogenic transfusion *(18)*. Many centers routinely bank autologous blood prior to surgery, which has been shown to decrease allogenic transfusion to less than 10% *(19)*.

LRP performed in centers of excellence has reduced blood loss significantly. Guillonneau et al. reported a mean EBL of 240 cc in the last 140 patients *(20)*. In a recent review of their last 550 cases, the transfusion rate was 5.27 % (a majority occurring early in their series). Similar results have been noted by Abbou et al. *(21)*. Our mean EBL is 175 cc after 70 cases. We have transfused one patient in our series, and only perform a type and screen preoperatively. Clearly, one of the benefits of the laparoscopic approach is the reduction in blood loss, which may reduce postoperative recovery. The pneumoperitoneum prevents the "venous leak" from smaller branches. Bipolar cautery and the harmonic scalpel may further contribute to a reduction in blood loss. Finally, the dorsal vein is ligated initially, but not divided until late in the procedure, which may create a stable thrombus thus reducing blood loss.

## ONCOLOGICAL RESULTS

At the time of this writing, LRP is still considered a novel technique. Long-term results are lacking, however, preliminary results are encouraging (Table 1). Before reviewing the most recent series, it is important to review the largest open series to date with respect to margin rates, recurrence, and progression. Han et al. recently reviewed Dr. Walsh's followup results for a cohort of 2494 men who underwent a retropubic RP at Johns Hopkins *(1)*. Of the 2404 men with followup, 17% had a recurrence of the disease after retropubic RP. The mean followup was 6.3 yr (range 1–17 yr). An isolated PSA was the only evidence of recurrence in 9.7%, 1.7% recurred locally without distant metastasis, and 5.8% had distant metastasis *(1)*. Finally, Kaplan-Meier analysis showed overall actuarial 5-, 10-, and 15-yr freedom from any type of recurrence of 84%, 74%, and 66%, respectively *(1)*. Moreover, their series as well as others demonstrated that recurrence is higher in those patients with advance clinical stage, Gleason score (especially 4 +3, and 8 to 10),

**Table 1**
**LRP Positive Margin Rates—Largest Series**

| | *Guillonneau et al. (11)* | *Turk et al. (12)* | *Rassweiler et al. (24)* | *Hoznek et al. (21)* | *Menon et al. (13)* |
|---|---|---|---|---|---|
| No. patients | 550 | 125 | 180 | 200 | 98 |
| | Positive Margin(%) | | | | |
| pT2a | 3.3% | 15.2% (incl. all pT2) | 2.3% (incl. all pT2) | 16.8% (incl. all pT2) | N/A |
| pT2b | 15% | | | | |
| pT3a | 33% | 38% | 15% | 48.8% (incl all pT3) | |
| pT3b | 47% | | 34% | | |
| Overall | | 26.4% | 16% | | 21% |

LRP = laparoscopic radical prostatectomy.

preoperative PSA, and pathological stage. Finally, positive margin rates for RP have declined since the late 1980s *(22)*. Rates as high as 41% were reported by centers of excellence in the early 1980s, which declined to 16% in the mid-1990s *(22)*. Epstein reported that during a 1 yr period (1994–1995) at Johns Hopkins, the positive margin rate fell to 8% in patients with T1C disease *(22)*. More recently, the overall positive margin rate for a single surgeon at Hopkins was 5.8%. These reductions are the product of tireless modifications and improvement in surgical technique.

Guillonneau and Vallancien reported on their results in 550 cases *(11)*. The positive margin rates in that series were 3.3% for pT2a, 15% for pT2b, 33% for pT3a, and 47% for pT3b (Table 1) *(11)*. When stratified by pathological stage, these results are certainly in line with other reported series. Guillonneau's series began in 1998 and mean followup is simply too short to draw any conclusions regarding the probability of recurrence, however, in an earlier series, 6% of patients with pT2 disease had a PSA above 0.1 ng/mL with a mean followup of 4.8 mo (range 1–18 mo) *(23)*. Abbou et al. reported on their series of 200 patients and found a 16.8% positive margin rate for patients with pT2 and 48.8% for pT3 disease. In that series, 89.6% of patients had a serum PSA below 0.1 ng/mL after a mean followup of 11 mo *(21)*. Rassweiler et al. had a 16% overall positive margin rate in their series of LRP *(24)*. There was a 2.3% positive margin rate for pT2 disease and 15% for patients with pT3 disease. Menon et al. utilized a novel technique of robotic-assisted LRP and report an overall 25% positive margin rate for the standard LRP and 17.5% overall positive margin rate for the robotic-assisted LRP *(13)*. Finally, we report similar results in our series of 70 patients. We note a 13% positive margin rate for pT2 disease and 45% for patients with pT3 disease *(14)*. Certainly, all of these results are comparable to open series reported on by Blute et al. and Soloway et al., respectively *(25,26)*. Soloway et al. reported an overall positive margin rate of 28% *(26)*. When comparing patients with pT2 disease, Blute's earlier series noted a 26% positive margin rate for pT2 *(25)*. When evaluating the 2518 patients in their open series, Blute et al. noted a 39% overall positive margin rate *(25)*. Variability in any surgeon's patient population may account for differences in positive margin rates as demonstrated by the examples described here. It is reasonable to note that the early laparoscopic series are at least comparable to most large open and perineal series. Finally, biochemical disease-free progression rates will be important to determine the efficacy of this procedure. Short-term data are similar to open series, but it is too early to make any meaningful statement regarding biochemical disease-free progression.

## PERIOPERATIVE OUTCOMES

### *Complications*

Intraoperative complication rates for the LRP and open/perineal procedures are quite comparable. In Guillonneau et al's most recent series, open conversion occurred in 1.2% of patients (*n*=567) *(27)*. No complications occurred in 470 patients (82.9%) and mean blood loss was 350 cc. Persistent anastomotic leak occurred in 10% of patients, requiring average catheter times of 12 d. The following complications also occurred: ureteral injury (0.5%), rectal injury (1.4%), and bladder injury (1.6%). Re-operation rates were 3.7% *(27)*. Abbou et al. reported two rectal injuries in their first 200 patients, four lymphoceles and one fistula. However, complication rates were directly related to surgeon experience with a 22.5% complication rate in the first 40 patients and 3.2% in the remaining number *(21)*. All series report small numbers of deep venous thrombosis (0.3%). Intraoperative bleeding is significantly lower in the LRP. This is due in part to meticulous dissection/cauterization using bipolar forceps, excellent control of the dorsal venous complex, and the pneumoperitoneum, which decreases the venous loss often associated with the open counterpart. These complication rates compare favorably with Lepor's series of 1000 consecutive cases *(18)*.

Ruiz-Deya et al. reviewed their series of 250 perineal RPs with less than a 24-h admission *(28)*. The incidence of rectal perforation was less than 2%, anastomotic stricture was 3%, perineal fistula was 0.4%, and blood transfusion was 11%. Interestingly, bowel dysfunction (diarrhea, soiled undergarments, or constipation) developed in 17% of patients. Of patients, 7% had persistent bowel dysfunction (9 out of 124 patients) *(28)*. In our series (*n* = 70), we have had two rectal injuries *(14)*. A majority of these complications occur early in each authors' series.

### *Incontinence*

A factor that has been, until recently, quite neglected is the patient's quality-of-life assessment as it relates to the new procedure. Emphasis in the past has been directed at impressions delivered by the caregiver, physician, insurance plan, or hospital. Patient participation and opinions have been somewhat secondary. This has been partly the result of inadequate and poorly defined instruments for assessment. The issue of urinary function, bother, and sexual function are important. The authors have used the UCLA cancer index as validated and published by Litwin to gain quality-of-life information on a prospective and longitudinal basis among patients having standard open RP by the retropubic route and those having LRP *(29)*. Fifty patients from each group were operated on during the same period. Pretreatment assessment for baseline along with 3-, 6-, and 12-mo quality-of-life assessments were obtained. In order to take the learning curve of the LRP into consideration, the 50 LRP cases were divided into two cohorts: grouped 1–25, and 26–50. The results of urinary function and bother are noted in Table 2 at 0, 1, 3, 6, and 12 mo. The UCLA Prostate Cancer index is scored in two steps. First, the response for each item is recoded with a value from 1 to 100. Second, an average value is calculated for the items in the functional (i.e., leaking) scales as well as the bother scales. As anticipated, baseline function is not at 100% in these men whose median age is 62 yr. The return to baseline for the first 25 cases of LRP in our series is inferior to the open cases at the measured time points but is quite comparable at 6 mo for the second 25 cases. At 6 mo, 74% of the open RP patients returned to their function baseline compared with 72% of our LRP series. Similarly, 83% of the open and LRP patients returned to their baseline or preoperative "bother" scores.

Other larger series report continence in a variety of ways. Olsson et al. found that at 1, 3, 6, and 12 mo, perfect diurnal continence (no pads or leaking) was 9.9%, 28.6%, 57.4%, and 56.8%, respectively *(30)*. No pads were used in 78.4% of patients at 12 mo. Guillonneau et al. reported an 82.3% continence rate (defined as no pads) at 12 mo *(11)*. These results are comparable to other open series.

### *Potency*

Initially, potency rates in most series were poor. The nerve-sparing approach was performed infrequently. However, more recent series from Guillonneau et al. note an 85% "spontaneous erection" rate in 47 consecutive patients that underwent the nerve-sparing approach *(11)*. Mean followup is short (less than 6 mo). Open series report a wide range of potency rates from 18 to 86% depending on bilateral/unilateral approaches and age of the patient at the time of surgery *(15,30,31)*. Although too early to make an accurate assessment, it appears that in the larger series, preservation of erectile function is possible. Moreover, as the open series continued to improve with experience, the same comment can be made for the LRP.

## CONTROVERSIAL ISSUES AND SHORTCOMINGS

LRP remains one of the most challenging procedures for urologist to date. The learning curve is steep (50 cases). Initial criticism from the urological community includes longer operative time, margin status, sexual function, hospital stay, and overall cost. Does a new procedure

Table 2
Results of Urinary Function and Bother

| | Month | | | | |
|---|---|---|---|---|---|
| | *0* | *1* | *3* | *6* | *12* |
| RRP (50) | 89%[a] | 27% | 64% | 74% | 76% |
| LRP1 (25) | 88% | 9% | 53% | 59% | 56% |
| LRP2 (25) | 88% | 27% | 56% | 72% | N/A |

[a]Each box represents the percentage return to baseline.

need to be better in all aspects of intraoperative, perioperative, and postoperative parameters in order to be accepted? If a procedure offers distinctive advantages in some aspects and is equivalent in others, can it be included as a viable surgical option? The urological community will answer these questions with respect to the LRP in time. However, when one looks at the retropubic RP and perineal RP approaches, one approach is not distinctly better than the other in published reports. Each offers its own unique features, and both are accepted as viable approaches. At this point, the LRP provides improved visualization, less blood loss, comparable cancer control, comparable continence, shorter catheter dwell times, and comparable complication rates to the open and perineal approaches. Disadvantages include the learning curve, early potency rates, and cost related to longer operative times. Cost may eventually be offset in earlier return to daily activities; however, the data is currently immature. Potency rates are at least comparable to some contemporary open and perineal series as noted earlier in this chapter, but not at the point reported by some centers of excellence.

One of the distinct disadvantages is the lack of tactile feedback during the LRP. The bladder neck, apex of the prostate, and rectum cannot be adequately assessed during the LRP. Whether this will affect operative results remains to be seen. The nerve-sparing approach is more difficult during the LRP. This may be a result of the poor tactile feedback or lack of precise instrumentation available to perform maneuvers necessary to preserve the nerves safely. Once again, long-term results and continued modifications will be necessary to resolve these issues.

The LRP is still in its infancy when compared to the open counterpart. The future of this procedure will be determined by long-term operative and postoperative results. Detailed assessments and prospective, randomized trials will help determine its place in the surgical armamentarium for adenocarcinoma of the prostate.

## REFERENCES

1. Han M, Partin AW, Pound CR, et al. Long-Term biochemical disease-free and cancer-specific survival following anatomic radical retropubic prostatectomy. Urol Clin N Am 2001; 28: 555–565.
2. Catalona WJ, Smith DS. Cancer recurrence and survival rates after anatomic radical retropubic prostatectomy for prostate cancer. J Urol 1998; 160: 2428–2434.
3. Schuessler WW, Schulam PG, Clayman RV, et al. Laparoscopic radical prostatectomy: initial short term experience. Urology 1997; 50: 854–857.
4. Guillonneau B, Vallancien G. Laparoscopic radical prostatectomy: The Montsouris Technique. J Urol 2000; 163: 1643–1649.
5. Abbou CC, Salomon L, Hoznek P, et al. Laparoscopic radical prostatectomy: Preliminary results. Urology 55(5): 630–634.
6. Rosenblum N, Lepor H. Radical Retropubic Prostatectomy. Urol Clin N Am 2001; 28(3): 499–507.
7. Sokoloff MH, Brendler CB. Indications and Contraindications for nerve-sparing radical prostatectomy. Urol Clin N Am 2001; 28(3): 535–543.
8. Stolzenburg JU, Do M, Pfeiffer H, et al. The endoscopic extraperitoneal radical prostatectomy (EERPE): technique and initial experience. World J Urol 2002; 20(1): 48–55.
9. Bollens R, Vanden Bossche M, Roumeguere, Th, et al. Extraperitoneal Laparoscopic Radical Prostatectomy. Eur Urol 2001; 40: 65–69.
10. Guillonneau B, Cathelineau X, Barret E, et al. Laparoscopic radical prostatectomy: Technical and oncological assessment of 40 operations. Eur Urol 1999; 36: 14–20.
11. Guillonneau B, Cathelineau X, Doublet J, et al. Laparoscopic radical prostatectomy: assessment after 550 procedures. Crit Rev Oncol Hematol 2002; 43(2): 123.
12. Turk I, Deger S, Winkelmann B, et al. Laparoscopic radical prostatectomy: technical aspects after experience with 125 cases. Eur Urol 2001; 40: 46–53.
13. Menon M, Shrivastava A, Tewari A, et al. Laparoscopic and robot assisted radical prostatectomy: Establishment of a structured program and preliminary analysis of outcomes. J Urol 2002; 168: 945–949.
14. Fabrizio MD, Turk I, Schellhammer PF. Laparoscopic radical prostatectomy: Reducing the learning curve using a mentor-initiated approach. J Urol 2002; 167 (Suppl 4) abstract 77.
15. Catalona WJ, Carvalhal GF, Mager DE, et al. Potency, continence and complication rates in 1870 consecutive radical prostactomies. J Urol 1999; 162: 433–438.
16. Zincke H, Bergstralh EJ, Blute MJ, et al. Radical prostatectomy for clinically localized prostate cancer: long term results of 1143 patients from a single institution. J Clin Oncol 1994; 12: 2254–2263.
17. Leandri P, Rossignol G, Gautier JR, et al. Radical retropubic prostatectomy: Morbidity and quality of life. Experience with 620 consecutive cases. J Urol 1992; 147: 883–887.
18. Lepor H, Nieder AM, Ferrandino MN. Introperative and postoperative complications of radical prostectomy in a consecutive series of 1000 cases. J Urol 2002; 166, 1729–1733.
19. Noldus J, Gonnermann D, Huland H. Autologous blood transfusion in radical prostatectomy: Results in 263 patients. Eur Urol 1995; 27: 213–217.
20. Guillonneau B, Cathelineau X, Doublet J, et al. Laparoscopic radical prostatectomy: the lessons learned. J. Endourol 2001; 15(4): 441–445.
21. Hoznek A, Salomon L, Olsson LE, et al. Laparoscopic radical prostatectomy: the Creteil experience. Eur Urol 2001; 40: 38–40.

22. Epstein JI. Pathologic assessment of the surgical specimen: Urol Clin N Am 2001; 28(3): 567–594.
23. Guillonneau B, Rozet F, Barrett E, et al. Laparoscopic radical prostactomy: assessment after 240 procedures. Urol Clin N Am 2001; 28(1): 189–202.
24. Rassweiler J, Sentker L, Seeman O, et al. Laparoscopic radical prostactomy with Heilbronn Technique: an analysis of the first 180 cases. J Urol 2001; 166, 2101–2108.
25. Blute ML, Bergstralh EJ, Iocca A, et al. Use of Gleason score, prostate specific antigen, seminal vesicle and margin status to predict biochemical failure after radical prostactomy. J Urol 2001; 165, 119–125.
26. Sofer M, Hamiliton-Nelson KL, Civantos F, et al. Positive surgical margins after radical retropubic prostatectomy: the influence of site and number on progression. J Urol 2002; 167(6): 2453–2456.
27. Guillonneau B, Rozet F, Cathelineau X, et al. Perioperative complications of laparoscopic prostactomy: The Montsouris 3-year experience. J Urol 2002; 167, 51–56.
28. Ruiz-Deya G, Davis R, Srivastav S, et al. Outpatient radical prostatectomy: Impact of standard perineal approach on patient outcome. J Urol 2001; 166, 581–586.
29. Litwin MS, Pasta DJ, Yu J. Urinary function and bother after radical prostatectomy or radiation for prostate cancer: a longitudinal, multivariate quality of life analysis from the Cancer of the Prostate Strategic Urologic Reseach Endeavor. J Urol 2000; 164(6), 1973–1977.
30. Olsson LE, Nadu SL, Hoznek A. Prospective patient -reported continence after laparoscopic radical prostatectomy. Urology 2001; 58(4): 570–572.
31. Walsh P, Marschke P, Ricker D, et al. Patient-reported urinary continence and sexual function after anatomic radical prostatectomy. Urology 2000; 55: 58–61.
32. Koa T, Cruess D, Garner D, et al. Multicenter patient self-reporting questionnaire on impotence, incontinence and stricture after radical prostatectomy. J Urol 2000; 163: 858.

# VI Bladder Cancer

# 15 Laparoscopic Radical Cystectomy

*Sidney C. Abreu,* MD
*and Inderbir S. Gill,* MD, MCh

*Contents*

Introduction
Patient Selection
Preoperative Patient Assessment and Preparation
Patient Positioning and Port Placement
Laparoscopic Radical Cystectomy in a Male
Laparoscopic Radical Cystectomy in a Female
Pelvic Lymph Node Dissection
Urinary Diversion
Conclusion
References

## INTRODUCTION

Localized muscle-invasive bladder cancer is most commonly treated by radical surgical removal of the bladder *(1)*. However, radical cystectomy is indeed a major abdominal surgery with a lengthy hospital stay and protracted recovery period *(2)*. With the advances in laparoscopy technique, most ablative surgeries in urology can be performed using a minimally invasive approach. Laparoscopic radical cystectomy can potentially preclude the significant postoperative morbidity inherent to the open procedure.

From: *Laparoscopic Urologic Oncology*
Edited by: J. A. Cadeddu © Humana Press Inc., Totowa, NJ

## PATIENT SELECTION

The selection criteria for a laparoscopic radical cystectomy follow the same principles of any laparoscopic transperitoneal approach. Generally, acute intraperitoneal infectious process and uncontrolled coagulopathy represent a contraindication for the laparoscopic approach. It is safer to exclude patients with multiple previous abdominal surgeries. Prior abdominal surgeries do not represent an absolute contraindication for the laparoscopic approach, but extra care should be taken during initial trocar insertion. Lysis of adhesions may also be required. Cold cut scissors should be used to avoid unintended thermal damage to bowel segments. Obesity is not, in itself, a contraindication to the laparoscopic approach. However, difficulty may be encountered while working in the deep pelvis in a patient with a thicker abdominal wall.

## PREOPERATIVE PATIENT ASSESSMENT AND PREPARATION

The preoperative assessment for patients undergoing laparoscopic radical cystectomy is similar to that done for the open procedure. In brief, patients undergo a complete physical exam, routine blood tests (complete blood count, renal panel, alkaline phosphatase, liver function tests, and calcium); a radiographic workup is also performed if required. Regarding the preoperative preparation, it is started on the day prior to the surgery. Because a urinary diversion follows the bladder removal, mechanical preparation is performed using 4 liters of GoLytley. Neomycin and metronidazole are used for the chemical preparation. Broad-spectrum intravenous antibiotics and subcutaneous low-molecular-weight-heparin (2500 units) are given prior to surgery.

## PATIENT POSITIONING AND PORT PLACEMENT

The patient is placed in the supine, modified low lithotomy position with thighs abducted and arms adducted to the sides. All bone prominences are carefully padded and bilateral sequential compression devices are applied to both calfs. The operative table is placed in a 45 Trendelenburg position. A Foley catheter is placed in the bladder after the patient is prepped and draped.

The surgeon is situated on the left of the patient. The first assistant is on the right of the patient and the second assistant is positioned next to the surgeon *(3,4)*.

A six-port transperitoneal approach is used (Fig. 1). A primary 10-mm port is placed at the umbilicus for the 0° laparoscope. Four secondary

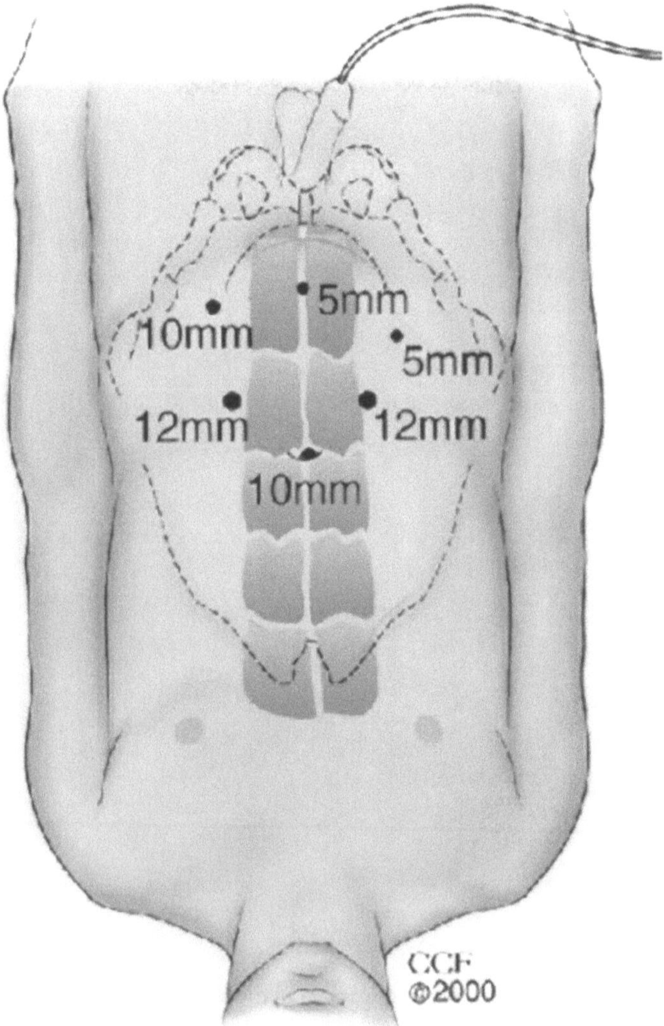


**Fig. 1.** Transperitoneal six-port approach (reprinted with permission, Cleveland Clinic Foundation).

ports are placed under visualization: a 12-mm port to the left of the umbilicus, lateral to the rectus muscle. A 10-mm and a 12-mm port are placed respectively in the left and right lower quadrants, approx 2 fingerbreadths to the ipsilateral anterior superior iliac spines. If an ileal conduit is the technique of choice for urinary diversion, another 12-mm port is placed at the preselected stoma site in the right rectus muscle. Otherwise, this 12-mm port is placed at the lateral border of the rectus

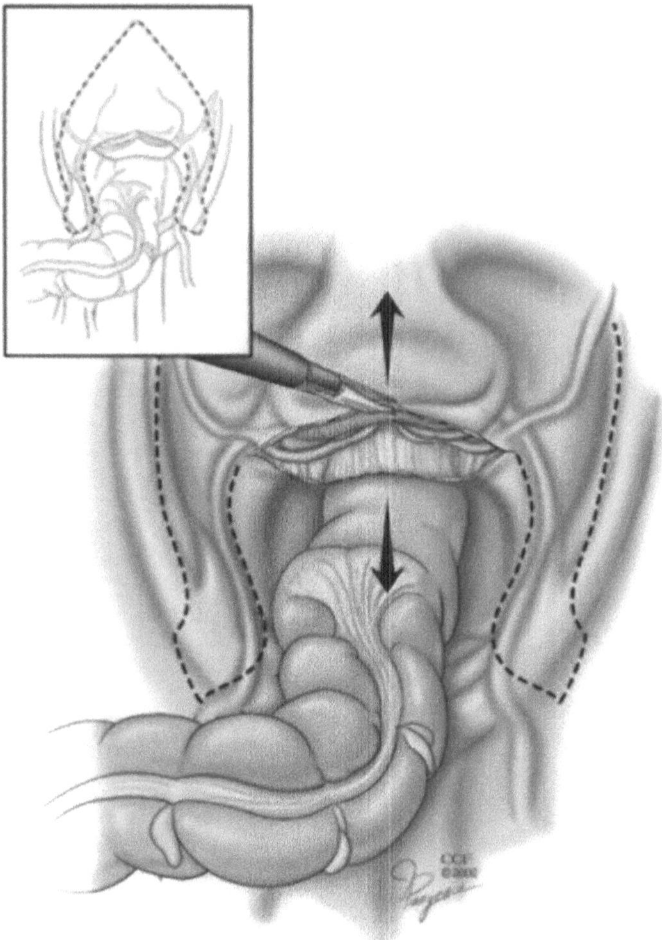

**Fig. 2.** Initial peritoneal incision is made in the rectovesical pouch. A plane is identified between the bladder and the rectum. Dashed line represents subsequent incision, laterally up to the common iliac. Inset represents extension of peritoneotomy onto the undersurface of the abdominal wall (reprinted with permission, Cleveland Clinic Foundation).

muscle approx 2 fingerbreadths caudal to the umbilicus. Finally, a 5-mm port is placed in the midline infra-umbilical location approx 2 fingerbreadths cephalad to the symphysis pubis *(3–8)*.

## LAPAROSCOPIC RADICAL CYSTECTOMY IN A MALE

The posterior peritoneal fold is incised posterior to the bladder in the rectovesical pouch and the pre-rectal plane is dissected (Fig. 2). The vasa deferentia are divided and dissection is continued along the posterior aspect of the seminal vesicles toward the bladder base. Denonvilliers fascia is incised and dissection along the anterior rectal surface is followed distally toward the apex of the prostate. On completion of the posterior dissection, the initial peritoneal incision is carried laterally on either side, up to the common iliac artery at the point of crossing of the ureter. Generous mobilization of the ureters is done bilaterally. Both ureters are mobilized down close to the bladder wall. Adequate mobilization of the left ureter is assured to allow subsequent tension-free retroperitoneal transfer to the right side for the ureteroileal anastomosis *(3,4)*.

The space of Retzius is entered by extending the peritoneal incisions onto the undersurface of the abdominal wall, extending lateral to the medial umbilical ligaments toward the umbilicus. The bladder is distended with 200 mL of saline and an inverted V incision is made in the anterior parietal peritoneum. The urachus is transected high, close to the umbilicus. The bladder is further mobilized from the abdominal wall and all the extraperitoneal perivesical fat is kept attached to the bladder *(3,4)*.

The lateral and posterior pedicles of the bladder are dissected (Fig. 3) with serial Endo-GIA firing (vascular 2.5-mm stapler, US Surgical, Norwalk, CT). Both ureters are clipped close to the bladder and divided. The distal ureteral margin is sent for frozen pathological examination. The endopelvic fascia is incised bilaterally and the dorsal venous complex is then controlled with either the Endo-GIA or by applying a suture *(3,4)*. The Foley catheter is removed and the urethra is transected using the Endoshears. The specimen is placed in a 15-mm Endocatch II bag (US Surgical, Norwalk, CT) for further extraction.

## LAPAROSCOPIC RADICAL CYSTECTOMY IN A FEMALE

In women, the uterus is retracted anteriorly, and the initial peritoneotomy is made in the rectovesical cul-de-sac. Further dissection is performed to develop a plane anterior to the rectum. The uterine broad ligaments and the vesical vascular pedicles are transected using Endo-GIA firing (vascular 2.5-mm stapler, US Surgical, Norwalk, CT). The urethra is sharply divided. The Foley catheter is delivered inside the abdominal cavity and used to retract the bladder cephalad. A sponge stick is inserted into the vagina to help with identification of the anterior vaginal wall and the subsequent plane of dissection *(9)*. The anterior vaginal wall is incised and the entire specimen along with uterus is extracted intact through the already open vaginal vault *(4,8,9)*. If an

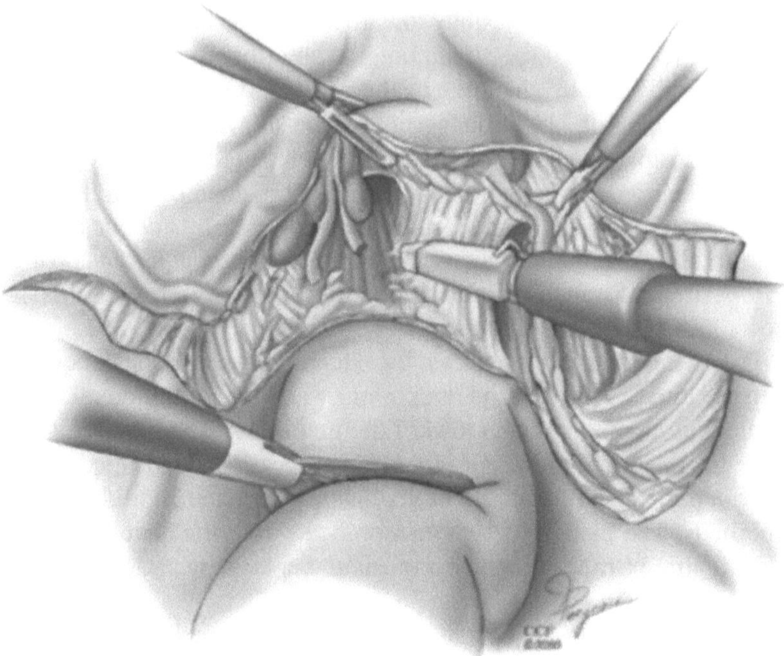

**Fig. 3.** Generous mobilization of the ureters is done. The lateral and posterior pedicles are secured with an Endo-GIA stapler (reprinted with permission, Cleveland Clinic Foundation).

orthotopic urinary diversion is not under consideration, the entire urethra is removed *en bloc* with the native bladder. Transverse closure of the vaginal wall defect is accomplished through the abdominal cavity with two running sutures *(8,9)*.

## PELVIC LYMPH NODE DISSECTION

Duplicating the open surgical principles, bilateral extended pelvic lymphadenectomy is performed including lymphatic tissue from the pubic bone distally to the bifurcation of the common iliac artery proximally *(7,9)*. The genitofemoral nerve laterally and the obturator nerve inferiorly are also landmarks for the pelvic lymph node dissection.

## URINARY DIVERSION

Laparoscopic continent and noncontinent techniques of urinary diversion have been performed clinically successfully. To date, ileal conduit, rectal sigmoid pouch, and orthotopic neobladder (Fig. 4) can be

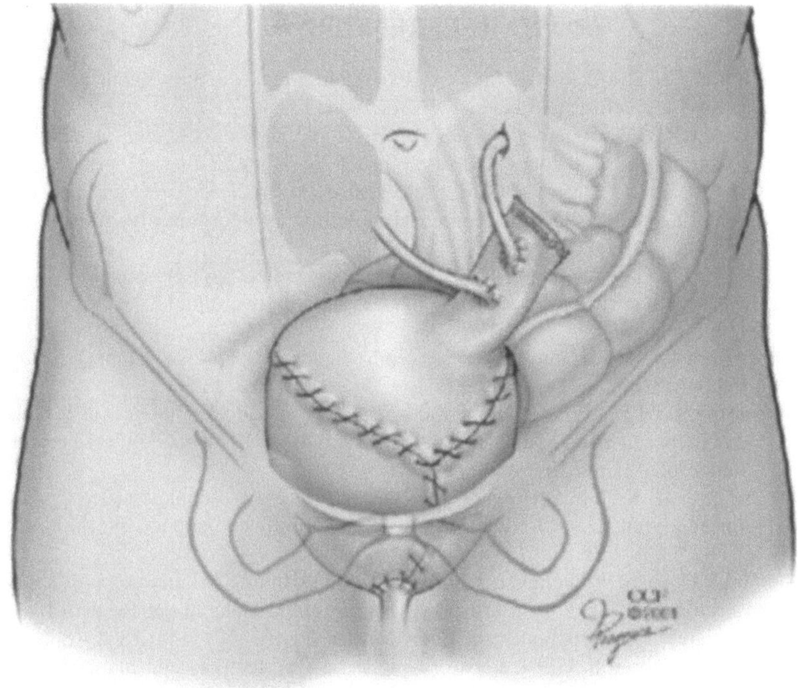

**Fig. 4.** Orthotopic neobladder urinary diversion following radical cystectomy. The entire procedure was performed completely intracorporeally (reprinted with permission, Cleveland Clinic Foundation).

constructed completely intracorporeally, using laparoscopic free-hand suturing exclusively *(3,4,8)*. Therefore, not only the ablative procedure (radical cystectomy), but also the reconstructive steps of the urinary diversion can be achieved by a minimally invasive approach.

## CONCLUSION

Laparoscopic radical cystectomy is an attractive treatment option for selected patients with localized muscle-invasive bladder cancer. It is indeed an advanced procedure; thus, should be attempted only by an experienced team *(3–9)*. Based on the significant morbidity of the open approach to radical cystectomy, the potential benefits from the laparoscopic approach should be considered. As in any surgical procedure, the established oncological principles must be followed. Critical evaluation of long-term surgical outcomes and comparison to standard open surgical techniques are essential.

## REFERENCES

1. Montie JE, Straffron RA, Stewart BH. Radical cystectomy without radiation therapy for carcinoma of bladder. J Urol 1984; 131: 477.
2. Bracken RB, McDonald MW, Johnson DE. Complications of single stage radical cystectomy and ileal conduit. Urology 1981; 28: 495–450.
3. Gill IS, Kaouk JH, Meraney AM, et al Laparoscopic radical cystectomy and continent ileal neobladder performed completely intracorporeally—the initial experience. J Urol 2002; 168(1): 13–18.
4. Gill IS, Fergany A, Klein EA, et al. Laparoscopic radical cystoprostatectomy with ileal conduit performed completely intracorporeally: the initial 2 cases. Urology 2000; 56: 26–30.
5. Kozminski M, Partamian K. Case report of laparoscopic ileal loop conduit. J Endourol 1992; 6: 147.
6. Sanchez de Badajoz E, Gallego Perales JL, Reche Rosado A, Gutierrez de la Cruz JM, Jimenez Garrido A. Laparoscopic cystectomy and ileal conduit: case report. J Endourol 1995; 9: 59–62.
7. Denewer A, Kotb S, Hussein O, El-Maadawy M. Laparoscopic assisted cystectomy and lymphadenectomy for bladder cancer: initial experience. World J Surg 1999; 23: 608–611.
8. Turk I, Deger S, Winkelmann B, Schonberger B, Loening SA. Laparoscopic radical cystectomy with continent urinary diversion (rectal sigmoid pouch) performed completely intracorporeally: the initial 5 cases. J Urol 2001; 165: 1863–1866.
9. Kaouk J, Abreu S, Gill I. Laparoscopic radical cystectomy and intracorporeal construction of orthotopic ileal neobladder in a female patient. J Endourol 2002; 16(Suppl 2) A210.

# 16 Laparoscopic Urinary Diversion

*James Borin,* MD *and Stephen J. Savage,* MD

*CONTENTS*

INTRODUCTION
INDICATIONS
CONTRAINDICATIONS
SURGICAL TECHNIQUE
RESULTS
CONTROVERSIAL ISSUES
SHORTCOMINGS OF LAPAROSCOPIC TECHNIQUE
SUMMARY
REFERENCES

## INTRODUCTION

Laparoscopic urologic oncology has progressed from simple, or essentially ablative procedures, to increasingly complex reconstructive procedures. Urinary diversion comprises what many urologists view as the most demanding reconstructive surgery. Herein, we describe the most recent progress in laparoscopic urinary diversion.

## INDICATIONS

The indications for laparoscopic urinary diversion are identical to those for open urinary diversion, including reconstruction after exenterative surgery of pelvic tumors, and palliation of advanced malignancy to alleviate severe urinary symptoms, obstruction, or fistula(e). However, when discussing the laparoscopic approach to urological disease, one must not only consider the indications for the

From: *Laparoscopic Urologic Oncology*
Edited by: J. A. Cadeddu © Humana Press Inc., Totowa, NJ

surgery, but also the risks and benefits of the laparoscopic approach over the open approach.

The first urological laparoscopic urinary diversion was performed in 1992 *(1)*, but subsequent experience has been limited until recently. As a result, one must discuss theoretical advantages that are merely partially substantiated in case reports and small retrospective reviews. Only increasing experience will allow more definitive statements on relative indications for the laparoscopic approach.

The well-established benefits of laparoscopic surgery include quicker recovery, decreased analgesic requirements, and better cosmesis *(2,3)*. Urinary diversion is typically performed on nutritionally depleted patients who often have prolonged recovery times *(4)*. As a result, the concept of reducing surgical stress and resultant perioperative morbidity via laparoscopy is increasingly attractive. Furthermore, those patients with malignancies that require urinary diversion are typically older patients who have a higher, although acceptable, rate of morbidity following radical cystectomy and urinary diversion *(5)*. These patients have already been shown to benefit from the laparoscopic approach to other malignant diseases *(6,7)*.

Interestingly, a 51% complication rate has been shown, 26% of the time, to be due to underlying medical illness. Many of these complications are cardiovascular in nature, and can potentially be attributed to the difficulty in managing such patients in the settings of the large fluid shifts that are known to occur after lengthy, open intra-abdominal procedures *(8)*. Laparoscopic urinary diversion often maintains a closed (or mostly closed) abdomen with minimal insensible losses and resultant decreased postoperative fluid shifts.

Similarly, many patients who require urinary diversion, both palliative and after cystectomy, will require some type of systemic therapy. Often, this cannot be provided until the patient recovers fully from the surgical intervention. It has been shown previously that patients are able to proceed to therapy more quickly after laparoscopic surgery *(9)*. Although this has not been definitively demonstrated following laparoscopic urinary diversion, it is clearly a plausible hypothesis.

## CONTRAINDICATIONS

As experience with laparoscopic surgery increases, absolute contraindications often become relative ones, and relative contraindications lead less often to an open surgical procedure. In general, contraindications for laparoscopic urinary diversion are the same as for other intraperitoneal procedures. In contrast to other urological laparoscopic procedures, urinary diversion typically requires a transperitoneal approach. As a result, one must consider the effect that previous treatments may have on the operative field.

Previous abdominal, and even pelvic, surgery is not, by itself, a contraindication to laparoscopic urinary diversion. Safe entry into the peritoneal cavity is of first importance, but a secondary consideration is the lysis of the many adhesions needed to approach the portion of the genitourinary tract to be diverted, as well as to mobilize the appropriate intestinal segment. Similarly, effects from prior irradiation may make surgical dissection considerably more complicated. Although the presence of adequate surgical planes aids laparoscopic surgery greatly, experience will gradually allow for more difficult dissections.

Obesity is another relative contraindication to laparoscopic urinary diversion. This is essentially due to two factors. First, the thickness of the abdominal wall makes the appropriate diversion more difficult, both in terms of creating a possible stoma, and in relation to the possible use of extracorporeal bowel anastomoses. Second, large amounts of intra-abdominal contents often need to be safely retracted to enter the retroperitoneum and mobilize the ureters. This, in turn, typically requires a greater amount of Trendelenburg, which can result in elevated peak insufflation pressures, and upper body edema.

Although the benefits of laparoscopy can be relatively greater in patients with significant comorbidities, one must be wary of systemic effects specific to $CO_2$ pneumoperitoneum, as well as the often slightly longer operative times that result from laparoscopy. The most common effects seen are related either to hemodynamic or pulmonary parameters, although some other less common effects have also been documented.

$CO_2$ pneumoperitoneum has been experimentally demonstrated to cause an increase in mean arterial pressure, pulmonary arterial wedge pressure, and partial $CO_2$ pressure. At the same time, cardiac output and arterial pH are significantly decreased *(10)*. Thus, patients with significant cardiac dysfunction and/or chronic obstructive pulmonary disease that result in baseline $CO_2$ retention may have difficulty tolerating laparoscopic urinary diversion. Once again, this is a relative contraindication, and with proper monitoring, these patients can often complete the laparoscopic diversion safely. Additionally, the surgeon should have a low threshold for elective open conversion in this setting.

Other scattered reports of possible sources of concern with laparoscopic surgery include transient elevation of hepatic function after pneumoperitoneum, thereby possibly excluding patients with severe liver dysfunction *(11)*. Experimentally, $CO_2$ pneumoperitoneum has had an adverse affect on patients with endotoxemia *(10)*. However, multiple clinical reports have demonstrated the feasibility of laparoscopy in the presence of sepsis, chiefly in patients with appendicitis or perforated duodenal ulcers *(12)*.

## SURGICAL TECHNIQUE

As with open surgical techniques, there is a seemingly infinite variety of approaches to laparoscopic urinary diversion. It is important to focus on a few basic concepts, which can then be adapted to personal preferences. The differences can essentially be defined as completely intracorporeal vs partially extracorporeal techniques, and continent vs noncontinent urinary diversion. Additionally, modifications with the ureterointestinal anastomosis are increasingly being described.

### *Port Placements*

Most laparoscopic urinary diversions will be performed after laparoscopic cystectomy, and, thus, those port sites (often five to six ports) will be used (Fig. 1). However, in the setting of nonorthotopic urinary diversion, the right para-median port site should be planned to coincide with the prelocalized stoma site. Although it is always recommended to place ports as orthogonally as possible, it is of even greater importance in this situation. If a urinary diversion without cystectomy is planned, the standard pelvic diamond configuration is satisfactory, with a supraumbilical port added as needed *(13)*.

### *Ureteral Mobilization*

In any diversion, one must take care to preserve an adequate length of ureter, as well as sufficient periureteral tissue. As with open surgery, the ascending and descending sigmoid colon must be reflected medially to access the retroperitoneum. The ureter can typically be identified either as it crosses the pelvic brim, or (in men) more distally next to the vas deferens. The advantage of laparoscopic urinary diversion over its open counterpart is that the ureter can be mobilized much closer to the bladder, thereby providing a greater amount of distal ureter. The ureter is subsequently clipped to allow for hydrodistention in preparation for subsequent ureterointestinal anastomosis while the ureteral margin is sent for frozen section analysis (Fig. 2). A stay suture in the ureter allows for facile traction during cephalad mobilization, as well as quick identification later in the procedure. Typically, the ureter should be mobilized until it can be brought to the contralateral abdominal wall (Fig. 3). This provides adequate length for subsequent intracorporeal or extra-

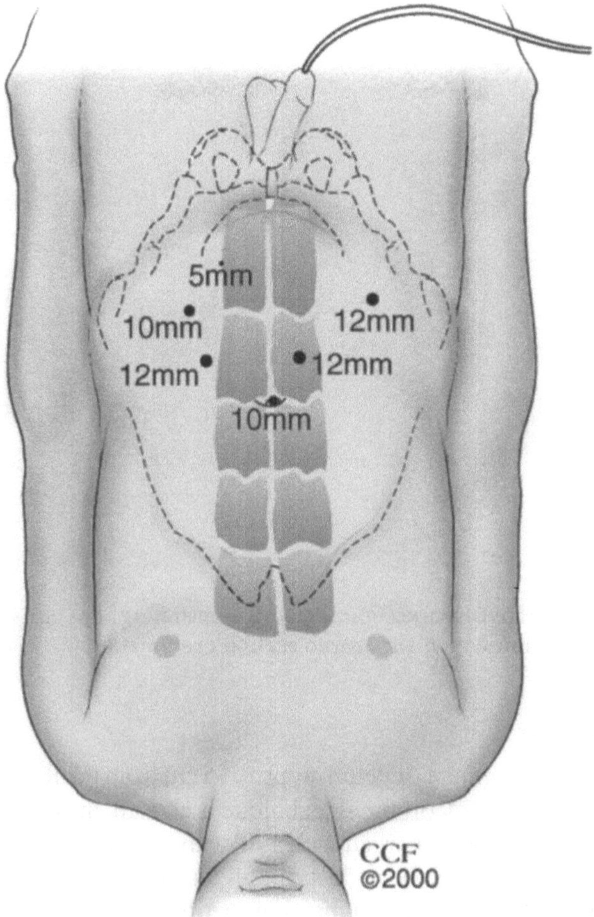


**Fig. 1.** Six-port configuration for laparoscopic cystectomy and urinary diversion. Note the right-sided 12-mm port, which is midrectus for future stoma site. (Courtesy of I. Gill, Cleveland Clinic Foundation.)

corporeal suturing. Finally, in the setting of a right-sided stoma (continent or noncontinent), the left ureter should be passed under the sigmoid mesentery (Fig. 4).

## *Diversion/Reservoir Formation*

### Ureterocutaneous Diversion

No further work is needed if a ureterocutaneous diversion is performed. A temporary single "J" stent can be placed after the ureter is brought out to the skin.

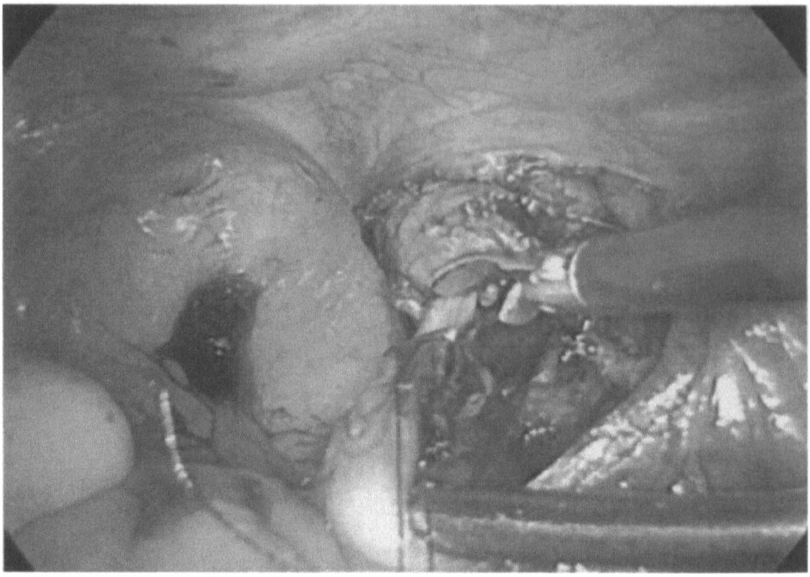

**Fig. 2.** Intraoperative laparoscopic image demonstrating clips on extreme distal ureter prior to transection and frozen section examination.

### Ileal Conduit

A 12–15 cm segment of ileum, approx 15 cm from the ileocecal valve is selected. If an extracorporeal technique is chosen, the distal aspect of the selected segment is marked with a silk stay suture. Once this is done, the ileum can either be brought through an extended port site (stoma site) or through the extraction incision (periumbilical). It is imperative to maintain the orientation of the bowel with appropriate atraumatic graspers so that the mesentery is not torsed. Once it is extracted, standard open techniques can be used to isolate the conduit segment.

If an intracorporeal technique is chosen, the isolated segment is marked at 12–15 cm using a paper ruler. The bowel is transected using the Endo-GIA stapler after dissection of a window in the mesentery. The mesentery can then be transected using either the Ligasure device (Valley Lab) or further firing of the Endo-GIA (Fig. 5). After appropriate orientation of the conduit is obtained, a side-to-side (functional end-to-end) anastomosis is obtained with two sequential firings of the Endo-GIA stapler (Fig. 6). The bowel can then be closed with either the Endo-GIA or a TA stapler. At all times, the surgical assistant must maintain a gentle, yet adequate, tension on the bowel during retraction. A stoma is subsequently formed in the standard fashion.

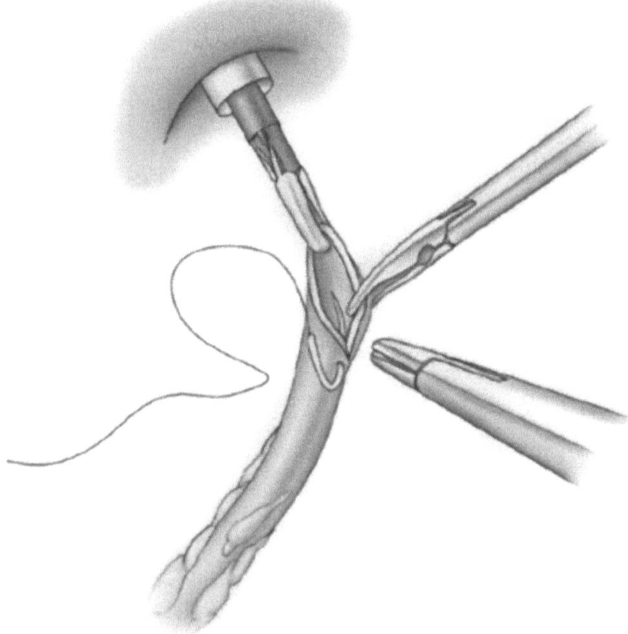

**Fig. 3.** Schematic demonstrating left ureter being brought across to contralateral abdominal wall to ensure adequate length prior to anastomosis. (Courtesy of I. Gill, Cleveland Clinic Foundation.)

## Continent Diversion

The most important aspect to laparoscopic continent urinary diversion is mobilization of the intestinal segment. If right colon is used, the entire hepatic flexure must be reflected so that the mesentery can easily reach the stoma site, and so that there is no tension on the ileocolonic anastomosis. Most frequently, extracorporeal techniques have been employed for pouch formation. However, free-hand suturing is clearly possible, mirroring what is accomplished during a laparoscopic orthotopic neobladder.

Another reported technique involves the creation of a rectal sigmoid pouch after radical cystectomy *(14)*. The antimesenteric border is incised for 10 cm in either direction from the rectosigmoid junction. The posterior walls of the rectum and sigmoid are opposed and sutured with a running absorbable suture. After the ureteral anastomosis is performed (discussed later) the anterior portion of the pouch is closed with a running suture.

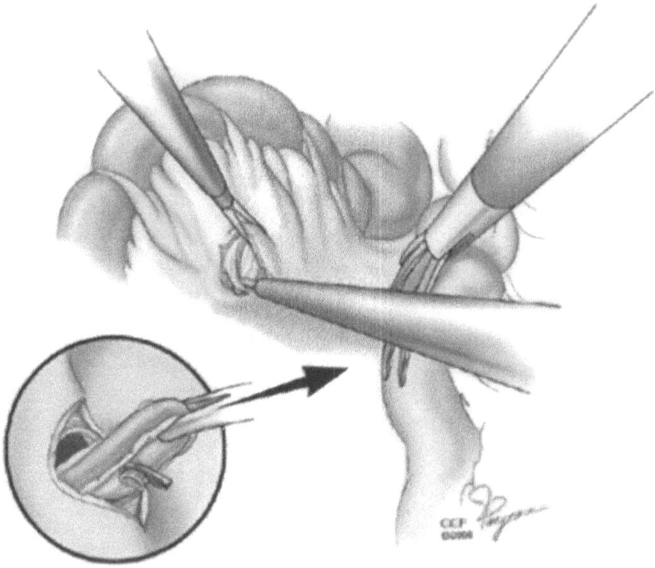

**Fig. 4.** Illustration demonstrating creation of window in sigmoid mesentery above sacral promontory. Inset demonstrates ureter being pulled through mesenteric window. (Courtesy of I. Gill, Cleveland Clinic Foundation.)

### Orthotopic Neobladder

The intestinal segment chosen for an orthotopic urinary diversion depends on surgeon preference. Just as with other laparoscopic urinary diversions, the orthotopic neobladder can be performed with or without some degree of extracorporeal surgery. In contrast to the other urinary diversions, a significant portion of the orthotopic neobladder requires laparoscopic reconstruction.

Gaboardi et al. *(15)* describe their technique of combined extracorporeal/intracorporeal orthotopic neobladder. They utilize a 5-cm supraumbilical extraction site to remove their cystectomy specimen, and exteriorize a 25-cm segment of ileum. After the segment is isolated using standard techniques, it is detubularized and the posterior portion of the U-plate is fashioned. The neobladder is replaced intracorporeally, and the posterior urethra is fixed to the neobladder. (It was noticed that this technique aided in the subsequent ureteral anastomosis.) After the ureters are attached, the anterior urethra is closed, followed by the anterior portion of the neobladder. Intracorporeal suturing is used for this portion of the operation.

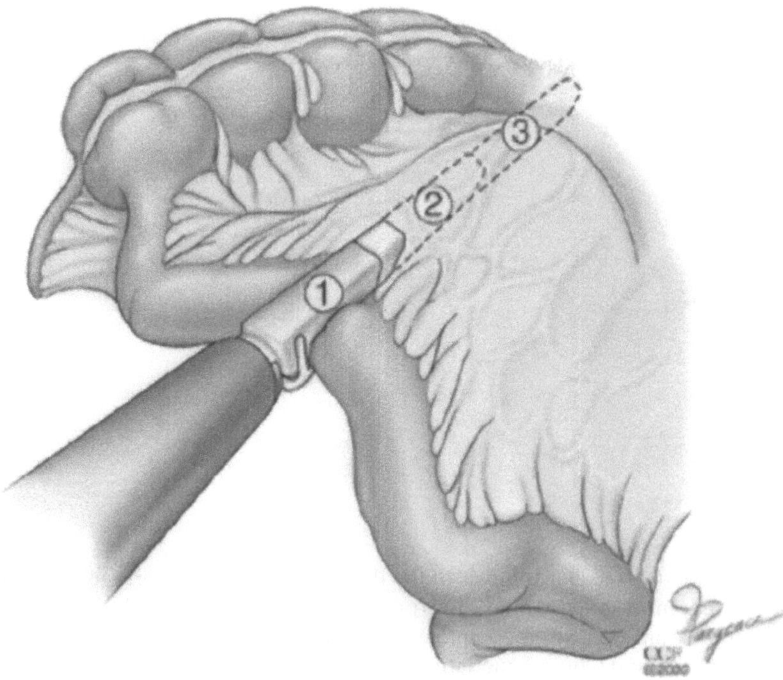


**Fig. 5.** Transection of mesentery of ileum to be used for conduit using sequential firings of Endo-GIA stapler. (Courtesy of I. Gill, Cleveland Clinic Foundation.)

Gill and colleagues *(16)* reported on their technique of intracorporeal creation of a Studer neobladder. To begin, in order to create the neobladder, the laparoscope is repositioned to the left lateral port, so that the surgeon is able to work through the midline infraumbilical and right pararectal ports[AM1]. A 65-cm segment of ileum, 15 cm from the ileocecal valve, is isolated in the usual fashion. The proximal 10 cm of ileum is maintained for the Studer limb, while the remaining 55 cm is detubularized along its antimesenteric border. The posterior plate is sutured and the Studer pouch is delivered to the pelvis. The laparoscope is placed once again at the umbilicus, and the most dependent portion of the posterior plate is selected as the site for urethroileal anastomosis. This is performed with two running sutures (Fig. 7), and a 22 French Foley catheter is inserted prior to completing the anterior portion of the anastomosis. The anterior portion of the neobladder is then closed with two running sutures after the Studer limb is prepared for the ureteral anastomosis.

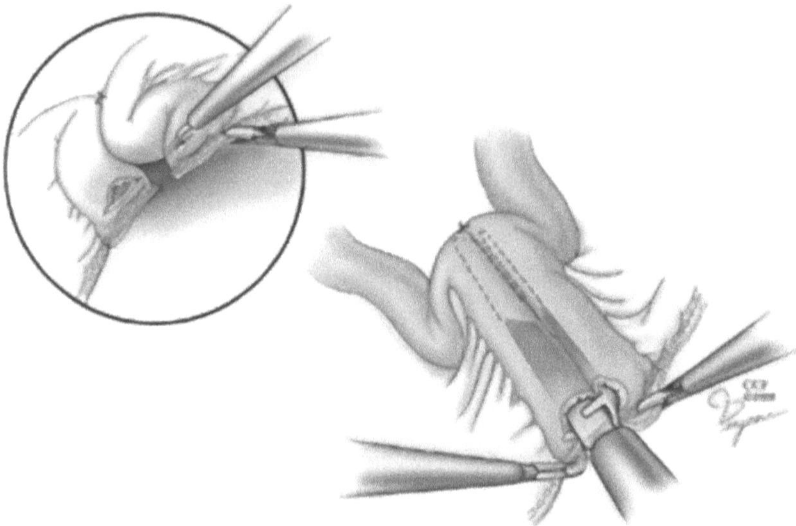

**Fig. 6.** Side-to-side anastomosis of the ileum performed similarly to the open procedure. Inset shows window into proximal and distal ends of the ileum, and side-to-side anastomosis is completed with the Endo-GIA stapler. (Courtesy of I. Gill, Cleveland Clinic Foundation.)

### *Ureterointestinal Anastomosis*

Once again, just as in open surgery, there are many options for performing the ureteral anastomosis. The majority of techniques simply duplicate open techniques using laparoscopic suturing. The most important point is to plan the time most appropriate for the placement of stents.

For ileal conduit formation, the stents are placed through the already formed stoma and through the enterotomy before the placement of anastomotic sutures *(13,17)*. After the posterior wall is sutured (Fig. 8), the stent is then advanced into the renal pelvis. Similar anastomotic techniques can be used in the Studer limb, although the stents are placed through stab incisions in the pouch prior to complete closure of the pouch *(16)* (Fig. 9). As an alternative, a nonrefluxing anastomosis can be created using an inverted nipple mechanism *(15)*.

The formation of a nonrefluxing anastomosis is facilitated through the use of a colonic segment for a continent urinary diversion. A 3-cm submucosal bed is created prior to placement of the ureters. A mucosa-to-mucosa anastomosis is then formed, the ureteral stents are placed, and the colonic mucosa is closed over the ureter, thereby creating a submucosal tunnel *(14)*. Just as in open surgery, care must be taken to mobilize mucosal flaps that can be closed over the ureter without tension.

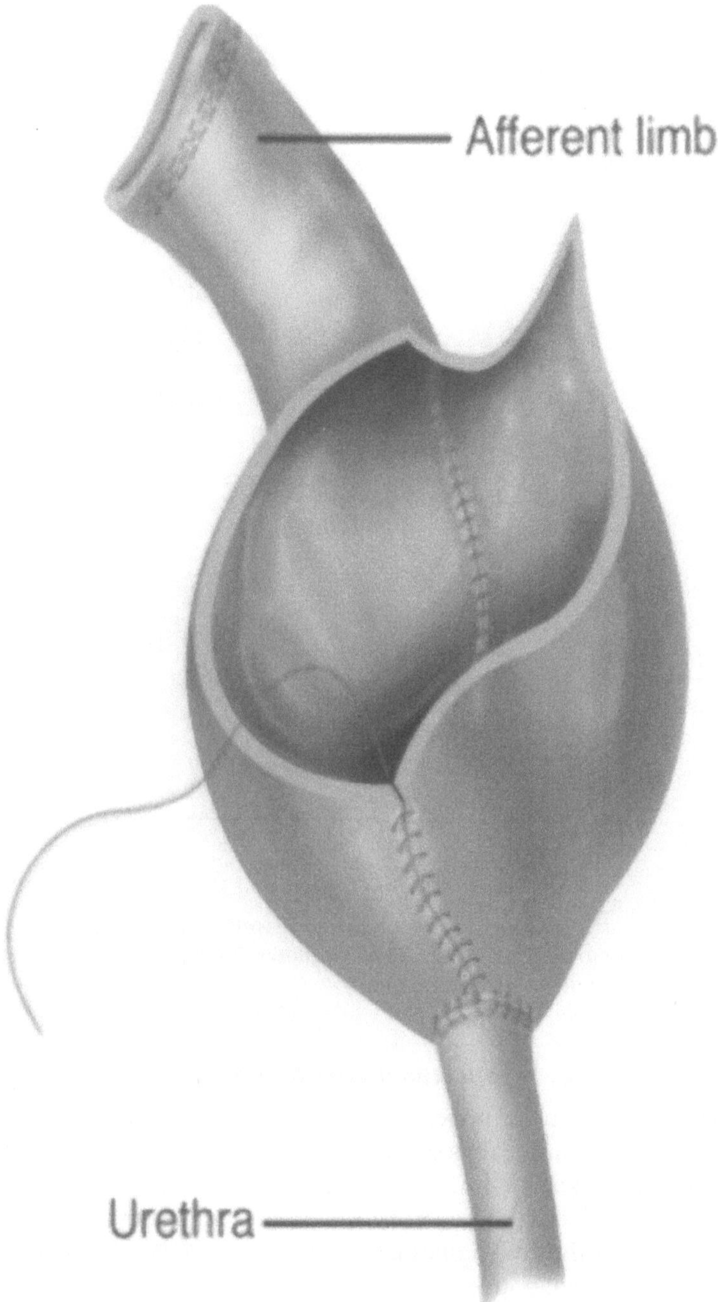


**Fig. 7.** Cartoon demonstrating Studer neobladder with closure of posterior plate, just after completion of urethral anastomosis. (Courtesy of E. McDougall, Vanderbilt University.)

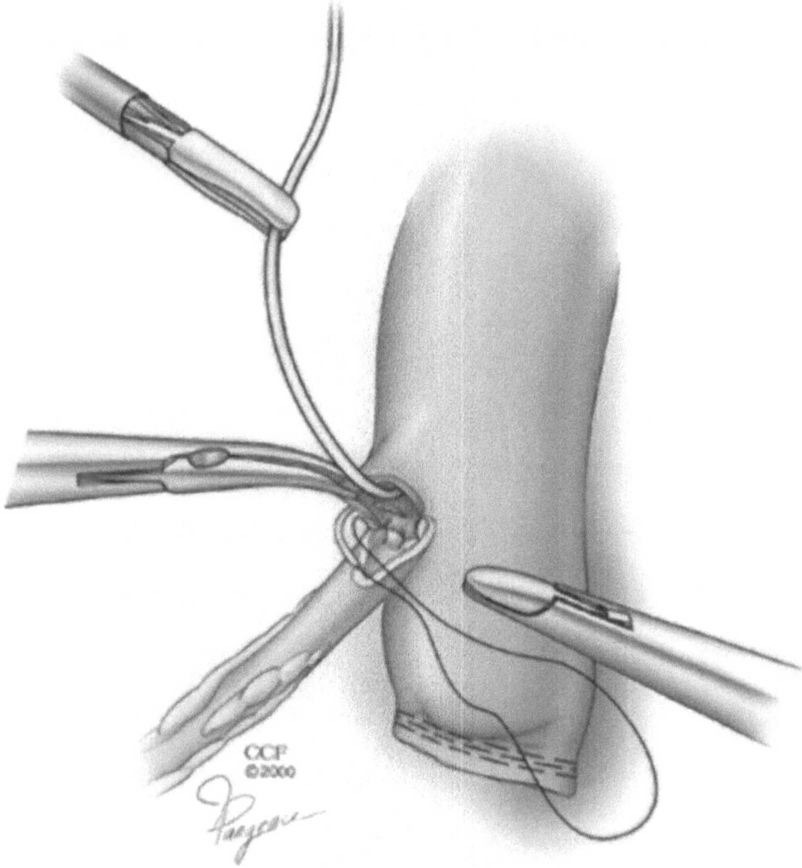


**Fig. 8.** Schematic showing closure of posterior wall of ureteroenteric anastomosis, just prior to placement of urinary diversion stent in the ureter. (Courtesy of I. Gill, Cleveland Clinic Foundation.)

## *Specimen Extraction*

In general, due to the propensity of transitional cell carcinoma to seed *(18)*, one should entrap a cystectomy specimen prior to removal through an extraction incision. In those situations in which some degree of extracorporeal dissection is performed, proper placement of the extraction incision will provide optimal exposure *(15,16,19)*. If completely intracorporeal urinary diversion is planned, it is important to choose a specimen extraction site that will interfere least with urinary diversion (i.e., vaginal extraction before ileal conduit or continent diversion *[20]*, or circum-umbilical incision after orthotopic neobladder *[16]*).

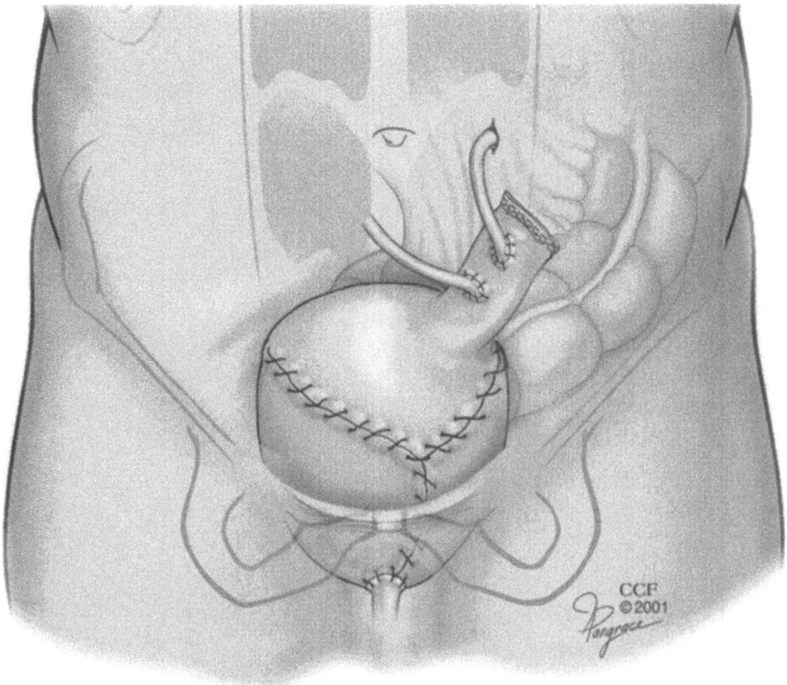


**Fig. 9.** Diagram of completed Studer neobladder with urinary diversion stents exiting the neobladder. (Courtesy of I. Gill, Cleveland Clinic Foundation.)

## RESULTS

As a result of the relative difficulty of laparoscopic urinary diversion, the overwhelming majority of reports have occurred only recently. As a result, it is difficult to comment on the long-term results. However, it is not unreasonable to compare the existing data with those from open counterparts. With any new technique, and laparoscopic techniques in particular, one must look at operative times, blood loss, hospital stay, complications, and length of followup. Although comparative studies are common in most other recent reports of laparoscopic urology, laparoscopic urinary diversion is so new that, to date, there have been none.

There have been 10 series (more than two patients) reported in the literature that are summarized in Table 1 *(14,19–26)*. The majority of these series of urinary diversion include concomitant cystectomy, which is expertly reviewed in Chapter 15. In contrast to cystectomy *(27)*, urinary diversion is performed with varying degrees of intra-corporeal and extracorporeal work. Although a wide range of operative times are

Table 1

| | *Gaboardi et al. (21)* | *Savage et al. (20)* | *Seth et al. (23)* | *Chiu et al. (24)* | *McGinnis et al. (22)* | *Abdel-Hakim et al. (19)* | *Turk et al. (14)* | *Puppo et al. (26)* | *Puppo et al. (27)* |
|---|---|---|---|---|---|---|---|---|---|
| Number of patients | 6 | 8 | 15 | 10 | 6 | 9 | 5 | 9 | 9 |
| Type of diversion | Orthotopic | Conduit (7)<br>Continent (1) | Conduit | Orthotopic | Conduit | Orhtotopic | Continent | Conduit | Ureterostomy |
| Operating room time (h) | 6.3<br>(5.3–8.7) | 11<br>(9–15) | 6.8 | 9.9 | 7.9<br>(7–9.5) | 8.3 | 7.4<br>(6.9–7.9) | — | 0.5–2.1 |
| Estimated blood loss (mL) | 310<br>(220–440) | — | 463 | 265<br>(30–750) | 450 | 150–500 | 245<br>(190–360) | — | — |
| Time to ambulate (d) | 3.5 | — | — | 2 | 2 | — | — | — | — |
| Time to oral intake (d) | 5.5 | 4.1<br>(2—11) | — | 4 | 4.5 | 3 | 3 | — | — |
| Length of hospital stay (d) | 7–9 | 9.4<br>(6–15) | — | — | 5.5 | 10 | 10 | 8.6 | 3–11 |
| Followup (mo) | — | 11.25 | 15.7 | 5.6 (4–8) | — | — | — | — | 10.8 |
| Complication rate (%) | — | 38 | — | 0 | 16 | — | 0 | 0 | 0 |
| Approach:<br>Intracorpreal (IC) or Extracorporeal (EC) | Combined IC/EC | 4 IC<br>4EC | 5 IC<br>10 EC | Hand-assisted EC | Hand-assisted EC | EC | IC | EC | IC |

reported, it appears that, in skilled hands, intracorporeal reconstructive work may take as much as twice as long as the open technique. This may be exacerbated by fatigue, which is inevitable after performing laparoscopic cystectomy. With increasing experience, however, authors note a rapid decrease in operative times.

In order to compare operative results with open series, one must also include the cystectomy, as it and urinary diversion are rarely separated in the literature. Additionally, it is difficult to find a contemporary series for comparison. As a result, two recently published single institution series have been used for comparison *(28,29)*. Furthermore, the laparoscopic urinary diversions reported on comprise a variety of approaches (continent/noncontinent intracorporeal/extracorporeal). The mean operative time in all combined series was 8.2 h, compared to a mean operative time of 5.5 h and 4 h, respectively, for the two open surgery groups. The two open surgery groups had a mean hospital stay of 13 d and 7.5 d, respectively, whereas the combined laparoscopic group had a mean hospital stay of 7.9 d.

There are few studies that comment on the longer term functionality of urinary diversions. One must look to the initial experimental data for more detailed physiological information. Fergany and colleagues *(30)*. reported on 10 survival pigs that had completely intracorporeal construction of an ileal conduit. Renal function was preserved and ureteroileal anastomoses were patent out to 3 mo. Six animals had stomal stenosis, which was attributed to porcine morphology. One animal was noted to have an internal hernia, which caused mortality. Following this study, the group performed porcine orthotopic neobladder *(31)*. Followup (1–3 mo) revealed adequate neobladder capacity (250–700 cc, $M = 420$) with low intravesical pressures (<20 cm $H_2O$) and stable serum creatinine, with no anastomotic strictures or leaks (Fig. 10).

Puppo et al. *(27)* reported on successful cutaneous ureterostomy, although infrequently performed, as a palliative urinary diversion with a mean followup of 10.8 mo. Clinically, a 5-yr followup of an isolated laparoscopic ileal conduit by intravenous (iv) urography revealed prompt, symmetric renal function without obstruction *(13)*. Gupta et al. *(32)* reported a 2-yr followup on five patients who underwent laparoscopic cystectomy and intracorporeal ileal conduit. All surviving patients had normal upper tracts on intravenous urography. However, one patient developed an internal hernia that required bowel resection and diverting ileostomy.

The remaining reports of laparoscopic ileal conduit in the literature comprise 28 patients *(20,22,23)*. The diversion-specific complication rate of the three series combined is 14%, including one early complication (ileus), and two minor late complications (nonobstructive pyelone-

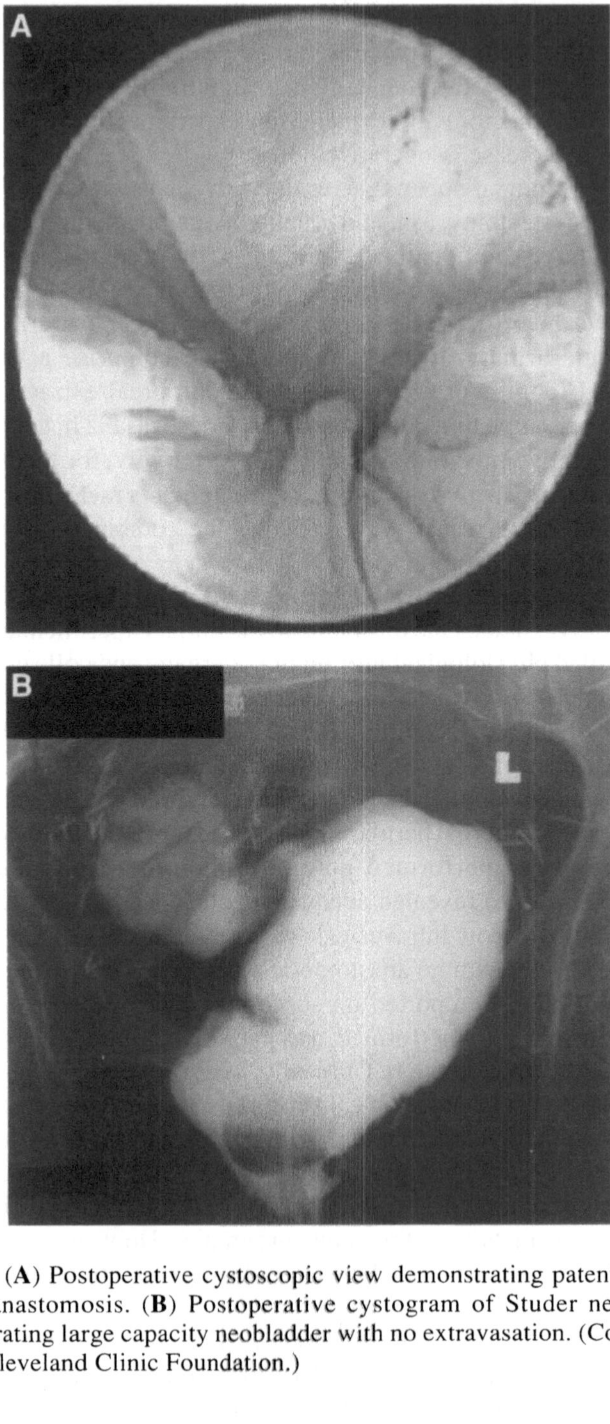


**Fig. 10.** (**A**) Postoperative cystoscopic view demonstrating patent urethroenteric anastomosis. (**B**) Postoperative cystogram of Studer neobladder demonstrating large capacity neobladder with no extravasation. (Courtesy of I. Gill, Cleveland Clinic Foundation.)

phritis), and one major late complication (entero-conduit fistula). It is notable that, to date, there are no reported ureterointestinal strictures (Fig. 11). These results compare well with open counterparts, which report perioperative diversion-specific complication rates between 10 and 18%. Interestingly, approx 5% of complications were wound-related, which contrasts with the known decrease in wound-related morbidity in laparoscopic surgery.

Minimal functional results are available for patients who have undergone continent urinary diversion. Of 10 patients who were reported to have rectal-sigmoid pouch, 8 had greater than 6-mo followup *(33)*. Patients were completely continent day and night, with voiding intervals between 2 and 6 h, and a mean pouch capacity of 376 cc. One patient had a pouch leak that required re-operation. The remainder of the series demonstrates the feasibility of the techniques, but does not comment on perioperative complications. As data mature, the complication rates must be compared with diversion-specific complications in recent continent diversion series (3.4%) *(29)* and orthotopic neobladder series (25%) *(28)*. These complications include those of renal, ureteroenteric, bowel, and calculus origin.

Certainly, there are a number of possible metabolic complications associated with removing a portion of bowel and incorporating it into the urinary tract. Although there is no basis to expect a difference in the incidence of these complications simply on the basis of the use of a laparoscopic approach, one must still be aware of the potential complications associated with each type of diversion.

## CONTROVERSIAL ISSUES

As with all newly developing laparoscopic procedures, laparoscopic urinary diversion requires validation as a viable alternative to standard open surgical approaches. Just as the continent diversion and orthotopic neobladder were proven to be initially feasible, and over time, often preferred over ileal conduit, urological surgeons need to demonstrate equivalent long-term functional results in all forms of urological diversion: conduit, continent diversion, and orthotopic diversion.

The often-voiced concern of the unknown effect of pneumoperitoneum on oncological surgery does not apply to urinary diversion. In general, laparoscopic urological surgery has evolved to the point where open techniques are reproduced faithfully. The danger would be in devising a new "laparoscopic" diversion that may not be equivalent to current standards (i.e., performing multiple cutaneous ureterostomies).

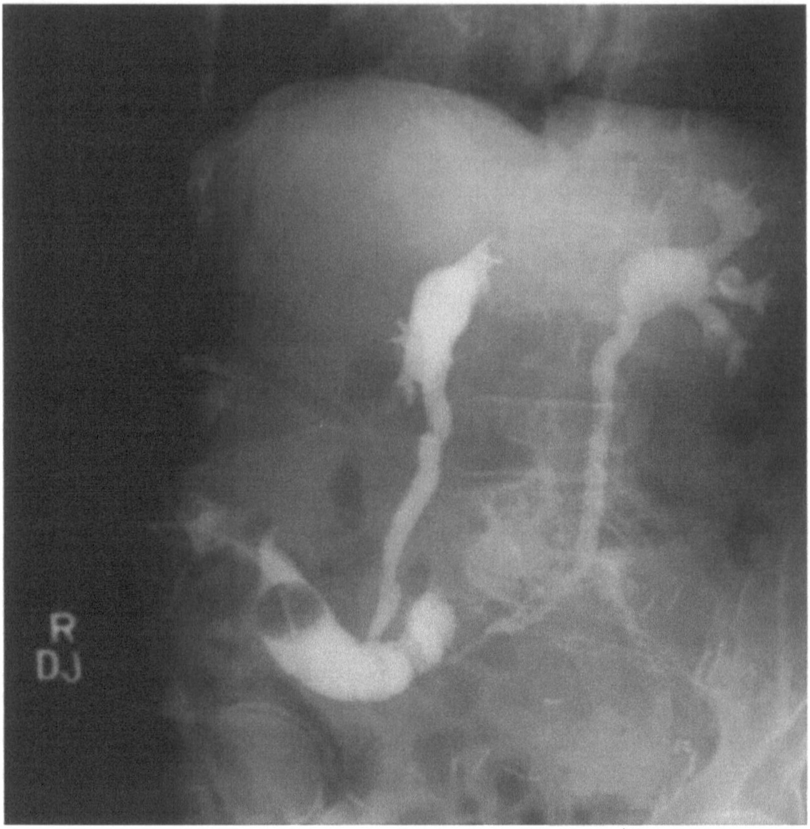


**Fig. 11.** Loopogram of laparoscopic ileal conduit demonstrating free reflux into both collecting systems. (Courtesy of I. Gill, Cleveland Clinic Foundation.)

## SHORTCOMINGS OF LAPAROSCOPIC TECHNIQUE

Not unlike its open counterpart, the greatest shortcoming of laparoscopic urinary diversion is its technical complexity. Because it is usually combined with laparoscopic cystectomy (a technically demanding surgery in its own right), its difficulty is often heightened by surgical fatigue. Furthermore, port sites and patient positioning that were planned for cystectomy may not be ideal for urinary diversion. Although increasing numbers of urological surgeons have become comfortable with laparoscopic ablative techniques, relatively few are at ease with complex reconstructive surgery. This is generally due to the limited degrees of freedom available for the necessary free-hand suturing. It is for that reason that many urological surgeons who are less familiar with laparoscopic techniques welcome the advantages provided by robotic surgical instrumentation.

Lengthy operative times are a direct result of surgical complexity. As a result, surgical complications related to prolonged anesthesia and pneumoperitoneum remain a shortcoming. However, as it is a relatively new laparoscopic procedure, its operative times are changing rapidly and will most likely become close to open operative times in the not-too-distant future.

Once functional equivalency is proven, the theoretical benefits of laparoscopic surgery (quicker recovery, decreased analgesia requirements, decreased blood loss) must overcome any disadvantages (steep learning curve, longer operative times, possible increased risk of thromboembolic disease) for both the urologist and the patient. How this will be accomplished has been a long-standing problem in the evolution of laparoscopic urological surgery. Ideally, prospective randomized trials could answer these questions. In the short term, however, the best answers will come in the form of appropriate surrogate endpoints that can be compared to those of contemporary open urinary diversion. Thus, although laparoscopic urinary diversion is in its infancy, proper patient selection and counseling is paramount.

## SUMMARY

Laparoscopic urinary diversion in all its forms (conduit, continent diversion, and orthotopic neobladder) is a rapidly evolving procedure. The ability to combine intracorporeal and extracorporeal surgical approaches will allow more urologists to begin performing laparoscopic diversions. Increasing experience with both complex urologic pelvic laparoscopy and reconstructive procedures will provide for improved operative times and results. Longer followup with functional results are necessary before it can be deemed equivalent to open urinary diversion.

## REFERENCES

1. Kozminski M, Partamian KO. Case report of laparoscopic ileal loop conduit. J Endourol 1992; 6: 147.
2. Gill IS, Sung GT, Hobart MG, et al. Laparoscopic radical nephroureterectomy for upper tract transitional cell carcinoma: the Cleveland Clinic experience. J Urol 2000; 164: 1513–1522.
3. Gill IS, Meraney AM, Schweizer DK, et al. Laparoscopic radical nephrectomy in 100 patients: a single center experience from the United States. Cancer 2001; 92: 1843–1855.
4. Terry WJ, Bueschen AJ. Complications of radical cystectomy and correlation with nutritional assessment. Urology 1986; 27: 229–232.

5. Stroumbakis N, Herr HW, Cookson MS, Fair WR. Radical cystectomy in the octagenarian. J Urol 1997; 158: 2113–2117.
6. McDougall EM, Clayman RV. Laparoscopic nephrectomy and nephroureterectomy in the octogenarian with a renal tumor. J Laparoendoscopic Surg 1994; 4: 233–236.
7. Hsu TH, Gill IS, Fazeli-Matin S, et al. Radical nephrectomy and nephroureterectomy in the octagenarian and nonagenarian: comparison of open and laparoscopic approaches. Urology 1999; 53: 1121–1125.
8. Wirthlin DJ, Cambria RP. Surgery specific considerations in the cardiac patient undergoing non-cardiac surgery. Prog Cardiovasc Dis 1998; 40: 453–468.
9. Walther MM, Lyme JL, Libutti SL, Linehan WM. Laparoscopic cytoreductive nephrectomy as preparation for administration of systemic interleukin-2 for treatment of metastatic renal cell carcinoma: a pilot study. Urology 1999; 53: 496–501.
10. Holthausedn UH, Nagelschmidt M, Troidl H. $CO_2$ pneumoperitoneum: what we know and what we need to know. World J Surg 1999; 23: 794–800.
11. Morino M, Giraudo G, Festa V. Alterations in hepatic function during laparoscopic surgery: an experimental clinical study. Surg Endosc 1998; 12: 968–972.
12. Targarona EM, Balague C, Knook MM, Trías M. Laparoscopic surgery and surgical infection. Br J Surg 2000; 87: 536–544.
13. Potter SR, Charambura TC, Adams JB, Kavoussi LR. Laparoscopic ileal conduit: five-year follow-up. Urology 2000; 56: 22–25.
14. Turk I, Deger S, Winkelmann B, Schonberger B, Loening SA. Laparoscopic radical cystectomy with continent urinary diversion (rectal sigmoid pouch) performed completely intracorporeally: the initial 5 cases. J Urol 2001; 165: 1863–1866.
15. Gaboardi F, Simonato A, Lissiani A, Gregori A, Bozzola A. Minimally invasive laparoscopic neobladder. J Urol 2002; 168: 1080–1083.
16. Gill IS, Kaouk JH, Meraney AM, et al. Laparoscopic radical cystectomy and continent orthotopic ileal neobladder performed completely intracorporeally: the initial experience. J Urol 2002; 168: 13–18.
17. Gill IS, Fergany A, Klein EA, et al. Laparoscopic radical cystoprostatectomy with ileal conduit performed completely intracorporeally: the initial 2 cases. Urology 2000; 56: 26–29.
18. Otani M, Irie S, Tsuji Y. Port site metastasis after laparoscopic nephrectomy: unsuspected transitional cell carcinoma within a tuberculous atrophic kidney. J Urol 1999; 162: 486–487.
19. Abdel-Hakim AM, Bassiouny F, Abdel-Azím MS, et al. Laparoscopic radical cystectomy with orthotopic neobladder. J Endourol 2002; 16: 377–381.
20. Savage SJ, McWilliams GW, Ky A, Droller MJ. Laparoscopic radical cystectomy and urinary diversion: the neglected minimally invasive frontier. J Endourol 2002; 16(Supp 1): A154.
21. Gaboardi F, Simonato A, Lissiani A, et al. Minimally invasive laparoscopic neobladder (M.I.L.A.N.): the initial experience. J Endourol 2002; 16(Supp 1): A125.
22. McGinnis DE, Hubosky SG, Bergmann LS. Hand-assisted laparoscopic radical cystoprostatectomy with ileal conduit in 6 consecutive patients. J Endourol 2002; 16(Supp 1): A153.
23. Seth A, Hemal AK, Kumar R, Gupta NP. Laparoscopic radical cystectomy: complications of initial 15 cases. J Endourol 2002; 16(Supp 1): A154.
24. Chiu AW, Huan SK, Chia-Hsiang L, et al. Hand assisted laparoscopic radical cystectomy with continent urinary diversion (ileal pouch). J Endourol 2002; 16(Supp 1): A154.

25. Denewer A, Kotb S, Hussein O, El-Maadawy M. Laparoscopic assisted cystectomy and lymphadenectomy for bladder cancer: initial experience. World J Surg 1999; 23: 608–611.
26. Puppo P, Ricciotti G. Videoendoscopically assisted transvaginal radical cystectomy. J Endourol 2001; 15: 411–413.
27. Puppo P, Ricciotti G, Bozzo W, Pezzica C, Geddo D, Perachino M. Videoendoscopic cutaneous ureterostomy for palliative urinary diversion. Eur Urol 1995; 28; 328–333.
28. Gburek BM, Lieber MM, Blute ML. Comparison of studer ileal neobladder and ileal conduit urinary diversion with respect to perioperative outcome and late complications. J Urol 1998; 160: 721–723.
29. Parekh DJ, Gilbert WB, Koch MO, Smith JA. Continent urinary reconstruction versus ileal conduit: a contemporary single-institution comparison of perioperative morbidity and mortality. Urology 2000; 55: 852–855.
30. Fergany AF, Gill IS, Kaouk JH, et al. Laparoscopic intracorporeally constructed ileal conduit after porcine cystoprostatectomy. J Urol 2001; 166: 285–288.
31. Kaouk JH, Gill IS, Meraney AM, et al. Laparoscopic orthotopic ileal neobladder. J Endourol 2001; 15: 131–142.
32. Gupta NP, Gill IS, Fergany A, Nabi G. Laparoscopic radical cystectomy with intracorporeal ileal conduit diversion: five cases with a 2-year follow-up. BJU Int 2002; 90: 391–396.
33. Tuerk IA, Davis JW, Deger S, et al. Follow-up after laparoscopic radical cystectomy and intracorporeal constructed rectum-sigmoid-pouch (Mainz pouch II). J Urol 2002; 164(Supp 4): 60.

# VII Complications of Laparoscopic Surgery

# 17 Management of Intra- and Postoperative Complications

*James R. Porter,* MD

*CONTENTS*

INTRODUCTION
LAPAROSCOPIC COMPLICATIONS
SPECIFIC COMPLICATIONS
POSTOPERATIVE COMPLICATIONS
SUMMARY
REFERENCES

## INTRODUCTION

The urologist performing laparoscopic surgical procedures is faced with several challenges. Although most urologists are familiar with working in a two-dimensional field due to endoscopic experience, the lack of depth perception and the degree of precision required in laparoscopy can pose significant problems. Laparoscopy requires familiarity with entirely new instrumentation and safe access to the peritoneal or retroperitoneal space may also present difficulty. The control of bleeding during laparoscopic procedures can be daunting, and diminished tactile feedback during laparoscopy may lead to tissue injury. Investigators have assessed the impact of training on acquisition of laparoscopic skills and it is clear that additional training beyond a weekend instructional course is required to perform laparoscopic procedures safely *(1)*. The teaching of laparoscopic skills in residency pro-

From: *Laparoscopic Urologic Oncology*
Edited by: J. A. Cadeddu © Humana Press Inc., Totowa, NJ

grams is early in its development, and laparoscopic training will be the mandate of academic medical centers in the future.

Laparoscopic urologic procedures have evolved from a basic diagnostic tool to an advanced ablative technique and recently to a reconstructive procedure. Although complications can occur during any laparoscopic procedure, as the complexity of the procedure increases so can the magnitude and scope of complications. As more sophisticated techniques are employed and new procedures are performed, previously unreported complications may occur.

If a complication occurs during a laparoscopic procedure, recognition is the key to bring prompt resolution and limit patient morbidity. However, recognition of complications may be hindered by issues such as bleeding, the limited field of view inherent with laparoscopic visualization, or unfamiliarity with tissue as seen through the laparoscope. Once a complication is recognized, successful management is affected by several factors including experience of the surgeon and assistant, availability of needed instrumentation, hemodynamic stability and body habitus of the patient, any pre-existing patient disease, and the particular anatomic structure that is injured. Of these variables, the experience of the operating surgeon and team is the most important factor in determining whether a complication can be managed laparoscopically or if open conversion will be required. It is important to realize that conversion to open surgery during a laparoscopic procedure is not a complication, and in almost every case, is a sign of good surgical judgment.

This review is intended to highlight the intraoperative and postoperative complications encountered during urologic laparoscopic procedures and their management. Although common complications encountered during routine laparoscopic procedures are covered, the emphasis of this review is on the management of complications associated with urologic laparoscopic oncologic procedures.

## LAPAROSCOPIC COMPLICATIONS

### *General Series*

It is useful to review laparoscopic complications from general laparoscopic urological series, because many of the complications in these reports will be observed in laparoscopic urologic oncology procedures. It has been stated that the complications associated with difficult laparoscopic procedures are similar to those for easier procedures because both types of procedures share the potential for access-related injuries, unrecognized bowel injuries, and dissection injuries *(2)*. Many of the general laparoscopic series include hundreds of patients so that both common and rare complications and their management are reported.

Table 1
Laparoscopic Complications from General Urologic Series

| *Author (reference)* | *Most common procedure* | *Cases* | *Overall compliaction rate* | *Most common complication* |
|---|---|---|---|---|
| Gill et al. *(3)* | Laparoscopic nephrectomy | 185 | 34 (18.4%) | Vascular injury |
| Peters et al. *(4)* | Pediatric laparoscopy | 5400 | 63 (1.18%) | Vascular injury |
| Gill et al. *(5)* | Retroperitoneal nephrectomy | 1043 | 49 (4.7%) | Vascular injury |
| Fahlenkamp et al. *(6)* | Lap varicocelectomy | 2407 | 107 (4.4%) | Vascular injury |
| Cadeddu et al. *(7)* | Laparoscopic nephrectomy | 738 | 88 (11.9%) | Neuropathy |

Considerable data exist regarding complications of laparoscopic urologic procedures (Table 1). Gill reported the results of a multi-institutional review of laparoscopic nephrectomy with the majority of procedures being performed for benign conditions *(3)*. The overall complication rate was 18.4% (34 of 185 patients). Intraoperative complications occurred in 7 patients (3.7%), with the most common complication being vascular injuries in 4 cases. Postoperative complications were noted in 27 patients (14.6%), with the most common complication being ileus in 4 patients. Peters reported his analysis of laparoscopic complications in the pediatric population, with 5400 laparoscopic procedures represented by the survey *(4)*. Based on returned questionnaires, the complication rates for both diagnostic and operative laparoscopic surgery cases were reported. (More than 5400 laparoscopic cases were represented by the survey.) The significant complication rate, as defined as injuries to the bowel, bladder, vascular structures, or abdominal herniations, was 1.18%. Bowel injury occurred in 0.17% of patients, bladder injury in 0.17%, and vascular injury in 0.43%. Peters noted that the strongest predictor of laparoscopic complication rate was practitioner experience. Complication rate for practitioners with fewer than 20 cases was 8.3%, whereas complication rate for practitioners with more than 100 cases was 2.8% (Fig. 1).

Laparoscopic complications associated with retroperitoneal and pelvic extraperitoneal procedures were pooled from 24 centers worldwide encompassing 1043 procedures *(5)*. The most common procedure in this

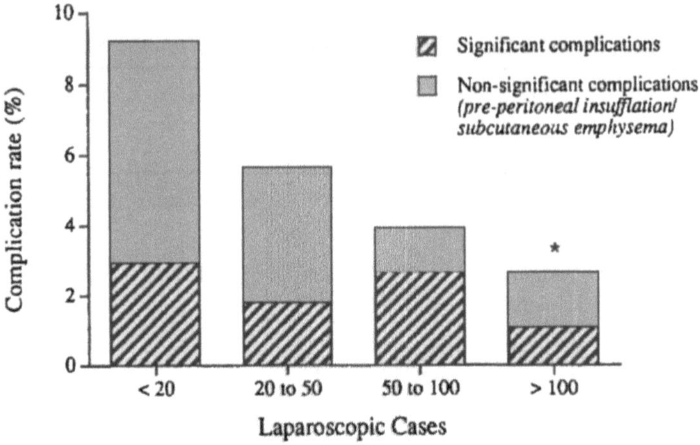


**Fig. 1.** Decreasing rate of complications for pediatric laparoscopic cases with increasing experience. Overall incidence is significantly lower for practitioners with more than 100 cases as compared to those with fewer than 20 cases ($p < 0.0035$). (From ref. *40*.)

series was simple nephrectomy followed by bladder neck suspension. Forty-nine patients (4.7%) experienced complications with vascular injuries comprising 47% of the injuries and the bladder was the most common organ injured. The laparoscopic working group of the German Urologic Association reported on complications in 2407 procedures at four centers *(6)*. The most common procedures performed were laparoscopic varicocelectomy (766) followed by pelvic lymph node dissection (PLND) (481). Overall, complications were noted in 107 patients (4.4%), with intraoperative complications in 67 (2.8%) and postoperative complications in 28 (1.4%). Again, the most common complication in the intraoperative period was vascular injury, and the majority of vascular injuries were due to errors of dissection. Wound-related issues were the most common morbidity during the postoperative period.

More recently, Cadeddu compiled the laparoscopic complications from urologists with advanced laparoscopic training who were early into clinical practice *(7)*. The survey reviewed 738 laparoscopic cases and the mean number of cases performed by each surgeon was 57. The most common procedure performed was nephrectomy. Complications occurred in 88 of 783 patients (11.9%) with the most common complications being neuropathy reported in 13 patients followed by urine leak in 9 patients.

Analysis of these series reveals that vascular injury, either due to access-related trauma or errors of disssection, is the most common intraoperative complication reported in most studies. Access-related injuries and errors of dissection are usually seen early in the experience of a laparoscopist and the surveys by Gill *(3,5)* and Fahlenkamp *(6)* encompassed the early experience for many of the centers reporting their results. This is in contrast to the survey reported by Cadeddu *(7)* where the most common injury was neuropathy most probably related to positioning injury. Those laparoscopists with advanced training benefited from exposure to proper access and dissection technique, essentially experiencing their learning curve during training and thereby decreasing the risk of vascular injuries.

## *Oncology Series*

Complications that accompany laparoscopic oncologic procedures may differ from those seen with laparoscopic procedures for benign conditions due to several factors. In malignant conditions, a wider field of dissection is required, which may lead to injury to surrounding structures. Gill noted that complications were three times more prevalent in procedures for malignant conditions (34%) as compared to benign conditions (12%) *(3)*. Malignant tissues are highly vascular and may contain neovascularity or parasitic vessels that can be difficult to control. Shoma found that kidneys with more vascularity were associated with a higher rate of open conversion than kidneys with poor blood flow *(8)*. Finally, some laparoscopic oncologic procedures require excision and reconstruction of the urinary tract, which may result in urine leak or strictures at anastomotic sites. Several recent series have reported the complications associated with laparoscopic oncologic procedures and these are listed in Table 2.

## *Laparoscopic Pelvic Lymph Node Dissection*

One of the first reports detailing the complications associated with laparoscopic urologic oncologic procedures was presented by Kavoussi. He authored a multi-institutional review of complications encountered during laparoscopic pelvic lymph node dissection (L-PLND) and reported 55 complications (14.8%) in 372 patients with 14 (3.8%) occurring intraoperatively and 41 (11.0%) in the postoperative period *(9)*. The most frequent intraoperative complication of L-PLND was vascular injury in 11 patients with 6 due to trocar injury and 5 due to dissection. The most frequent postoperative complications of L-PLND

Table 2
Laparoscopic Complications from Urologic Oncologic Series

| *Author (reference)* | *Procedure* | *Cases* | *Overall complications* | *Intraoperative complications* |
|---|---|---|---|---|
| Kavoussi et al. *(9)* | L-PLND | 372 | 55 (14.8%) | 14 (3.8%) |
| Cadeddu et al. *(10)* | LRN | 157 | 16 (10.2%) | 3 (1.9%) |
| Dunn et al. *(11)* | LRN | 60 | 23 (37.7%) | 6 (10%) |
| Ono et al. *(12)* | LRN | 100 | 13 (13%) | 10 (10%) |
| Gill et al. *(13)* | LNU | 42 | 5 (12%) | 2 (4.8%) |
| Gill et al. *(15)* | LPN | 50 | 6 (12%) | 2 (4%) |
| Nelson et al. *(16)* | L-RPLND | 29 | 4 (13.8%) | 2 (6.9%) |
| Guillonneau et al. *(18)* | LRP | 567 | 105 (18.5%) | 25 (4.4%) |

L-PLND = laparoscopic pelvic lymph node dissection; LRN = laparoscopic radical nephrectomy; LNU = laparoscopic nephroureterectomy; LPN = laparoscopic partial nephrectomy; L-RPLND = laparoscopic retroperitoneal lymph node dissection; LRP = laparoscopic radical prostatectomy.

were bowel related with prolonged ileus in 5, small bowel obstruction in 2, and delayed recognition of bowel injury in 2 patients.

### *Laparoscopic Radical Nephrectomy*

A mult-institutional experience with laparoscopic radical nephrectomy (LRN) was reported by Cadeddu in which 157 LRN procedures were performed *(10)*. All patients were clinical stage T1-2, N0,M0 with negative metastatic workup. Complications occurred in 16 of 157 patients (10.2%) with one intraoperative death thought to be due to pulmonary embolus, and another death 1 mo after surgery due to congestive heart failure. The most common complication was postoperative ileus noted in four patients. There were six open conversions either due to adhesions or to control hemorrhage.

A detailed comparison of complications between LRN and open radical nephrectomy (ORN) was presented by Dunn *(11)*. This study compared 60 LRNs to 33 patients undergoing ORN, and comparison between the two groups was based on tumor size. Complications occurred in 23 patients in the LRN group (37.7%) with 21 minor and 2 major complications. The major complications involved ligation of the superior mesenteric artery in one patient and persistent back bleeding from the renal vein side of a staple line. There were 5 vascular injuries in the LRN group and transfusions were required in 7 patients (12%). The ORN group experienced complications in 18 patients (55%) with 14 minor and 4 major complications. Major complications included injury to the superior mesenteric artery requiring reanastomosis in one patient and colonic injury requiring repair in another. Another patient experienced significant intraoperative hemorrhage requiring a 4-unit blood transfusion. This patient also developed a pulmonary embolus. The final major complication involved significant retroperitoneal hemorrhage requiring re-exploration and ultimately required dialysis for chronic renal failure. The transfusion rate for the ORN group was 15%.

Ono presented his experience with LRN, which included 100 cases over 8 yr *(12)*. Complications were reported in 13 (13%) patients with intraoperative complications in 10 and postoperative complications in 3. Of the 10 intraoperative complications, 6 involved vascular injury, with 4 of those requiring open conversion to gain vascular control. Blood transfusions were required in 5 patients (5%). Ono compared the LRN group to 46 ORNs and noted complications in 4 of 46 (8.7%) patients. Of the two intraoperative complications, one involved injury to the renal vein and the other was a splenic injury. The two postoperative complications were both ileus: one was treated conservatively and one required exploration for lysis of adhesions. Transfusion was required in four patients (8.7%).

### *Laparoscopic Nephroureterectomy*

The complications associated with laparoscopic nephroureterectomy (LNU) were presented by Gill and compared to an open nephroureterectomy cohort *(13)*. Of the 42 patients undergoing LNU, complications occurred in 5 (12%) compared to 10 complications out of 35 patients (28.6%) in the open group. Two intraoperative complications occurred in the laparoscopic group: fluid extravasation during endoscopic release of the distal ureter and one renal vein injury necessitating open conversion for control. Another open conversion was performed electively because of concerns regarding adequate tumor excision with the laparoscopic approach. The remaining three complications in the laparoscopic group were due to atelectasis. The 10 complications in the open group presented in the postoperative period with 4 patients having atelectasis, 5 with ileus, and 1 patient sustaining a pneumothorax.

### *Laparoscopic Partial Nephrectomy*

The application of laparoscopic techniques to nephron-sparing surgery and standardization of the procedure is the latest challenge for urologists performing laparoscopic surgery. Many techniques have been employed to control bleeding *(14)*, however, the principles of vascular control as practiced in open nephron surgery appear to be the most successful. Gill recently published his experience with laparoscopic partial nephrectomy (LPN) with an emphasis on recreating the open technique *(15)*. Complications were seen in 6 of 50 patients (12%) with three major and three minor complications. Minor complications included atelectasis, atrial fibrillation, and a serosal tear of the bowel. Major complications consisted of intraoperative hemorrhage in one patient due to incomplete control of the renal hilum, which was eventually controlled laparoscopically. Another patient developed recurrent, delayed hemorrhage from the resection bed, which required open nephrectomy for control. The final complication was a urine leak, which resolved with internal stenting.

### *Laparoscopic Retroperitoneal Lymph Node Dissection*

For patients with stage 1 nonseminomatous germ cell testicular tumors (NSGCT), open retroperitoneal lymph node dissection (RPLND) has been standard therapy for patients at high risk for lymph node metastasis. However, the morbidity of the open RPLND is substantial, leading many to choose chemotherapy. In an effort to decrease the morbidity of the open RPLND, investigators have reported their experience with laparoscopic RPLND for the staging of NSGCT. Nelson reviewed their initial experience with laparoscopic RPLND for clinical stage 1 NSGCT and cited 4 complications in the series of 29 *(16)*. Intraoperative bleeding due to venous injury occurred in two patients, both requiring open conversion for repair. The other two complications developed in the postoperative period with one lymphocele and another patient suffering flank compartment syndrome from positioning.

Laparoscopic RPLND has been extended to treat stage IIB testicular cancer patients with residual masses after chemotherapy *(17)*. Twenty-four patients were treated, and there were no open conversions reported. Intraoperative bleeding was encountered in five patients but it was managed laparoscopically without problem. The only complications noted were postoperative chylous ascites in five patients, and 1 patient developed a lymphocele. All episodes of chylous ascites resolved with low fat diet. No re-operations were necessary.

### *Laparoscopic Radical Prostatectomy*

The standardization of laparoscopic radical prostatectomy (LRP) has brought widespread interest in this procedure as an alternative treatment for localized prostate cancer. The technique requires skill with laparoscopic reconstruction, and it is distinctive with regard to anatomic location and surrounding structures. Because of these factors, many of the complications associated with LRP are unique to this procedure.

Guillonneau et al. presented the complications associated with LRP during their initial 3-yr experience with the technique *(18)*. The overall complication rate was 18.5% with 105 complications noted in 97 patients out of 567. Open conversion was performed in 7 of the initial 70 patients: 3 for uncontrolled bleeding and 4 for difficult dissection. Re-operation to correct complications was required in 20 patients. The most common complication was prolonged urine leakage from the vesicourethral anastomosis seen in 57 patients (10%), and all but one patient healed with prolonged catheter drainage. There were eight rectal injuries: six were repaired primarily without sequelae. Other bowel injuries included two ileal injuries and one sigmoid injury all three unrecognized at surgery and presenting on postoperative d 3. All three injuries were repaired with bowel diversion as were the two rectal injuries that did not heal primarily.

Ureteral complications developed in four patients, with two of the injuries presenting postoperatively as persistent urinary ascites. These two injuries were thought to be due to delayed necrosis of the ureter during lateral dissection of the bladder. One injury responded to ureteral stenting, whereas the other required re-implantation. Another ureteral injury occurred during transection of what was thought to be the vas deferens, and this was repaired laparoscopically without incident. The final ureteral injury presented as anuria, and during re-exploration, the anastomotic sutures included the ureter causing obstruction. This was corrected by revision of the vesicourethral anastomosis.

The remaining major complications included wound dehiscence in four patients; all repaired at re-operation. Five patients developed postoperative pelvic hematoma: one due to venous injury during laparoscopic PLND, two cases due to postoperative anticoagulant therapy, and two cases with no obvious cause. All five patients required re-operation for resolution.

## SPECIFIC COMPLICATIONS

### *Vascular Injury*

Vascular injuries are the most common injuries reported during urologic laparoscopic surgery *(6)* and they may be access-related or caused

Table 3
Laparoscopic Vascular Injuries from Urologic Series

| *Author (reference)* | *Procedure* | *Cases* | *Vascular Injury* | *Type* |
|---|---|---|---|---|
| Gill et al. *(3)* | Laparoscopic nephrectomy | 185 | 3 (1.6%) | 2/3 Dissection injury |
| Fahlenkamp et al. *(6)* | Multiple | 2407 | 40 (1.7%) injury | 40 Dissection |
| Thiel et al. *(19)* | Transperitoneal laparoscopy | 274 | 6 (1.7%) | 6 Dissection injury |
| Meraney et al. *(20)* | Retroperitoneal laparoscopy | 404 | 7 (1.7%) | 5/7 Dissection injury |
| Rassweiler et al. *(21)* | Laparoscopic nephrectomy | 482 | 22 (4.6%) | Not reported |

by errors in dissection. Several series have reported their experience with vascular injury during urologic laparoscopic procedures; however, some studies failed to distinguish vascular injury caused by dissection from that caused by access injuries. The occurrence of vascular injury is reported from 1.6 to 4.6% of laparoscopic procedures (Table 3) *(3,6,19–21)*. Gill noted vascular injuries in 3 (1.6%) of 185 patients undergoing laparoscopic nephrectomies with two of the three injuries due to error in dissection *(3)*. Fahlenkamp reviewed the German experience with laparoscopic complications and found 40 vascular injuries in 2407 patients *(6)*. Vascular injuries were the most frequent complication in that report. Thiel noted six major vascular injuries during 274 transperi-toneal laparoscopic cases *(19)*. All were venous dissection injuries, and the authors noted that vessel injury was more likely to occur during complex laparoscopic procedures in patients who had undergone previous surgery in the region. This concept was supported by a recent report by Meraney who reviewed the complications of retroperitoneal laparoscopic surgery and noted seven vascular injuries in 404 patients *(20)*. Five of the seven vascular injuries occurred during dissection and the majority of vascular injuries in this series occurred in patients who had previous abdominal surgery. Rassweiler reported 22 vascular injuries out of 482 laparoscopic nephrectomies for a rate of 4.6% *(21)*.

Although the rate of vascular injury is low, these injuries tend to be the most common intraoperative complication *(3,6,9,12,21,22)* and in many reports, vascular injury during dissection is the most frequent cause for emergent open conversion *(3,16,20–22)*. Vascular injuries tend to occur during procedures where dissection is required around large vessels as in laproscopic nephrectomy or laparoscopic RPLND *(16)* but are rare in cases such as LRP, where large vessels are rarely encountered *(18)*. In 567 LRPs, Guillonneau noted only three bleeding episodes significant enough to require open conversion *(18)*. Although this appears to be the trend, there are exceptions. In the multicenter study by Cadeddu involving 157 LRNs, there was not a single vascular injury due to dissection *(10)*.

The need for open conversion to control vascular injury appears to occur early in the laparoscopic experience of the surgeon. Meraney noted that open conversion was required in three of their first four vascular injuries, however their three subsequent vascular injuries were controlled using laparoscopic techniques, and open conversion was not required to control vascular complications during their last 200 cases *(20)*. Guillonneau reported seven open conversions for LRP in the first 70 patients, with three due to bleeding, but no conversions in the subsequent 497 cases *(18)*. Thiel noted successful laparoscopic repair of four consecutive venous injuries after open repair of the first *(19)*.

Rarely, vascular injuries have occurred due to malfunctioning of endoscopic stapling devices. Chan et al. reported 10 occurrences of stapler malfunction in 565 cases for a rate of 1.7% *(23)*. In 5 of the 10 cases, malfunctioning of the staple device was due to application of the stapler over previously placed metal clips, which caused the stapler to misfire. Others have reported similar problems with the endoscopic stapling device *(3,22,24)*.

The majority of vascular injuries during laparoscopy are due to errors in dissection. Most commonly this is due to inadequate exposure of the vascular structure leading to either direct sharp injury or thermal injury to the vessel. The principle of dissecting from superficial to deep structures (from known to unknown) must be followed in order to avoid this type of injury. Control of the bleeding vessel may be a challenge due to several factors. First, bleeding from a vessel quickly obscures the source as blood pools around the injured vessel. Second, the injured vessel is often not completely exposed as the dissection injury often occurs during exposure of the vessel. Third, unlike open surgery the application of manual direct pressure is difficult, and depending on the laparoscopic instrument in the abdomen, the quick application of pressure to the bleeding vessel may be impossible.

Once a vascular injury has occurred, an immediate assessment is required to determine whether an attempt at laparoscopic repair should be performed or if open conversion is necessary. If the surgeon is inexperienced, or if this is a case early in the learning curve, then immediate open conversion should be performed. However, if the surgeon is more experienced and the necessary instrumentation is available, then a laparoscopic repair may be attempted. The first principle is to provide tamponade to the bleeding area with the available instrument that is in the abdomen at the time of injury. Additional ports may be required to provide exposure and suction as needed. The pneumoperitoneum should be maintained because this may decrease venous bleeding *(19)*. Once the area of bleeding has been identified, further exposure of surrounding structures should be carefully performed to allow complete visualization of the region. After adequate exposure has been obtained, the area of entry may be identified and repaired either with intracorporeal suturing or judicious placement of clips. On occasion, an injury may be repaired by firing a vascular stapling device *(20)*. Failure to control hemorrhage by any of these measures, or the occurrence of hemodynamic instability in the patient, should prompt immediate open conversion. It is important in any laparoscopic procedure to have an open laparotomy tray open and available in the room in the event that emergent laparotomy is required.

### *Access-Related Injury*

Access-related injuries to abdominal viscera or retroperitoneal vascular structures are estimated to occur at a rate between 0.05 and 2.8% *(25,26)*. Although these are rare injuries, when they do occur, the consequences can be devastating with a mortality rate of 13% *(27)*. A review by Chadler of insurance claims and Food and Drug Administration Medical Device Reports of access-related injuries over a 2-yr period revealed bowel and retroperitoneal vascular injury comprised 76% of all injuries incurred in the process of establishing a primary port *(27)*. The small bowel was the most common organ injured and nearly 50% of both large and small bowel injuries were unrecognized for 24 h or longer. Delayed recognition, along with age greater that 59 yr and major vascular injury, were each independent predictors of death. Shielded pyramidal cutting trocars were the most common trocar type associated with access injuries, and trauma from Veress needles accounted for 18% of the injuries. Injuries were also observed with open, Hasson-type, blunt cannulas, which were associated with two deaths: one from unrecognized bowel injury and another from retroperitoneal vascular injury. The authors concluded that no entry technique or device is absolutely safe and that access injuries to abdominal viscera and vessels may be more common than is currently reported in the literature *(27)*.

Laparoscopic access injuries in the urologic literature are reported as one of three injuries: visceral organ or vascular trauma, abdominal wall vessel laceration, or port-site herniation. Kavoussi reported 10 (2.7%) trocar-related injuries in 372 patients treated with laparoscopic PLND *(9)*. Four of the injuries were due to laceration of the epigastric vessels, three were bladder injuries, two were due to injury to a superficial abdominal wall vessel, and one was a small bowel injury. Gill noted four (2.2%) trocar injuries in 185 laparoscopic nephrectomy patients *(3)*. There were two port-site hernias, one abdominal wall hematoma, and one trocar injury to the kidney resulting in open laparotomy. In a survey of pediatric urological laparoscopy, Peters noted abdominal wall herniations in 0.15% of patients *(4)*. He also noted that significant complications occurred more frequently in patients in which the Veress needle was used (2.55%) compared to the Hasson technique (1.19%, $p < 0.006$). Although the type of access technique was found to be significant, the most important factor in predicting the occurrence of complications in this study was practitioner experience *(4)*.

A recent review of laparoscopic nephrectomy revealed the potential risks involved in using optical trocars to gain primary port access into the peritoneal cavity. After insufflation is performed with a Veress needle, an optical trocar is used to visually pass through each layer of the abdominal wall. The idea is that direct visualization while passing the trocar should allow identification of intra-abdominal structures and thereby decrease the risk of injury to viscera. Siqueira et al. reported three access-related injuries in the series of 213 patients *(22)*. One injury involved laceration of the inferior epigastric artery, which resolved with conservative treatment. The other two injuries involved liver injury while passing an optical trocar. Both injuries were managed conservatively. Injury while using optical trocars has also been confirmed in the gynecologic literature *(28)*.

The open technique of gaining laparoscopic access is not without complication as noted in a report by Peters *(29)*. The injury involved a segment of small bowel that had been included in the purse-string suture placed around the access incision. Inspection of the primary access site from a secondary trocar identified the trapped bowel and the serosal defect was repaired. The conclusions of this case report were that care must be used when placing a purse-string suture, and the initial access site should be inspected from a secondary trocar site to look for injury.

It is clear from the experience of many that there is no perfect access technique and no method is risk free. With this concept in mind, the man-

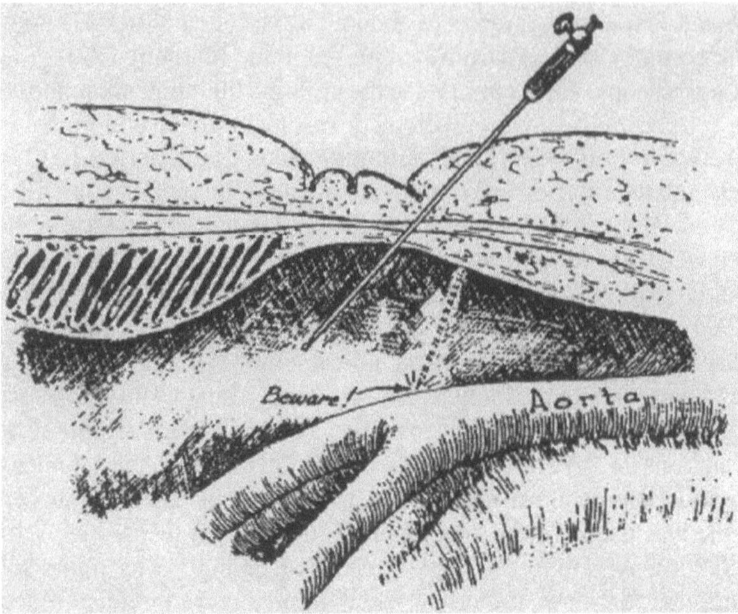


**Fig. 2.** Proximity of the umbilicus to the aortic bifurcation during Veress needle placement. (From ref. *29a*.)

agement of access injuries should focus on prevention and recognition. If a closed entry technique is employed using a Veress needle and blind primary trocar, then prevention requires clear knowledge of the underlying anatomy and their proximity to landmarks on the skin (Fig. 2) *(29a)*. The distance from the abdominal skin surface at the umbilicus to the ventral surface of the aorta can be less than 5 cm in a thin woman *(27)*. Some have suggested avoiding midline access altogether because of the potential risks, and advocate primary access in the left upper quadrant *(30)*. If a patient has an incision from previous surgery, this area should be avoided and primary access should be obtained in a location remote from the incision, or an open access technique should be employed.

Although the Veress needle may be smaller than a trocar, complications can occur with this device, and the Veress needle accounted for 18% of access-related injuries in a recent report *(27)*. Veress needle placement was perceived as the most difficult aspect of laparoscopy as noted in a review by See *(31)*. When the Veress needle is passed, the adbominal wall should be elevated with penetrating towel clips and the Veress needle should be left open to permit air to enter the peritoneal space and allow the bowel and omentum to fall away (Fig. 3). Before

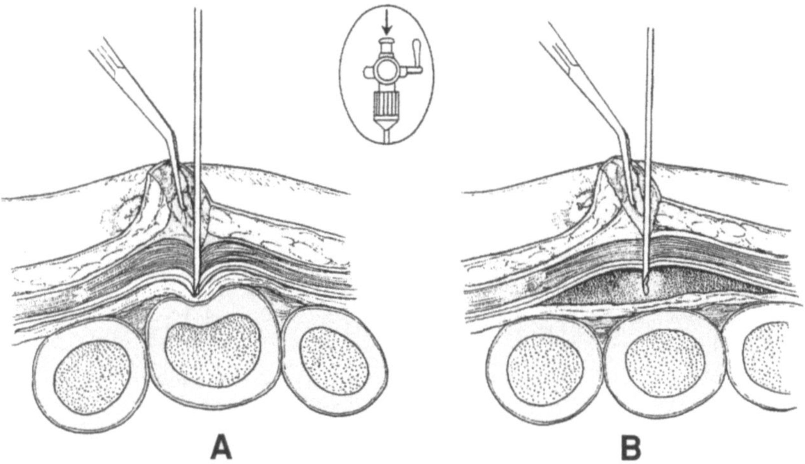


**Fig. 3.** Visceral deformation or displacement (**A**), and the importance of having an open stopcock for air entry (**B**) to allow omentum and bowel to drop away from the elevated ventral abdominal wall. (From ref. *27*.)

$CO_2$ insufflation, aspiration, irrigation, re-aspiration, and drop test should confirm the location of the needle. Any question as to the location of the needle should prompt removal. Once the needle is felt to be in the correct position, $CO_2$ insufflation should be started at low flow (1–3 L/min) and the initial pressure reading from the needle should be noted. A pressure reading greater than 8–10 mm Hg or an occlusion reading from the insufflator should prompt the slow retraction of the needle until the pressure reading is acceptable. It is also important to communicate with the anesthesiologist at this time to inform him or her that insufflation is underway so that close monitoring can be performed. Any sudden change in the hemodynamics of the patient or end tidal $CO_2$ reading should lead to cessation of insufflation.

Prevention of primary trocar injury requires knowledge and control of the axial forces at work during application of the trocar. Some have suggested temporary overinflation of the abdomen with the Veress needle to 20–25 mm Hg to maximize the space between abdominal wall and viscera as well as increase abdominal wall resistance *(32)*. If a shielded, cutting-type trocar is used, the skin incision must be wide enough to allow the trocar to pass easily. The abdominal wall should be stabilized with towel clips and the angle of passage should take into account underlying anatomy. Axial force control at this point is key and can be degraded by positioning that requires more muscle recruitment to exert a given amount of force (i.e., having the table too high, or

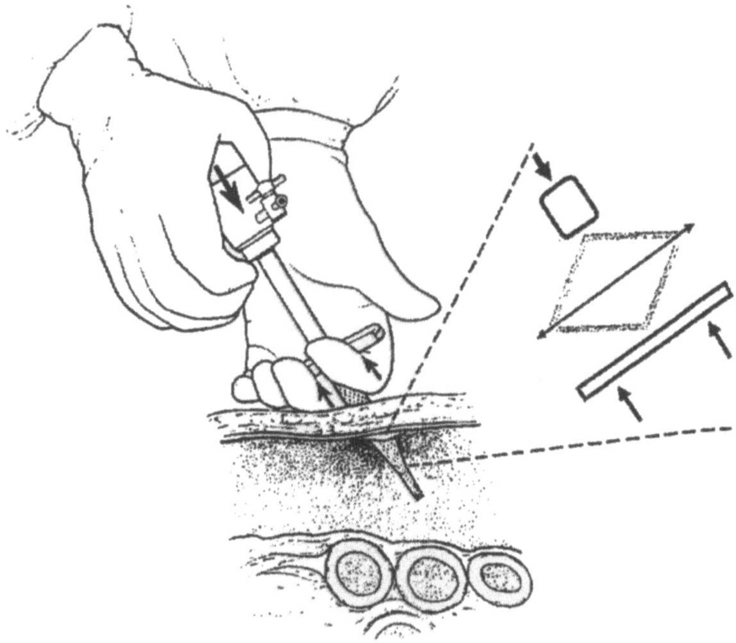

**Fig. 4.** Radially dilating trocar converts axial force to a radical vector by diamond-shaped, skeletal elements embedded in an expandable sheath. (From ref. *27*.)

reaching across the patient to put in a lateral port) *(27)*. Once the primary trocar is placed, its position should be confirmed immediately by passing the laparoscope through and observing for underlying injury. Secondary trocars are passed under direct vision, but care must be exercised during this procedure as injuries have occurred with secondary trocars, including injury to retroperitoneal vascular structures *(27)*. Once a secondary trocar is in place, the primary entry site should be viewed to look for injury. In an effort to redirect axial force during trocar placement, radially expanding trocars (Fig. 4) have been developed and have been shown to be safe with a very low incidence of injury *(27,33)*.

If the open, or Hasson, technique is used to gain access, care must be taken to avoid underlying bowel during the creation of the incision as exposure is limited. One of the criticisms of the Hasson technique is that there is loss of $CO_2$ from the cannula site, which can decrease the working space. Some surgeons have attempted to solve this problem by placing a purse-string suture around the cannula site. However, care must be exercised as complications have been reported with this technique as noted previously *(29)*.

If vascular of bowel injury is suspected during Veress needle or primary trocar placement, immediate conversion to an open procedure should be performed. Although a bowel injury may be recognized laparoscopically, the full extent of the injury may be underappreciated by the view from the laparoscope and combined injury of bowel and vascular structures are well documented *(27)*. A high index of suspicion is required to recognize bowel injury owing to trocar placement, as nearly half of all bowel injuries (47% for small bowel and 49% for colon) went undetected for at least 24 h, and delayed recognition of injury was an independent predictor of mortality *(27)*.

Complications secondary to insufflation can lead to cardiopulmonary disturbance, hypercarbia with subsequent acidosis, and occasionally pulmonary gas embolism. If cardiac arrhythmias or hemodynamic changes occur during insufflation, the pneumoperitoneum should be released, and the anesthesiologist should be consulted regarding measures to correct the cardiac changes. These measures include decreasing the anesthetic concentrations, rapid administration of intravenous fluid, and appropriate drug therapy to correct persistent cardiovascular abnormalities *(34)*. Presentation of hypercarbia and acidosis can sometimes be corrected by increasing the minute ventilation by adjusting the respiratory rate or tidal volume. If the hypercarbia persists, laparoscopy may need to be aborted in favor of open surgery. If $CO_2$ gas embolus is suspected, the pnemoperitoneum should be released, and if possible, the patient should be placed in the left lateral decubitus position and in slight Trendelenburg in an attempt to keep the gas embolus from entering the pulmonary circulation. Some anesthesiologists will have transesophageal echocardiography available in the operating room, and this can be used to visualize the gas embolus and possibly assist with aspiration of the gas with a central venous catheter.

Injury to abdominal wall vasculature during trocar placement can be minimized by a thorough understanding of the anatomy of the anterior abdominal wall. The inferior epigastric artery courses on the posterior surface of the rectus muscle, upward and medially on a line from the midpoint of the inguinal ligament toward the umbilicus. At the level of the semilunar line, it changes course and heads cephalad running between the midline and lateral boarder of the rectus muscle (Fig. 5). The inferior epigastric vessels can be avoided by placing trocars in the midline, lateral to the boarder of the rectus muscle, or with direct visualization of the vessel from inside the abdomen. In thin patients, transillumination of the abdominal wall may allow the inferior epigastric vessels to be seen and this maneuver is also helpful to identify and avoid superficial vessels. If the epigastric artery is injured attempts at cautery

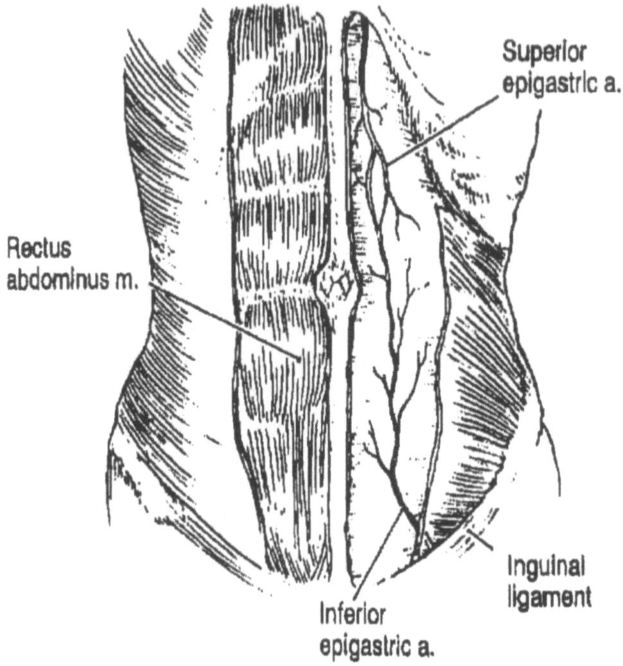


**Fig. 5.** Course of the epigastric vessels in relation to surface anatomy. (From ref. *35*.)

are usually unsuccessful and the best method of control is suture ligation. This can be performed laparoscopically using a small-caliber piercing needle such as a Carter-Thomasen needle or a Stamey needle *(35)*. The suture is passed on both sides of the bleeding site perpendicular to the vessel. The suture may be tied on the skin over a gauze bolster or under the skin surface if the suture was passed within the trocar incision.

Port-site herniation can occur at any trocar site, however it is rarely seen with 5-mm trocars and tends to occur more frequently below the level of the umbilicus. Most laparoscopists recommend closure of any trocar site greater than 5 mm especially those below the umbilicus *(36)*. Closure can be accomplished with needle devices and the suture should be placed under direct vision to ensure that the port site is closed. This can be especially challenging in obese patients. An exception to the 5-mm port-site closure rule involves the recently introduced radially expanding trocars that do not cut fascia and therefore leave a smaller fascial defect *(33)*. In the author's experience, we have placed more than 500, 11-mm and 12-mm radially dilating trocars and have yet to identify a trocar-site hernia despite not closing the port sites.

Table 4
Laparoscopic Bowel Injuries from Urologic Series

| *Author (reference)* | *Procedure* | *Cases* | *Bowel injury* | *Delayed recognition* |
|---|---|---|---|---|
| Kavoussi et al. *(9)* | L-PLND | 372 | 3 (0.8%) | 2/3 |
| Fahlenkamp et al. *(6)* | Multiple | 2407 | 6 (0.2%) | 6/6 |
| Guillonneau et al. *(18)* | LRP | 567 | 11 (1.9%) | 4/11 |
| Bischoff et al. *(37)* | Multiple | 915 | 10 (1.1%) | 4/10 |
| Parra et al. *(38)* | Multiple | 221 | 1 (0.4%) | 1/1 |

L-PLND = laparoscopic pelvic lymph node dissection; LRP = laparoscopic radical prostatectomy.

## *Bowel Injury*

The occurrence of laparoscopic bowel injury in the general surgical and gynecologic literature is approx 0.13% *(37)*. Fifty percent were due to electrocautery injury and 69% were not recognized at the time of injury. The mortality rate for unrecognized bowel injury was 3% (8 of 266 patients).

In the urologic literature, bowel injury is reported from 0.2% to 1.9% (Table 4) *(6,9,18)*. Kauvoussi reported three (0.8%) bowel injuries in 372 L-PLNDs *(9)*. One injury was recognized and repaired by open laparotomy. The other two injuries presented postoperatively and resolved after repair: one small bowel injury repaired on postoperative d 6 and a colonic injury that presented 4 mo after surgery in a patient who received prior radiotherapy to the pelvis. In the German Urologic Association review, bowel injury occurred in 6 (0.2%) of 2407 cases and one patient with a colonic perforation died from a pulmonary embolus during hospitilization for treatment *(6)*. Electrocautery injury was implicated in 12 of 20 visceral injuries, but it is unclear how many bowel injuries were attributable to cautery.

Guillonneau noted 11(1.9%) bowel injuries in 567 LRPs *(18)*. There were eight rectal injuries due to direct laceration with seven of these injuries recognized and repaired laparoscopically. One of the seven repairs broke down, requiring re-operation and diverting colostomy. One rectal injury presented after surgery on postoperative d 3, and required open repair and diverting colostomy. There were two ileal injuries, which presented 3 d after surgery and both were repaired with diverting ileostomies. There was one sigmoid injury that also presented on postoperative d 3 and was repaired at laparotomy with diverting colostomy. The cause of the sigmoid injury and one of the ileal injuries were unknown but thought to be due to stray monopolar electrocautery.

From these studies, it is apparent that many bowel injuries go unrecognized at the initial laparoscopic procedure. There also appears to be a relationship between stray electrocautery energy and the development of bowel injury. A comprehensive review of laparoscopic bowel injury was presented by Bishoff in which these issues were addressed *(37)*. He reported eight (0.8%) bowel injuries in 915 cases, and included two bowel injuries from outside referral in the series. Of the 10 injuries, 4 bowel perforations presented in a delayed manner, and these patients presented in an atypical fashion. The presentation included severe, single trocar-site pain, abdominal distension, diarrhea, and leukopenia. Of the four patients, two died of sepsis within 4 d of the original laparoscopic procedure. Six of 10 patients had bowel abrasions, which were oversewn in 5. The single patient with an abrasion that was not sutured developed an abscess and enterocutaneous fistula. Clearly, from this review, many bowel injuries go unrecognized and can have devastating consequences if not detected. The presenting signs of laparoscopic bowel injuries are not the classic presentation observed with open surgical bowel perforations. Finally, even bowel abrasions, especially those due to electrocautery, should be repaired to prevent delayed bowel leakage. Parra also noted delayed presentation of a cecal perforation due to thermal injury from cautery *(38)*.

As with access-related injuries, the best management of bowel injuries involves prevention and recognition. Preventing inadvertent perforation from sharp laparoscopic instruments requires experience and spatial orientation between underlying bowel and port sites. Until this experience is attained, it is wise to track the movement of all sharp instuments with the laparoscope as they are placed inside the abdomen. If the bowel is overly distended due to gas, then special care should be employed to prevent inadvertent perforation or consideration should be given to rescheduling the procedure once bowel distension is resolved. If bowel perforation is in question, the segment of interest should be thoroughly evaluated to look for signs of entry. Electrocautery injuries can be prevented by inspecting the insulation on the outside of the instrument to check for breaks. The surgeon must be aware that any part of an instrument may allow stray energy to be transferred to tissue, including portions of the instrument that are out of the field of view. The tissue being cauterized must be isolated from surrounding structures to prevent thermal spread from the application site.

Rectal injuries during LRP can occur even with significant experience. Guillonneau recorded two rectal injuries between case number 501 and 567 *(18)*. Use of a rectal bougie during the procedure may help with identifying the rectal tissue plane, but more likely it allows rapid recognition of rectal entry when it occurs. Most rectal injuries recongized at the time of injury may be repaired primarily in two layers without a diverting colostomy *(18)*. If the patient had prior radiation or if the primary repair is questionable, then consultation with a general surgeon is appropriate. The same management principle applies to colonic and small bowel injuries. If the injury is recognized, an attempt at primary repair is indicated. Laparoscopic repair of bowel injury has been reported to be safe and bowel diversion can be avoided in most cases *(39)*. If there is any question as to the integrity of the repair, then open repair should be considered. Bowel injuries that are discovered in the postoperative period should be treated by open laparotomy with bowel diversion.

## POSTOPERATIVE COMPLICATIONS

The incidence of postoperative complications in laparoscopic urological procedures shows wide variation (Table 5). Kavoussi reported 41 (11%) postoperative complications in 372 pelvic lymph node dissections with 6 of the 41 complications requiring operative repair *(9)*. The most common complication reported was urinary retention. The review by Gill of laparoscopic nephrectomy revealed 25 (13.5%) postoperative complications in 185 cases *(3)*. Six of the complications involved the gastrointestinal tract, whereas six others were cardiac complications. The German Urologic Association Working Group on Laparoscopy reported 15 (3.1%) postoperative complications out of 482 patients *(21)*. Of the 15 complications, 7 were delayed bleeding episodes, 4 were due to abscess formation, and 2 presented as intestinal stenosis. There was 1 trocar-site hernia and 1 pancreatic fistula. The re-intervention rate for the first 20 cases for each surgeon in this series was 7% but fell to 1.7% for all procedures after the 20th case.

The majority of complications reported in the review by Cadeddu were postoperative, with 14 of 16 complications occurring after surgery *(10)*. The most common complication was ileus (4) followed by urinary

**Table 5**
**Postoperative Complications from Laparoscopic Urologic Series**

| *Author (reference)* | *Procedure* | *Cases* | *Postoperative complication* | *Most common complication (no.)* |
|---|---|---|---|---|
| Kavoussi et al. *(9)* | L-PLND | 372 | 41 (11.0%) | Urinary retention (7) |
| Gill et al. *(3)* | Laparoscopic nephrectomy | 185 | 25 (13.5%) | Ileus (4) |
| Rassweiler et al. *(21)* | Laparoscopic nephrectomy | 482 | 15 (3.1%) | Delayed bleeding (7) |
| Cadeddu et al. *(10)* | LRN | 157 | 14 (8.9%) | Ileus (4) |
| Fahlenkamp et al. *(6)* | Multiple | 2407 | 28 (1.1%) | Subcuateous emphysema (6) |
| Dunn et al. *(11)* | LRN | 61 | 17 (27.9%) | Fever/atelectasis (5) |
| Guillonneau et al. *(18)* | LRP | 567 | 78 (13.7%) | Anastomotic leak (57) |

L-PLND = laparoscopic pelvic lymph node dissection; LRN = laparoscopic radical nephrectomy; LRP = laparoscopic radical prostatectomy.

tract infection (2) and pulmonary embolus. Fahlenkamp reported 28 (1.1%) postoperative complications out of 2407 procedures and noted 6 cases of subcutaneous emphysema, 5 wound infections, 5 trocar hernias, 4 lymphoceles, 4 fevers, 2 episodes of epididymitis, and 2 patients suffering pulmonary embolus *(6)*.

Postoperative complications were noted in 17 patients (27.9%) out of 23 complications in a series by Dunn who reviewed 61 LRNs *(11)*. All of the postoperative complications were characterized as minor with the most common complication being fever/atelectasis in 5 patients. All postoperative complications were self-limited and resolved without intervention. Siqueira reported 4 (1.8%) postoperative complications out of 213 laparoscopic nephrectomies *(22)*. Three complications involved the bowel with one sigmoid perforation, one case of colonic ischemia and one duodenal stress ulcer. The remaining complication was postoperative respiratory failure requiring reintubation. A recent review of complications in LRP revealed postoperative complications in 78 patients (13.7%) out of 567 procedures *(18)*. The most common postoperative complication was persistent urine leak from the anastomosis in 57 patients followed by ileus in 6 and hemoperitoneum in 5.

A review of the postoperative complications in these series reveals that the vast majority resolve with expectant management. However, some postoperative complications can be anticipated and recognized if a high index of suspicion is maintained. Postoperative bleeding resulting in abdominal wall ecchymoses or intra-abdominal hematoma can be prevented by close observation for bleeding at the conclusion of the procedure. Every port site should be observed during removal of the port to observe for bleeding and secured with a closure device as described previously *(36)*. The area of dissection in the abdomen must be thoroughly evaluated to discover bleeding vessels, and the intra-abdominal pressure should be lowered to approx 5 mm Hg to identify venous bleeding that may be tamponaded by the pneumoperitoneum.

Postoperative ileus occurs mainly in the setting of laparoscopic nephrectomy and the true cause is unknown. It may be due to residual blood, urine, or other peritoneal irritants or possibly how the colonic mesocolon is handled during bowel mobilization. Excessive traction on the mesocolon, which contains nerves and blood vessels supplying the colon, may be a cause of delayed bowel function. During retroperitoneal laparoscopy the colon is not manipulated, but is close to the area of dissection. There was not a single report of ileus in a review of 1043 retroperitoneal and extraperitoneal procedures *(5)* or in a recent review of retroperitoneal vascular and bowel complications *(20)*.

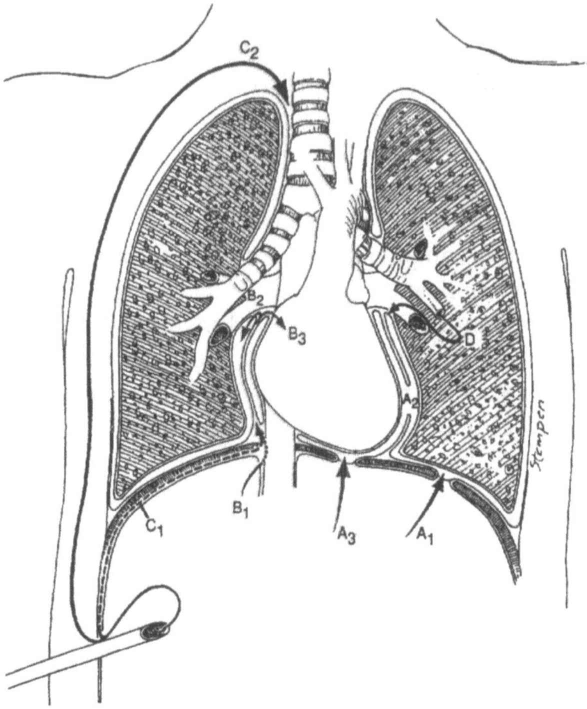


**Fig. 6.** Possible routes of $CO_2$ escape into the thoracic spaces leading to pneumomediastinum and pneumothorax. Route B represents tracking along the great vessels through the diaphragmatic hiatus. (From ref. *40*.)

The development of subcutaneous emphysema can result from preperitoneal insufflation with the Veress needle or dissection of $CO_2$ in tissue planes during retraction of a laparoscopic cannula from the peritoneum *(40)*. Subcutaneous emphysema is commonly seen in association with retroperitoneal laparoscopy and was present in 94% of patients during retroperitoneal procedures compared to 71% for transperitoneal procedures *(41)*. Although most cases of subcutaneous emphysema are clinically insignificant, some occurrences may predispose to hypercapnia if extensive *(40)*. Subcutaneous emphysema is also associated with pneumothorax and pnemomediastinum, especially during extra-peritoneal surgery *(41)*. Gill noted six cases of pneumothorax and four cases of pneumomediastinum in review of retroperitoneal laparoscopy *(5)*. During extraperitoneal surgery, $CO_2$ can move along the great vessels through the diaphragm hiatus and into the chest (Fig. 6). Pneumothoraces due to $CO_2$ should readily reabsorb and tube thoracostomy should not be required unless direct lung injury from a trocar is suspected or there is clinical evidence of pulmonary compromise.

The urinary complications reported in laparoscopic series may be unique to the patient population or the procedure itself. The high rate of urinary retention in the series of L-PLND may be related to the fact that men who are being staged for prostate cancer probably have associated bladder outlet obstruction and are at higher risk for retention. This factor combined with general anesthesia, intravenous fluid replacement, and possibly pelvic pain could account for the episodes of retention. The urine leaks noted after LRP are due to non-watertight vesicourethral anastomoses and are treated with drainage of the pelvis and prolonged urethral catheterization. Rarely, revision of the anastomosis is needed for a persistent leak *(18)*. Ureteral injuries are rare, and when recognized at the initial surgery, can be repaired primarily without difficulty *(18)*. However, ureteral injuries may be due to thermal damage secondary to electrocautery resulting in delayed presentation as a urinoma near the site of injury *(18,38)*.

## SUMMARY

Although laparoscopic urologic procedures have become more complex, the complications associated with these techniques are similar to those for simple procedures. Obtaining access to the peritoneal or retroperitoneal space requires careful planning and knowledge of the underlying anatomy to prevent potentially catastrophic injury. Vascular dissection injuries, although rare, are a leading cause of open conversion. Bowel injuries during laparoscopic procedures are difficult to recognize and they may present with atypical signs and symptoms that may cause greater delay in recognition.

Each laparoscopic procedure may also be associated with a complication unique to that particular operation, and therefore, a high index of suspicion will be needed to detect these events. Prevention and recognition are the key to management of laparoscopic complications, and with experience and attention to detail, a successful outcome will be obtained.

## REFERENCES


1. Clayman RV. Editorial. J Urol 1999; 162: 770.
2. Vallencien G, Cathelineau X, Baumert H, Doublet JD, Guillonneau B. Complications of transperitoneal laparoscopic surgery in urology: review of 1,311 procedures at a single center. J Urol 2002; 168: 23–26.
3. Gill IS, Kavoussi LR, Clayman RV, et al. Complications of laparoscopic nephrectomy in 185 patients: a multi-institutional review. J Urol 1995; 154: 479–483.

4. Peters CA. Complications in pediatric urological laparoscopy: results of a survey. J Urol 1996; 155: 1070–1073.
5. Gill IS, Clayman RV, Albala DM, et al. Retroperitoneal and pelvic extraperitoneal laparoscopy: an international perspective. Urology 1998; 52: 566–571.
6. Fahlenkamp D, Rassweiler J, Fornara P, Frede T, Loening SA. Complications of laparoscopic procedures in urology: experience with 2,407 procedures at 4 German centers. J Urol 1999; 162: 765–770.
7. Cadeddu JA, Wolfe JS Jr, Nakada S, et al. Complications of laparoscopic procedures after concentrated training in urological laparoscopy. J Urol 2001; 166: 2109–2111.
8. Shoma AM, Erkay I, El-Kappany H. Laparoscopic nephrectomy: prediction of outcome in relation to the preoperative risk factors in two approaches. J Endourol 2001; 15: 517–522.
9. Kavoussi LR, Sosa E, Chandhoke P, et al. Complications of laparoscopic pelvic lymph node dissection. J Urol 1993; 149: 322–325.
10. Cadeddu JA, Ono Y, Clayman RV, et al. Laparoscopic nephrectomy for renal cell cancer: evaluation of efficacy and safety: a multicenter experience. Urology 1998; 52: 773–777.
11. Dunn MD, Portis AJ, Shalhav AL, et al. Laparoscopic versus open radical nephrectomy: a 9-year experience. J Urol 2000; 164: 1153–1159.
12. Ono Y, Kinukawa T, Hattori R, et al. The long-term outcome of laparoscopic radical nephrectomy for small renal cell carcinoma. J Urol 2001; 165: 1867–1870.
13. Gill IS, Sung GT, Hobart MG, et al. Laparoscopic radical nephroureterectomy for upper tract transitional cell carcinoma: the Cleveland Clinic experience. J Urol 2000; 164: 1513–1522.
14. Gill IS, Munch LC, Clayman RV, et al. A new renal tourniquet for open and laparoscopic partial nephrectomy. J Urol 1995; 154: 1113–1116.
15. Gill IS, Desai MM, Kaouk JH, et al. Laparoscopic partial nephrectomy for renal tumor: duplicating open surgical techniques. J Urol 2002; 167: 469–477.
16. Nelson JB, Chen RN, Bischoff JT, et al. Laparoscopic retroperitoneal lymph node dissection for cllinical stage 1 nonseminomatous germ cell testicular tumors. Urology 1999; 54: 1064–1067.
17. Janetschek G, Hobisch A, Hittmair A, et al. Laparoscopic retroperitoneal lymphadenectomy after chemotherapy for stage IIB nonseminomatous testicular carcinoma. J Urol 1999; 161: 477–481.
18. Guillonneau B, Rozet F, Cathelineau X, et al. Perioperative complications of laparoscopic radical prostatectomy: the Montsouris 3-year experience. J Urol 2002; 167: 51–56.
19. Thiel R, Adams JB, Schulam PG, Moore RG, Kavoussi LR. Venous dissection injuries during laparoscopic urological surgery. J Urol 1996; 155: 1874–1876.
20. Meraney AM, Samee AA, Gill IS.:Vascular and bowel complications during retroperitoneal laparoscopic surgery. J Urol 2002; 168: 1941–1944.
21. Rassweiler J, Fornara P, Weber M, et al. Laparoscopic nephrectomy: the experience of the laparoscopy working group of the German Urologic Association. J Urol 1998; 160: 18–21.
22. Siqueira TM, Kuo RL, Gardner TA, et al. Major complications in 213 laparoscopic nephrectomy cases: the Indianapolis experience. J Urol 2002; 168: 1361–1365.
23. Chan D, Bishoff JT, Ratner L, Kavoussi LR, Jarret TW. Endovascular gastrointestinal stapler device malfunction during laparoscopic nephrectomy: early recognition and management. J Urol 2000; 164: 319–321.

24. Deng DY, Meng MV, Nguyen HT, Bellman GC, Stoller ML. Laparoscopic linear cutting stapler failure. Urology 2002; 60: 415–419.
25. Harkki-Siren P. The incidence of entry-related laparoscopic injuries in Finland. Gyn Endo 1999; 8: 335.
26. Hulka JF, Levy BS, Parker WH, Phillips JM. Laparoscopic-assisted vaginal hysterectomy: American Association of Gynecologic Laparoscopists' 1995 membership survery. J Am Assoc Gyn Laparosc 1997; 4: 167–171.
27. Chandler JG, Corson SL, Way LW. Three spectra of laparoscopic entry access injuries. J Am Coll Surg 2001; 192: 478–490.
28. Sharp HT, Dodson MK, Draper ML, et al. Complications associated with optical-access laparoscopic trocars. Ob Gyn 2002; 99: 553–555.
29. Sadeghi-Nejad H, Kavoussi LR, Peters CA. Bowel injury in open technique laparoscopic cannula placement. Urology 1994; 43: 559–560.
29a. Hulka JF. Complications. In: Textbook of laproscopy (Hulka JF, ed.), Grune & Straton, New York, 1985.
30. Hunter JG. Invited commentary on "Three spectra of laparoscopic entry access injuries." J Am Coll Surg 2001; 192: 490.
31. See WA, Fisher RJ, Winfield HN, Donovan JF. Laparoscopic surgical training: effectiveness and impact on urological surgical practice patterns. J Urol 1993; 149: 1054–1057.
32. Phillips G, Garryu R, Kumar C, Reich H. How much gas is required for initial insufflation at laparoscopy? Gyn Endo 1999; 8: 369.
33. Shekarriz B, Gholami SS, Rudnick DM, Duh Q, Stoller M. Radially expanding laparoscopic access for renal/adrenal surgery. Urology 2001; 58: 683–687.
34. Monk TG, Weldon BC. Anesthetic Considerations for Laparoscopic Surgery. J Endourol 1992; 6: 89.
35. Green LS, Loughlin KR, Kavoussi LR. Management of epigastric vessel injury during laparoscopy. J Endo 1992; 6: 99.
36. Capelouto CC, Kavoussi LR. Complications of laparoscopic surgery. Urology 1993; 42: 2–12.
37. Bishoff JT, Allaf ME, Kirkels W, et al. Laparoscopic bowel injury: incidence and clinical presentation. J Urol 1999; 161: 887–890.
38. Parra RO, Hagood PG, Boullier JA, Cummings JM, Mehan DJ. Complications of laparoscopic urological surgery: experience at St. Louis University. J Urol 1994; 151: 681–684.
39. Reich H. Laparoscopic bowel injury. Surg Laparosc Endo 1992; 2: 74.
40. Wolf JS, Stoller ML. The physiology of laparoscopy: basic principles, complications and other considerations. J Urol 1994; 152: 294–302.
41. Wolf JS, Monk TG, McDougall EM, McVlennnan BL, Clayman RV. The extraperitoneal approach and subcutaneous emphysema are associated with greater absorption of corbon dioxide during laparoscopic renal surgery. J Urol 1995; 154: 959–963.

# Index

**A**

Abdomen, exiting, 14-15, 104
Abdominal wall injuries and trocar placement, 345
Access-related injuries, 340-346
Adjuvant techniques
  in renal tumor ablation, 118-119
  in upper urinary tract urothelial carcinoma, 157
Adrenal adenomas, benign, 207
Adrenalectomy, bilateral, 219
Adrenal tumors, 221-222. *See also* Laparoscopic adrenalectomy
Adrenal vein, securing, transperitoneal radical/total nephrectomy, 10
Adrenocortical carcinoma, 220-221
Aldosteronoma, 215-216
Anastomoses
  obesity and bowel anastomoses, 307
  uterointestinal anastomosis, laparoscopic urinary diversion, 314-316, 320
  uterovesical anastomosis, LRP, 282-284
Androgen-deprivation therapy and prostate cancer, 265, 267
Anterior bladder neck, division of (LRP), 280-282

**B**

Balloon dilation, use in retroperitoneoscopic nephroureterectomy, 162
Balloon dissection, requirements of in renal cyst management, 88
Bilateral adrenalectomy, 219
Bioheat equation, 137-140
Bipolar electrocautery, use in LPN, 98
Bladder
  anterior bladder neck, division of in LRP, 280-282
  freeing from abdominal wall (LPN), 277-278
  laparoscopic nephroureterectomy, 162-166, 167
  laparoscopic urinary diversion, orthotopic neobladder, 312-314
  Studer neobladder, creation of, 313, 314-316, 317, 320
Bladder cancer. *See* Laparoscopic radical cystectomy
Bosniak classification of renal cysts, 72, 73, 74
Bowel injuries, 44, 347-349, 351, 352

**C**

Cable tie, use in LPN, 98-99, 100
Carcinoma. *See also* laparoscopic adrenalectomy; renal cell carcinoma
  adrenocortical, 220-221
  metastatic, 27-33, 245-247
  upper urinary tract urothelial, 155, 157
Cluster electrode described, 137
Complications. *See also individual procedures by name*
  access-related injuries, 340-346
  bowel injuries, 44, 347-349, 351, 352
  cryotherapy, 124-125
  general laparoscopic series, 330-333
  history of, 329-330
  morcellation, 44-45
  postoperative, 349-353
  radiofrequency techniques, 124-125, 148
  vascular injury, 337-340
  Veress needles, injuries involving, 342-343, 345, 352
Computed tomography scanning
  adrenocortical carcinoma, use in, 221
  aldosteronoma, use in, 216

and clinical tumor staging, 45
cryotherapy and radiofrequency techniques, 118, 125, 127, 149
detection of incidental adrenal masses, 203, 205, 207, 210
diagnosis of excess cortisol production, 218, 219
HALRN, 53
percutaneous RFA, 143, 144, 149
renal protocol contrast, use in renal cyst management, 82
CO2 pneumoperitoneum
and bowel injuries, 352
and laparoscopic urinary diversion, 307-308
Cortisol production. *See* excess cortisol production
Costs
HALRN, 68-69
laparoscopic adrenalectomy, 225
laparoscopic nephrectomy, 24-25
laparoscopic pelvic lymph node dissection, 261-262
laparoscopy vs open surgery, 261-262
morcellation, 44
transperitoneal radical/total nephrectomy, 24-25
Cryotherapy in renal tumor ablation
adjuvant techniques, 118-119
computed tomography scanning, 118, 125, 127, 149
controversies surrounding, 130-131
fluoroscopy, use in, 125, 127
histologic changes, 129-130
history of, 111-112
indications and contraindications, 112-114
limitations of, 118
magnetic resonance imaging, 118, 125, 127, 149
mechanism of action, 114
morbidity and complications, 124-125
radiographic changes, 125-129
results, 119-122, 124
surgical technique, 114-118
thermocouple technology, 118
ultrasonography, 118, 125, 127, 149
CT scanning. *See* Computed tomography scanning
Cushing's syndrome
described, 216-217
diagnosis, 217-218
results, 219-220
treatment, 218-219, 225
Cytoreductive laparoscopic radical nephrectomy
contraindications for, 28
controversial issues regarding, 30, 32-33
indications for, 28
limitations of, 33
results, 32
surgical technique, 29-32

**D**

Dorsal vein complex, ligation of in LRP, 278-279
Double loop tourniquet, use in LPN, 99-100
Duodenum, laparoscopic view of, 9

**E**

Electrical prostrate morcellator (EPM), 40
Emphysema, 352
Endocatch system, use in morcellation, 39
Endotoxemia and CO2 pneumoperitoneum, 308
Energy deposition in RFA, 137-140
Entrapment
for intact removal, transperitoneal radical/total nephrectomy, 13
for morcellation, transperitoneal radical/total nephrectomy, 11-12
Epigastric vessels, course of, 346
Excess cortisol production
described, 216-217
diagnosis, 217-218
results, 219-220

treatment, 218-219
Extraperitoneal laparoscopic technique, laparoscopic adrenalectomy, 202-203

F

Fine needle aspiration, use in tumor identification, 208-209
Flouroscopy, use in cryotherapy and radiofrequency techniques, 125, 127
Forecast ablation described, 127, 129

G

Gelport, description of, 59, 60
Gonadal vein, securing, transperitoneal radical/total nephrectomy, 9, 15-16

H

HALNU. *See* Hand-assisted laparoscopic nephroureterectomy
HALRN. *See* Hand-assisted laparoscopic radical nephrectomy
Hand-assisted laparoscopic nephroureterectomy, 159-160
Hand-assisted laparoscopic partial nephrectomy (HALPN), 97. *See also* Laparoscopic partial nephrectomy
Hand-assisted laparoscopic radical nephrectomy
  anathestic considerations of, 53
  application of, 51-52, 95
  costs, 68-69
  general discussion, 65-69
  hand access devices, description of, 59
  indications and contraindications for, 52
  postoperative care, 65
  preparation for, 53-56
  surgical technique, 59-65
  trocars and hand port placement, 56-59
HandPort, description of, 59
Hasson technique and access injuries, 344
Hemostasis, major issue of LPN, 98
Hyperaldosteronism, primary and hypertension, 215

I

Incidentaloma in laparoscopic adrenalectomy, 203, 205, 207-211
Incisional hernias and morcellation, 45
Intact specimen removal
  entrapment, transperitoneal radical/total nephrectomy, 13
  morcellation vs, 42-47
  postoperative assessment, 42-44
Intra-corporeal free-hand suturing, use in LPN, 96
Intraoperative laparoscopic ultrasound, 125
IOLUS. *See* Intraoperative laparoscopic ultrasound

L

Laparoscopic adrenalectomy
  adrenal tumors, metastatic, 221-222
  adrenocortical carcinoma, 220-221
  aldosteronoma, 215-216
  carcinoma, metastatic, 27-33, 245-247
  carcinoma, primary
    contraindications, 236-237
    controversies, 247
    history of, 235-236
    results, 243-245
    surgical technique
      access, 237
      left adrenalectomy, 206-211, 237-239
      right adrenalectomy, 239-241
      specimen retrieval/closure, 241-242
      variations, 242-243
  costs, 225
  extraperitoneal laparoscopic technique, 202-203
  history of, 195-196
  incidentaloma in, 203, 205, 207-211
  indications and contraindications, 196-197, 226
  morbidity and recovery, 223-225

needlescopic adrenalectomy, 222
partial adrenalectomy, 222-223
pediatric adrenalectomy, 222
pheochromocytoma, 212-215, 223, 226, 236
surgical technique
extraperitoneal laparoscopic technique, 202-205
lateral transperitoneal technique, 198-202
overview, 197-198
Laparoscopic nephrectomy
complications of, 331-332, 334-335, 338-339, 341, 349-351
costs, 24-25
history of, 3, 51-52
morbidity, 23-24
morcellation and, 37-38
results, 20-22, 23
role of in metastatic renal cell carcinoma, 27-33
surgical technique
access, 4-7
left side, 15-18
overview, 4
right side, 7-15
Laparoscopic nephroureterectomy
complications, 334, 335
distal ureter, management of, 161-162
hand-assisted, 159-160
history of, 155-156
indications, 156-157
morcellation, use of, 156-157, 169
preoperative preparation, 157
results, 166-171
retroperitoneoscopic nephroureterectomy, 161, 162
technique, choosing, 157
transperitoneal LNU, 157-159
ureteral dissection after nephrectomy
laparoscopic extravesical cuff with bladder closure, 165-166
open ureteral resection, 165
transvesical bladder cuff-one port, 166, 167
ureteral dissection before nephrectomy
pluck technique, 162-163
transvesical bladder cuff technique-two ports, 163-164
ureteral intussusception technique, 164-165
ureteral unroofing with laparoscopic bladder cuff stapling, 162-163
Laparoscopic partial adrenalectomy, 222-223
Laparoscopic partial nephrectomy
complications, 336
controversial issues, 106, 108
history of, 93-94
indications for, 94
morbidity, 104-106
oncologic results, 106-107
surgical procedure
bipolar electrocautery, 98
cable tie, use of, 98-99, 100
double loop tourniquet, 99-100
exiting and closing of abdomen, 104
hand-assisted laparoscopic partial nephrectomy (HALPN), 97
microwave coagulation, 101-102
open surgery, duplication of, 95-97
overview of, 94-95
preoperative preparation, 95
radiofrequency coagulation, 102-103
resection and hemostasis, 95
ultrasonic shears, 100-101
water-jet dissection, 101
technical challenges of, 108
Laparoscopic pelvic lymph node dissection
complications, 332, 333-334, 341, 347, 349-350, 353
controversies of, 262-265
costs, 261-262
history of, 251-252
indications and contraindications, 252-253, 275

limitations of procedure, 266-267
morbidity, 265-266
oncologic efficacy of treatment, 254-259
perioperative data
open PLND, 259
transperitoneal approach, 256-257
procedural efficiency, 260-261
results, 253-254
separate staging PLND, indications for, 263
surgical technique, 253
Laparoscopic radical cystectomy
history of, 297
indications, 298
patient preparation, 298
pelvic lymph node dissection, 302
port placement, 298-300
surgical technique, female, 301-302
surgical technique, male, 300-301
urinary diversion, 302-303
Laparoscopic radical prostatectomy
complications of, 337, 339, 347-348, 349, 353
extraperitoneal technique, 285
history of, 273-274
indications and contraindications, 274-275
limitations of, 290-291
oncological results, 286-288
operative results, 285-286
perioperative outcomes, 289-290
robotically assisted, 285, 288
surgical technique
anterior bladder neck, division of, 280-282
bladder, freeing from abdominal wall, 277-278
dorsal vein complex, ligation of, 278-279
nerve-sparing approach, 280-281, 290
prostate, exposure of, 278
trocar placement, 275-276
uterovesical anastomosis, 282-284
vas deferens, incising, 276-277
Laparoscopic retroperitoneal lymph node dissection
complications of, 186, 334, 336, 339
as diagnostic tool, 187
history, 177-178
indications, 178-179, 180
postoperative care, 186
results
post chemotherapy, stage II or III disease, 189
stage I NSGCT's, 186-187, 188
surgical techniques
left-side transperitoneal laparoscopic RPLND, 184
post chemotherapy, stage II or III disease, 185
preoperative preparation, 179-181
retroperitoneal approach, using, 185-186
right-side transperitoneal, 181-184
Laparoscopic ultrasound and tumor identification, 95, 203
Laparoscopic urinary diversion
controversies, 321
history of, 305
indications and contraindications, 305-308
limitations of, 322-323
results, 317-321
specimen extraction, 316-317
surgical technique
diversion/reservoir formation
continent diversion, 311-312
ileal conduit, 310-311
orthotopic neobladder, 312-314
uterocutaneous diversion, 309
port placements, 308-309
specimen extraction, 316-317
ureteral mobilization, 308-309
uterointestinal anastomosis, 314-316, 320

Laparoscopy
advantages of, 306
complications, 330-333
costs vs open surgery, 261-262
evolution of, 330
limitations of, 267
LapDisc, 59
LapSac, 12, 38-39
Lateral transperitoneal technique, laparoscopic adrenalectomy, 198-202
Ligasure device, laparoscopic view of, 17
LNU. *See* Laparoscopic nephroureterectomy
L-PLND. *See* Laparoscopic pelvic lymph node dissection
LPN. *See* Laparoscopic partial nephrectomy
LRP. *See* laparoscopic radical prostatectomy
L-RPLND. *See* Laparoscopic retroperitoneal lymph node dissection

M

Magnetic Resonance Imaging
adrenocortical carcinoma, 221
aldosteronoma, 216
cryotherapy and radiofrequency techniques, 118, 125, 127, 149
detection of incidental adrenal masses, 203, 205, 207-208
diagnosis of excess cortisol production, 218
in-phase/opposed phase chemical shift imaging, for differentiating adrenal tumors, 207
MEN2. *See* Multiple endocrine neoplasia 2
Metastatic adrenal tumors, 221-222
Metastatic carcinoma, 27-33, 245-247
Microwave coagulation, LPN, 101-102
Minimally invasive surgery
advantages of, 255, 260
progression of as surgical advance, 93
Morcellation
bowel injury, 44
complications, 44-45
defined, 37
devices used in, 38-41
electrical prostrate morcellator (EPM), 40
Endocatch system, 39
incisional hernias and, 45
and laparoscopic nephrectomy, 37-38
laparoscopic nephroureterectomy, use in, 156-157, 169
methodology, 41-42
Morce-power, 40, 41
operative time, 44
Serrated Edge Macro Morcellator (SEMM), 40, 41
Steiner electromechanical morcellator, 40, 41
transperitoneal radical/total nephrectomy, 14
and tumor control, 47
and tumor recurrence, 47
and tumor staging, 45-47
vs intact specimen removal, 42-47
X-tract morcellator, 40, 41
MRI. *See* Magnetic Resonance Imaging
Multiple endocrine neoplasia 2
and partial adrenalectomy, 222
and pheochromocytoma, 212

N

Necrosis zone, increasing, 139
Needlescopic adrenalectomy, 222
Nephron-sparing surgery, 93, 112
Nephropexy in renal cyst management, 86
Nerve-sparing approach, LRP, 280-281, 290
Nitrous oxide and HALRN, 53
NP-59, use in identifying adrenal lesions, 208
NSGCT. *See* testicular cancer, management of
NSS. *See* Nephron-sparing surgery

## O


Obesity and bowel anastomoses, 307
Omniport, description of, 59
Open surgery, duplication of in LPN, 95-97
Organ sacks, 38-39


## P


Pararenal dissection, transperitoneal radical/total nephrectomy, 7-9, 15
Partial adrenalectomy, laparoscopic, 222-223
Pediatric adrenalectomy, 222
Pediatric laparoscopy, complications of, 331, 341
Pelvic lymph node dissection, laparoscopic radical cystectomy, 302
Percutaneous radiofrequency tumor ablation. *See also* Radiofre-quency techniques in renal tumor ablation
  available systems and applications, 141-144
  complications of, 148
  history of, 135-136
  indications for, 141, 145-146
  limitations of, 148-149
  local tissue interactions, 140-141
  mechanism of action, 136-141
  and MRI, 118, 125, 127, 149
Perineal radical prostatectomy, operative results, 285-286
Peripelvic cysts, 79-80, 87-88
Peritoneal incisions, transperitoneal radical/total nephrectomy, 7-9, 15
Pheochromocytoma, 212-215, 223, 226, 236
Plasma DHEA sulfate levels, as tumor marker, 221
Pnemothorax and emphysema, 352
Pneumomediastinum and emphysema, 352
Pneumosleeve, description of, 59
Port sites
  access-related injuries, 340
  bowel injuries and, 351
  cytoreductive LRN, 31
  hand-assisted laparoscopic radical nephrectomy (HALRN), 56-59
  herniation of, 346
  laparoscopic radical cystectomy, 298-300
  laparoscopic urinary diversion, 308-309
  left-side transperitoneal laparoscopic RPLND, 184
  left transperitoneal adrenalectomy, 204
  retroperitoneal radical nephrectomy, 19
  right-side transperitoneal laparoscopic RPLND, 183
  right transperitoneal adrenalectomy, 199
  right transperitoneal nephrectomy, 5, 6
  transperitoneal laparoscopic nephroureterectomy, 157-159
  tumor recurrence, 47, 169, 255
Postoperative assessment, intact extraction, 42-44
Prostate, exposure of in LRP, 278
Prostate cancer. *See also* Laparoscopic pelvic lymph node dissection; Laparoscopic radical prostatectomy
  androgen-deprivation therapy and, 265, 267
  and tumor aggressiveness, 255
Prostate Cancer Index, UCLA, 290


## R


Radical nephrectomy, history of, 51-52
Radiofrequency ablation, 103, 146
Radiofrequency coagulation, 102-103, 147
Radiofrequency techniques in renal tumor ablation. *See also* Percutaneous radiofrequency tumor ablation
  adjuvant techniques, 118-119

controversies surrounding, 130-131
flouroscopy, use in, 125, 127
hematuria, use in, 147
histologic changes, 129-130
history of, 111-112
imaging, importance of, 146-147
indications and contraindications, 112-114
limitations of, 118
mechanism of action, 114
morbidity and complications, 124-125, 148
and MRI, 118, 125, 127, 149
radiographic changes, 125-129
results, 119-121, 123-124
surgical technique, 114-118
Radionics 200 Watt generator, use in percutaneous RFA, 141
Rectal sigmoid pouch, creation of, 311-312
Renal cell carcinoma. *See also* renal cysts, management of
and the adrenal gland, 245, 246
computed tomography, use in, 143, 144, 149
defined, 27
imaging, importance of, 146-147
metastatic
laparoscopic nephrectomy, role in, 27-33
percutaneous radiofrequency tumor ablation, use in
available systems and applications, 141-144
complications of, 148
hematuria, use in, 147
history of, 135-136
indications for, 141, 145-146
limitations of, 148-149
local tissue interactions, 140-141
mechanism of action, 136-141
radiofrequency techniques in renal tumor ablation
adjuvant techniques, 118-119
controversies surrounding, 130-131
hematuria, use in, 147
histologic changes, 129-130
history of, 111-112
imaging, importance of, 146-147
indications and contraindications, 112-114
limitations of, 118
mechanism of action, 114
morbidity and complications, 124-125
overview of surgical technique, 114-118
radiographic changes, 125-129
results, 119-121, 123-124
ultrasound and, 143
Renal cysts, management of. *See also* renal cell carcinoma
Bosniak category I cysts, 81
Bosniak category II cysts, 82
Bosniak category III cysts, 83
general discussion, 71-74
intermediately complex renal cysts, 74-75
laparoscopic treatment data, 76-78
peripelvic cysts, laparoscopic treatment of, 79-80
surgical techniques
general discussion, 80, 82-84
peripelvic cysts, 87-88
retroperitoneal approach, 88-89
transperitoneal approach, 84-87
Renal hilum
control of, LPN, 96
transperitoneal radical/total nephrectomy, 10-11, 17-18
Renal pelvic tumors and the ureteral intussusception technique, 164
Retroperitoneal approach, renal cysts, 88-89
Retroperitoneal radical nephrectomy, surgical technique, 18-20
Retroperitoneoscopic nephroureterectomy, 161, 162

Retropubic radical prostatectomy, 285, 286, 289, 291
RFA. *See* Radiofrequency techniques

S

Serrated Edge Macro Morcellator (SEMM), 40, 41
Specimen freezing, transperitoneal radical/total nephrectomy, 11
Spoon/cup biopsy forceps, use of for tumor retraction, 29
Staging issues, morcellation vs intact specimen removal, 45-47
Steiner electromechanical morcellator, 40, 41
Studer neobladder, creation of, 313, 314-316, 317, 320
Subcutaneous emphysema, 352

T

Testicular cancer, management of
  complications of, 186
  history, 177-178
  indications, 178-179, 180
  postoperative care, 186
  results
    post chemotherapy, stage II or III disease, 189
    stage I NSGCT's, 186-187, 188
  surgical techniques
    left-side transperitoneal, 184
    post chemotherapy, stage II or III disease, 185
    preoperative preparation, 179-181
    retroperitoneal approach, 185-186
    right-side transperitoneal, 181-184
Thermocouple technology, use in cryotherapy and radiofrequency techniques, 118
Tissue heating, influencing, 137
Transperitoneal approach, renal cysts, 84-87
Transperitoneal laparoscopic nephroureterectomy, 157-159
Transperitoneal radical/total nephrectomy
  costs, 24-25
  morbidity, 23-24
  results, 21-23
  surgical technique
    access, 4-7
    left side, 15-18
    overview, 4
    right side, 7-15
Trocars
  access injuries involving, 340, 341, 343-344, 345
  hand-assisted laparoscopic nephroureterectomy (HALNU), use in, 160
  hand-assisted laparoscopic radical nephrectomy (HALRN), 56-59
  laparoscopic adrenalectomy, 237
  laparoscopic radical prostatectomy, 275-276
  use of, 6-7
Tumor aggressiveness, 255
Tumor control, 47
Tumor identification
  computed tomography scanning, 203, 205, 207, 210
  DHEA sulfate levels, 221
  fine needle aspiration, 208-209
  magnetic resonance imaging, 203, 205, 207-208
  morcellation and, 46-47
  NP-59, 208
  ultrasonography, 95, 203
Tumor markers, 221
Tumor recurrence, 47, 169, 255

U

UCLA Prostate Cancer Index, 290
Ultrasonic shears, use in LPN, 100-101
Ultrasonography
  intraoperative laparoscopic ultrasound, 125
  renal cell carcinoma, 143

use in cryotherapy and radiofrequency techniques, 118, 125, 127, 149
use in detection of incidental adrenal masses, 203
use in localization of adrenal gland, 202
use in percutaneous RFA, 143, 149
Umbrella array electrode described, 137-138
Ureter, securing, transperitoneal radical/ total nephrectomy, 9, 11, 16
Ureteral dissection
after nephrectomy
laparoscopic extravesical cuff with bladder closure, 165-166
open ureteral resection, 165
transvesical bladder cuff-one port, 166, 167
before nephrectomy
pluck technique, 162-163
transvesical bladder cuff technique-two ports, 163-164
ureteral intussusception technique, 164-165
ureteral unroofing with laparoscopic bladder cuff stapling, 162-163
Ureteral intussusception technique and renal pelvic tumors, 164
Urinary diversion, laparoscopic
controversies, 321
history of, 305
indications and contraindications, 305-308
limitations of, 322-323
results, 317-321
specimen extraction, 316-317
surgical technique
diversion/reservior formation
continent diversion, 311-312
ileal conduit, 310-311
orthotopic neobladder, 312-314
uterocutaneous diversion, 309
port placements, 308
uterointestinal anastomosis, 314-316, 320
techniques, reconstructive, 302-303
Urothelial carcinoma, upper urinary tract, 155, 157. *See also* Laparoscopic nephroureterectomy
Uterointestinal anastomosis, laparoscopic urinary diversion, 314-316, 320
Uterovesical anastomosis, LRP, 282-284

**V**

Vascular injury complications, 337-340
Vas deferens, incising in LRP, 276-277
Veress needles, injuries involving, 342-343, 345, 352
VHL disease. *See* von Hippel-Lindau disease
von Hippel-Lindau disease
and partial adrenalectomy, 222
and pheochromocytoma, 212
treatment of, 136, 146

**W**

Water-jet dissection, use in LPN, 101

**X**

X-tract morcellator, 40, 41

**Z**

Zone of necrosis, increasing, 139

FSC
www.fsc.org
MIX
Papier aus verantwortungsvollen Quellen
Paper from responsible sources
FSC® C105338

If you have any concerns about our products,
you can contact us on
**ProductSafety@springernature.com**

In case Publisher is established outside the EU,
the EU authorized representative is:
**Springer Nature Customer Service Center GmbH**
**Europaplatz 3, 69115 Heidelberg, Germany**

Printed by Libri Plureos GmbH
in Hamburg, Germany